Clinical
Electromyography

Guest Editor

DEVON I. RUBIN, MD

NEUROLOGIC
CLINICS

www.neurologic.theclinics.com

Consulting Editor
RANDOLPH W. EVANS, MD

May 2012 • Volume 30 • Number 2

SAUNDERS an imprint of ELSEVIER, Inc.

W.B. SAUNDERS COMPANY
A Division of Elsevier Inc.

1600 John F. Kennedy Boulevard • Suite 1800 • Philadelphia, Pennsylvania 19103-2899

http://www.theclinics.com

NEUROLOGIC CLINICS Volume 30, Number 2
May 2012 ISSN 0733-8619, ISBN-13: 978-1-4557-4224-0

Editor: Donald Mumford

Neurologic Clinics (ISSN 0733-8619) is published quarterly by Elsevier Inc., 360 Park Avenue South, New York, NY 10010–1710. Months of issue are February, May, August, and November. Periodicals postage paid at New York, NY, and additional mailing offices. Subscription prices are $285.00 per year for US individuals, $470.00 per year for US institutions, $140.00 per year for US students, $359.00 per year for Canadian individuals, $564.00 per year for Canadian institutions, $397.00 per year for international individuals, $564.00 per year for international institutions, and $199.00 for Canadian and foreign students/residents. To receive student/resident rate, orders must be accompanied by name of affiliated institution, date of term, and the *signature* of program/residency coordinator on institution letterhead. Orders will be billed at individual rate until proof of status is received. Foreign air speed delivery is included in all *Clinics* subscription prices. All prices are subject to change without notice. **POSTMASTER:** Send address changes to *Neurologic Clinics*, Elsevier Health Sciences Division, Subscription Customer Service, 3251 Riverport Lane, Maryland Heights, MO 63043. **Customer Service: Telephone: 1-800-654-2452 (U.S. and Canada); 314-447-8871 (outside U.S. and Canada). Fax: 314-447-8029. E-mail: journalscustomerservice-usa@elsevier.com (for print support); journalsonlinesupport-usa@elsevier.com (for online support).**

Reprints. For copies of 100 or more of articles in this publication, please contact the Commercial Reprints Department, Elsevier Inc., 360 Park Avenue South, New York, New York, 10010-1710; Tel.: (+1) 212-633-3812; Fax: (+1) 212-462-1935, and E-mail: reprints@elsevier.com.

Neurologic Clinics is also published in Spanish by Nueva Editorial Interamericana S.A., Mexico City, Mexico.

Neurologic Clinics is covered in *Current Contents/Clinical Medicine, MEDLINE/PubMed (Index Medicus), EMBASE/Excerpta Medica, and PsycINFO, and ISI/BIOMED.*

Printed and bound by CPI Group (UK) Ltd, Croydon, CR0 4YY
Transferred to Digital Print 2012

Contributors

CONSULTING EDITOR

RANDOLPH W. EVANS, MD
Clinical Professor, Department of Neurology, Baylor College of Medicine, Houston, Texas

GUEST EDITOR

DEVON I. RUBIN, MD
Associate Professor of Neurology, Department of Neurology, Mayo Clinic,
Jacksonville, Florida

AUTHORS

NEIL BUSIS, MD, FAAN
Chief, Section of Neurology, Division of Medicine; Director, Neurodiagnostic Laboratory,
UPMC Shadyside Hospital, Pittsburgh, Pennsylvania

WILLIAM S. DAVID, MD, PhD
Associate Professor of Neurology, Department of Neurology, Harvard Medical School,
Boston, Massachusetts

ELLIOT L. DIMBERG, MD
Assistant Professor of Neurology, Department of Neurology, Mayo Clinic,
Jacksonville, Florida

RACHEL DITRAPANI, MD
Department of Neurology, Mayo Clinic, Jacksonville, Florida

MARK A. FERRANTE, MD
Director, EMG Laboratory, Guadalupe Regional Medical Center, Seguin, Texas; Clinical
Professor, Department of Neurology, University of Tennessee Health Science Center,
Memphis, Tennessee

VERA FRIDMAN, MD
Instructor of Neurology, Harvard Medical School, Department of Neurology,
Boston, Massachusetts

LYELL K. JONES Jr, MD
Department of Neurology, Mayo Clinic, Rochester, Minnesota

VERN C. JUEL, MD
Associate Professor of Medicine (Neurology), Duke University School of Medicine;
Associate Director, Electromyography Laboratory, Duke University Medical Center,
Durham, North Carolina

KATHLEEN D. KENNELLY, MD, PhD
Assistant Professor of Neurology, Department of Neurology, Mayo Clinic, Jacksonville, Florida

DAVID LACOMIS, MD
Professor of Neurology and Pathology, Division of Neuromuscular Diseases, University of Pittsburgh School of Medicine, UPMC- Presbyterian, Pittsburgh, Pennsylvania

KERRY H. LEVIN, MD
Chairman, Department of Neurology; Director, Neuromuscular Center, Cleveland Clinic; Professor of Medicine (Neurology), Cleveland Clinic Lerner College of Medicine, Cleveland, Ohio

MARK A. ROSS, MD, FAAN
Professor of Neurology, Director, EMG Laboratory, Department of Neurology, Mayo Clinic Arizona, Scottsdale, Arizona

DEVON I. RUBIN, MD
Associate Professor of Neurology, Department of Neurology, Mayo Clinic, Jacksonville, Florida

ERIC J. SORENSON, MD
Associate Professor of Neurology, Department of Neurology, Mayo Clinic, Rochester, Minnesota

JAMES C. WATSON, MD
Consultant and Assistant Professor of Neurology, Mayo Clinic, Rochester, Minnesota

Contents

As a fundamental component of the electrodiagnostic evaluation, nerve conduction studies provide valuable quantitative and qualitative insights into neuromuscular function. Nerve conduction studies are useful in the identification and characterization of several neuromuscular disorders, particularly disorders of peripheral nerve. Abnormalities of nerve conduction studies may anticipate specific pathologic processes, such as demyelination or axonal loss, and may provide precise localization of focal nerve lesions. As with other elements of the electrodiagnostic evaluation, nerve conduction studies must be performed with careful attention to technique and must be interpreted in a clinical context.

Needle electromyography (EMG) records electrical signals generated from muscle fibers and interprets the signals to characterize underlying pathologic changes that are occurring in motor units within muscles. Different types of spontaneously firing waveforms and motor unit potential changes occur with different neuromuscular disorders. The performance of reliable EMG studies depends on the technical skills of the physician in inserting, moving, recording with a needle electrode, and analyzing electric signals recorded from muscle. This article reviews the technique of needle EMG and recognition and interpretation of various EMG waveforms. The author presents several demonstrative videos at www.neurologic.theclinics.com.

CTS is a clinically defined syndrome; however, there is value added by an evidence-based electrodiagnostic approach to (1) efficiently confirm the diagnosis (particularly before invasive interventions), (2) to identify neurogenic mimickers or superimposed processes that may influence the response to treatment, and (3) to stratify the degree of neurogenic injury to help the clinician make management decisions in conjunction with the severity of the clinical symptoms. The literature on the electrodiagnostic diagnosis of CTS is reviewed and an evidence based diagnostic algorithm is proposed. Confounders to CTS electrodiagnostic diagnosis are discussed (crossovers, peripheral neuropathy, and recurrent symptoms after surgical release).

Upper extremity mononeuropathies are some of the common disorders seen in neurophysiology laboratories. Electrophysiologic studies rely on accurate localization based on knowledge of applicable anatomy and features of history and physical examination. Careful electrodiagnostic studies provide an accurate diagnosis, help localize the lesion site, exclude alternate diagnoses, reveal unsuspected diagnoses, determine pathophysiology of lesions, and assess severity, timeframe, and prognosis of lesions. This article discusses the electrodiagnostic approach to ulnar neuropathy, proximal median neuropathy, radial neuropathy, musculocutaneous neuropathy, axillary neuropathy, suprascapular neuropathy, and long thoracic neuropathy. Pertinent aspects of the history and physical examination, nerve conduction studies, and electromyography are presented.

This article discusses the anatomy of lower limb mononeuropathies and reviews the general approach to evaluating patients in the electrodiagnostic laboratory with suspected mononeuropathies of the lower limb. Through illustrative cases of patients presenting with a floppy foot, buckling knee, or painful foot, the approaches using nerve conduction studies and needle electromyography are reviewed, and the pattern of findings of peroneal, tibial, sciatic, femoral, and obturator neuropathies is shown.

Electrodiagnostic studies are an important component of the evaluation of patients with suspected peripheral nerve disorders. The pattern of findings and the features that are seen on the motor and sensory nerve conduction studies and needle electromyography can help to identify the type of neuropathy, define the underlying pathophysiology (axonal or demyelinating), and ultimately help to narrow the list of possible causes. This article reviews the electrodiagnostic approach to and interpretation of findings in patients with peripheral neuropathies.

The brachial plexus is one of the largest and most complex structures of the peripheral nervous system and, as such, cannot be studied by a single nerve conduction study (NCS) or muscle sampled by needle electrode examination (NEE). Typically, the screening sensory NCS is used and expanded to identify the region of involvement, the motor NCS is applied to determine the severity of the process, and the NEE is used to further characterize the lesion. Our approach to the electrodiagnostic assessment of the brachial plexus is the focus of this article; 3 electrodiagnostic cases with discussion follow this article.

Radiculopathy is a common neurologic disorder. Electrodiagnosis can provide a physiologic assessment of the localization, degree of axon loss, severity, and chronicity of the intraspinal canal lesion, and distinguish it from other neuromuscular disorders. This article reviews electrodiagnostic aspects related to evaluating patients with suspected radiculopathies.

The motor neuron diseases are a set of disorders associated with the selective degeneration of motor neurons. Amyotrophic lateral sclerosis (ALS) is the most common and confers the gravest prognosis. Although ALS occurs with known genetic causes in a small minority, other motor neuron disorders have well-defined genetic mutations. Electrodiagnostic testing is important to distinguish these various disorders. Electrodiagnostic testing is also crucial for distinguishing potential mimic syndromes, such as multifocal motor neuropathy and inclusion body myositis. Newer neurophysiology techniques have been developed in the past several years. What role these techniques will play in clinical practice is currently unknown.

Neuromuscular junction (NMJ) disorders may be demonstrated using repetitive nerve stimulation (RNS) testing and single-fiber electromyography (SFEMG). RNS testing with low frequency stimulation reduces the safety factor of neuromuscular transmission (NMT) and may elicit decrementing compound muscle action potential (CMAP) responses. Exercise or tetanic nerve stimulation may potentiate acetylcholine release in presynaptic NMT disorders with CMAP facilitation. SFEMG is a selective recording technique assessing MFAPs within the same motor unit. Jitter is increased in NMJ disorders, and is the temporal variability between these MFAPs. Impulse blocking reflects failure of NMT. RNS and SFEMG findings in NMJ disorders are reviewed.

Electrodiagnostic testing is a useful component of the approach to a patient with suspected myopathy. It follows the history and is guided by the neurologic examination findings. Uncovering various electrodiagnostic patterns (eg, fibrillation potentials with short-duration motor unit potentials, short-duration motor unit potentials without fibrillation potentials, myotonic discharges, and short-duration motor unit potentials with complex repetitive discharges) can lead to more targeted laboratory testing and a refined differential diagnosis. Electromyography may also be used to detect subclinical myopathy, assess disease activity, and help select a suitable muscle for biopsy.

THE CLINICS ARE NOW AVAILABLE ONLINE!

Access your subscription at:
www.theclinics.com

Preface

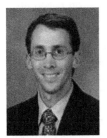

Devon I. Rubin, MD
Guest Editor

Neuromuscular disorders are commonly encountered in general and specialty neurologic practices. In some instances the diagnosis of a specific neuromuscular condition can be made entirely on clinical grounds, such as a patient who consistently leans on his elbow and develops tingling in his 5th and half of his 4th digits, indicating an ulnar neuropathy. Unfortunately, in many cases the presenting symptoms are nonspecific and could be the result of several possible etiologies, such as a patient with generalized weakness that may be the result of a myopathy, neuromuscular junction disorder, or motor neuron disease. Therefore, in practice, electrodiagnostic testing is an integral and complementary component of the evaluation of patients with suspected neuromuscular conditions.

The techniques of nerve conduction studies and needle EMG are seemingly simple, straightforward, and widely performed by neurologists; however, in reality, these studies are complicated and require expert training and experience to perform and interpret appropriately. Accurate performance and interpretation of EMG studies requires a solid understanding of the normal and abnormal physiology of nerve, neuromuscular junction, and muscle, an understanding of technical issues that can affect the recorded responses, and knowledge of the changes that occur on the various electrodiagnostic studies in different pathologic conditions.

In this issue of *Neurologic Clinics*, a group of experts in electrodiagnostic medicine concisely review a number of important and practical aspects related to the performance and interpretation of electrodiagnostic studies. The beginning articles review the concepts of nerve conduction studies and needle examination and focus on the general changes or findings that occur with different types of conditions. The next group of articles are separated according to specific problems or disorders that may be encountered in the electrodiagnostic laboratory, ranging from common conditions such as carpal tunnel syndrome or peripheral neuropathies to uncommon conditions such as brachial plexopathies and neuromuscular junction disorders. Each article reviews the approaches and considerations taken when evaluating each type of problem, and illustrative cases are included within individual articles as well as in

Neurol Clin 30 (2012) xi–xii
doi:10.1016/j.ncl.2011.12.015
0733-8619/12/$ – see front matter © 2012 Elsevier Inc. All rights reserved.

neurologic.theclinics.com

a separate article dedicated to case studies. An additional article discusses technical issues that must be considered when performing and interpreting the studies, since many technical problems can mimic abnormalities. Finally, an article on billing and coding of electrodiagnostic studies—including the recent changes to coding for electrodiagnostic studies—completes the issue.

The goal and hope of this issue are that it will assist physicians who are learning or performing EMG in their practices by helping to solidify the approaches that they take when performing EMG studies, assist in their understanding of the findings that are expected in different conditions, and ultimately lead to improvements in diagnostic accuracy and patient care.

I wish to thank all of the expert authors who have dedicated their time and efforts to contributing to the issue. I would also like to thank Donald Mumford, *Clinics* developmental editor for Elsevier, who provided editorial assistance throughout the development of this issue.

Devon I. Rubin, MD
Department of Neurology
Mayo Clinic
4500 San Pablo Road
Jacksonville, FL 32224, USA

E-mail address:
rubin.devon@mayo.edu

Nerve Conduction Studies: Basic Concepts and Patterns of Abnormalities

Lyell K. Jones Jr, MD

KEYWORDS

- Nerve conduction studies • Sensory conduction studies
- Motor conduction studies • F waves • H reflexes
- Clinical neurophysiology • Neuromuscular disease

As a fundamental component of the electrodiagnostic evaluation, nerve conduction studies (NCSs) provide valuable quantitative and qualitative insight into neuromuscular function.[1] Typically paired with needle electrode examination, NCS may direct the clinician to definitive diagnostic testing or provide the sole substantiation of a neuromuscular diagnosis. The clinical value of NCS is tempered by a variety of potential sources of technical error that can be mitigated with careful attention to technique.[2] Like all elements of the electrodiagnostic evaluation, NCS must be interpreted with the clinical scenario in mind, and, in this manner, they serve as a useful extension of the neurologic examination.

The goals of this article are to review the neurophysiologic underpinnings of NCS, to outline the technical factors associated with the performance of NCS, and to demonstrate characteristic NCS changes in the setting of various neuromuscular conditions.

BASIC CONCEPTS
Anatomic Considerations

The responsiveness of the peripheral nervous system to electrical stimulation has been recognized since at least the eighteenth century.[3] In the simplest terms, modern clinical NCSs consist of stimulating a peripheral nerve and recording the response elsewhere on contiguous nerve or from a skeletal muscle innervated by that nerve. Although a variety of methods may be used for stimulus or recording,[4] most NCSs currently are performed with cutaneous, or surface, stimulating and recording electrodes. As a result, it is

The author has nothing to disclose.
Department of Neurology, Mayo Clinic, 200 First Street SW, Rochester, MN 55905, USA
E-mail address: Lyell@mayo.edu

Neurol Clin 30 (2012) 405–427
doi:10.1016/j.ncl.2011.12.002
0733-8619/12/$ – see front matter

important for the electrodiagnostician to understand that all surface points of stimulation, points of recording, and measurements thereof are approximations of the locations of their subcutaneous targets. This principle is important in terms of understanding that surface measurements may not precisely reflect underlying anatomy and that uncertainty of sites of stimulation or recording limits the value of the study.[5] A useful rule of thumb is that an NCS is useful insomuch as the examiner is certain what is being stimulated and what is being recorded.

For example, surface electrical stimulation of deeper nerves (such as the lower trunk of the brachial plexus) often requires large amounts of current. As a result, nearby neural structures (in this case, other elements of the brachial plexus) are likely to be incidentally stimulated. This may introduce doubt as to the generator of recorded responses elsewhere on the limb. Conversely, recording from proximal muscles that are adjacent to large similarly innervated muscles leads to a degree of uncertainty as to the source of a surface-recorded response.

For these reasons, NCS of proximal structures is technically challenging and performed much less commonly than NCS of more distal, and therefore easier to isolate, limb structures.[6] With careful attention to technique, the examiner can approach a reasonable degree of certainty of selective stimulation and recording of distal nerves and muscles.

Stimulation

Stimulation methods can be tailored to the desired target (eg, needle electrodes may be used to stimulate proximal spinal nerves), but, in general, nerve stimulators consist of a handheld bipolar probe comprising an anode and a cathode. The cathode is typically oriented distally or in the direction of the intended action potential recording. Skin at anticipated sites of stimulation should be cleaned to minimize impedance. The stimulus may be delivered at either a constant current (in milliamperes) or a constant voltage (in volts), generally the former. It is important to ensure that at each site of nerve stimulation all elements of the nerve are depolarized as completely as possible; this is achieved with successive stimuli using increasing levels of current until a point at which the current is increased but the size of the recorded potential does not change. This is referred to as supramaximal stimulation. In practice, this stimulation is performed with small incremental increases in current (around 10 mA with each increase) until an intermediate response is detected. Then the stimulating electrodes are adjusted positionally in a technique called sliding to ensure that the optimal point of nerve stimulation has been isolated.[7] Current is subsequently increased until supramaximal stimulation is obtained. The duration of the stimulus is generally 0.1 milliseconds (ms) but may be increased to up to 1.0 ms if a supramaximal response cannot be obtained with up to 100 mA of current. Motor and larger sensory axons have lower depolarization thresholds (in other words, they are stimulated with smaller amounts of current) than small-diameter sensory fibers,[7] a physiologic feature that has clinical relevance discussed later.

Recording

Recording electrodes consist of an active (or G1) electrode and an inactive (reference or G2) electrode placed at some distance from G1. The spatial relationship between the recording electrodes is important because the distance between them allows for the difference in charge (or voltage) that generates the recorded potential.[8] A compromise must be reached when determining the distance between G1 and G2 recording sites. Electrodes that are too close to one another may lack sufficient electrical distinction, resulting in spuriously small responses, and electrodes placed too far apart enhance the recording of unwanted environmental or physiologic artifacts. As with stimulation, recording methods are also adapted to the target at hand. Metal or self-adhesive active and reference recording electrodes may be used for muscle or nerve recording, and digital nerves may be recorded using ring electrodes. A surface ground electrode is required and may be placed between the stimulation and recording sites; self-adhesive ground electrodes may suffice, although large lead grounds may be necessary at times to minimize environmental electrical artifact. Skin preparation at all points of recording is crucial, particularly for smaller-amplitude sensory responses, and, with metal electrodes, a conducting gel is required to minimize impedance. The recorded potentials are measured as a function of time and voltage (generally in a range from microvolts to millivolts, depending on the structure recorded). Normal values for commonly performed NCS should be established within each laboratory's practice, or, when use of published normal values is required, careful adherence to normative technique must be observed.[9,10] Uncommonly performed NCSs may need to be compared with contralateral studies to determine normality (in the setting of clinically unilateral processes).[11]

TYPES OF NCSs

NCSs may generally be divided into motor studies (where skeletal muscle is the recording target) and sensory studies (where peripheral nerve is the recording target) (**Fig. 1**). Recordings from the nerve can reflect depolarization of sensory elements alone or of both sensory and motor (mixed) elements of the nerve.[12] Other techniques such as F-wave and H-reflex recording follow similar principles and are reviewed here. Common and uncommon motor and sensory NCSs are listed in **Tables 1–4**.

Motor Conduction Studies

The G1 recording electrode in motor NCSs is placed over the innervation point of the muscle of interest, also known as the end plate or motor point.[13] Often, but not exclusively, this point is located over the midbelly of the muscle. The G2 reference electrode is generally placed distally; typically, this is over the inserting tendon of the muscle. Supramaximal stimulation of the innervating nerve is then performed over at least 2 points on the nerve.

At each site of stimulation, a nerve action potential is generated that propagates in both directions along the nerve. Via neuromuscular transmission, the distal-traveling nerve action potential generates an action potential in the innervated muscle. The recorded potential represents the summated and largely synchronous depolarization of nearly all the muscle fibers in the muscle and is appropriately termed a compound muscle action potential (CMAP, in some settings called an M wave).

Various attributes of the CMAP are of clinical interest, and it is worthwhile to consider the "anatomy" of the waveform (**Fig. 2**). The initial deflection of this biphasic waveform is upward (counterintuitively described as a negative deflection), reflecting the placement of the G1 electrode over the point of depolarization of the muscle. The CMAP amplitude, measured from the baseline to the negative peak, is an invaluable measure and generally occurs on the order of millivolts (mV). Owing in part to the relatively uniform size and action potential propagation rate of peripheral motor axons, CMAP amplitudes are generally similar between distal and proximal sites of stimulation (more proximally generated CMAPs are slightly smaller).[6] The documented CMAP amplitude may be taken from proximal or distal stimulation sites, although the chosen site should be consistent within an electrodiagnostic practice. The distal

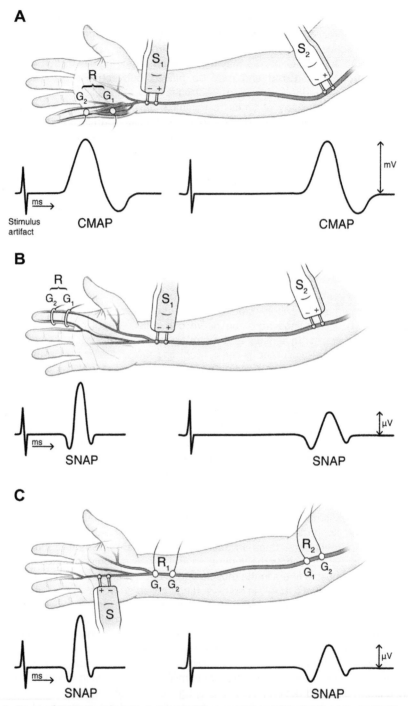

Fig. 1. Types of NCSs. An ulnar motor study (*A*), a median antidromic sensory study (*B*), and a median orthodromic sensory study (*C*). Note the lower SNAP amplitude with more distant stimulation compared with the preserved CMAP amplitude at both stimulation sites. R, recording site; S, stimulation site.

Table 1
Commonly performed motor NCSs

Nerve	Proximal Stimulation Site	Distal Stimulation Site	Recorded Muscle
Upper limb			
Median	Elbow (antecubital fossa)	Wrist (between PL and FCR tendons)	Abductor pollicis brevis
Ulnar	Elbow (several centimeters proximal to the medial epicondyle)	Wrist (medial to the FCU tendon)	Abductor digiti minimi
Lower limb			
Peroneal	Knee (medial to the tendon of the biceps femoris)	Ankle (lateral to AT tendon)	Extensor digitorum brevis
Tibial	Knee (popliteal fossa)	Ankle (behind the medial malleolus)	Abductor hallucis

Abbreviations: AT, anterior tibialis; FCR, flexor carpi radialis; FCU, flexor carpi ulnaris; PL, palmaris longus.

latency of the CMAP, measured in milliseconds from the time of stimulation at a distal site to the initial deflection of the waveform, is measured and recorded. The difference in latency between proximal and distal sites of stimulation divided by the distance between those sites yields the conduction velocity.

Table 2
Uncommonly performed motor NCSs

Nerve	Proximal Stimulation Site	Distal Stimulation Site	Recorded Muscle
Bulbar			
Facial	—	Stylomastoid foramen or anterior to the tragus	Nasalis
Spinal accessory	—	Posterior border of the SCM	Trapezius
Upper limb			
Suprascapular	—	Suprascapular notch	Infraspinatus
Axillary	—	Erb point	Deltoid
Musculocutaneous	Erb's point	Anterior axillary fold	Biceps brachii
Radial	Spiral groove	Proximal forearm (medial to BR)	Extensor digitorum communis or extensor indicis proprius
Lower limb			
Femoral	—	Inguinal ligament	Rectus femoris
Peroneal	Knee (medial to the tendon of the biceps femoris)	Fibular head	Anterior tibialis
Tibial	Knee (popliteal fossa)	Ankle (behind the medial malleolus)	Abductor digiti minimi pedis

Abbreviations: BR, brachioradialis; SCM, sternocleidomastoid.

Table 3
Commonly performed sensory NCSs

Nerve	Proximal Stimulation Site	Distal Stimulation Site	Recording Site	Proximal Recording Site
Upper limb				
Antidromic				
Median	Elbow (antecubital fossa)	Wrist (between PL and FCR tendons)	Second digit (ring electrodes)	—
Ulnar	Elbow (several centimeters proximal to the medial epicondyle)	Wrist (medial to the FCU tendon)	Fifth digit (ring electrodes)	—
Radial	—	Lateral forearm	Wrist (as the nerve crosses the EPL tendon)	—
Orthodromic				
Median	—	Palmar crease	Wrist (between PL and FCR tendons)	Elbow (antecubital fossa)
Ulnar	—	Palmar crease	Wrist (medial to the FCU tendon)	Elbow (several centimeters proximal to the medial epicondyle)
Lower limb				
Antidromic				
Sural	—	3 sites along the nerve in midleg and distal leg	Ankle (behind the lateral malleolus)	—
Superficial peroneal	—	Anterior leg	Ankle (lateral to the AT tendon)	—
Orthodromic				
Medial plantar	—	Arch of the foot	Ankle (behind medial malleolus)	—

Abbreviations: AT, anterior tibialis; EPL, extensor pollicis longus; FCR, flexor carpi radialis; FCU, flexor carpi ulnaris; PL, palmaris longus.

Table 4
Uncommonly performed sensory NCSs

Nerve	Proximal Stimulation Site	Distal Stimulation Site	Recording Site
Bulbar			
Greater auricular	—	Lateral neck	Anterior to mastoid process
Upper limb			
Antidromic			
Dorsal ulnar cutaneous	—	Medial forearm	Mediodorsal hand
Lateral antebrachial cutaneous	—	Lateral to biceps brachii tendon	Lateral forearm
Medial antebrachial cutaneous	—	Medial to biceps brachii tendon	Medial forearm
Radial	—	Lateral forearm	First digit (ring electrodes)
Median	Elbow (antecubital fossa)	Wrist (between PL and FCR tendons)	First or third digit (ring electrodes)

Abbreviations: FCR, flexor carpi radialis; PL, palmaris longus.

$$\text{Conduction velocity} = \frac{\text{proximal latency} - \text{distal latency}}{\text{distance}}$$

The conduction velocity is measured in meters per second. This method, as opposed to calculating the velocity only with distal stimulation and dividing by the distance to the G1 electrode, allows for measurement of conduction over a longer segment of nerve and dilutes the effects of any distance measurement errors.

These quantitated features of the CMAP are the most commonly measured and provide valuable information regarding the speed of conduction of the nerve (distal latency and conduction velocity) and overall integrity of the motor unit (amplitude). Other less commonly measured attributes include the area under the CMAP and the duration of the CMAP.[5] In addition to these quantified measures, it is crucial for the electrodiagnostician to visually inspect the waveforms for accurate marking, as well as for qualitative abnormalities that are lost in the automated measures included on most electrodiagnostic software platforms.

Sensory Conduction Studies (Including Mixed Nerve Studies)

Stimulation of a sensory or mixed nerve also generates a bidirectionally propagating action potential that can be recorded and measured at other accessible points along the nerve.[12] The recorded potentials are called sensory nerve action potentials (SNAPs) and represent the summated depolarization of all nerve fiber action potentials; although these responses represent summated nerve action potentials and are therefore technically "compound" in nature, this term is not generally applied. When the stimulation and recording is performed on a mixed nerve, both sensory and motor fibers are depolarized, but, in general, the larger, more heavily myelinated, and faster-conducting sensory fibers are the primary constituents of the recorded potential.[7] For this reason, mixed nerve studies are discussed here and may generally be viewed in the same category as pure sensory nerve studies, although historically they have also

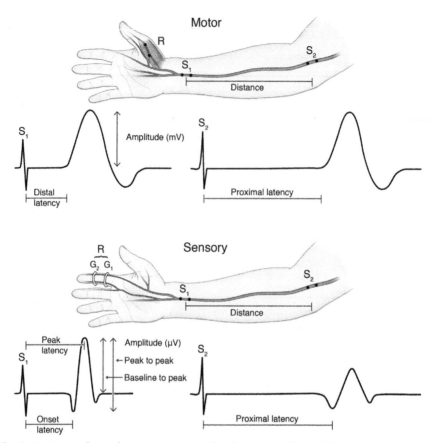

Fig. 2. Anatomy of waveforms. In motor studies (*upper panel*), the CMAP amplitude (mV) is measured from baseline to negative (*uppermost*) peak and the distal latency (ms) is measured to the initial deflection with distal stimulation. In contrast, the SNAP (*lower*) amplitude (μV) is measured from the positive peak to the negative peak, and the distal latency (ms) is measured to the negative peak of the distally acquired waveform. The conduction velocity (m/s) for both is taken as the time difference between distal-onset latency and proximal latency divided by the distance. R, recording site; S, stimulation site.

been considered separately.[14] Small nerve fibers, which as outlined earlier, have higher stimulation thresholds, do not generate a meaningful contribution to the surface-recorded SNAP. Conventional sensory studies therefore primarily assess large sensory fibers.

The principles of stimulation are similar to those outlined earlier for motor studies. In terms of recording electrodes, it is worth reemphasizing the importance of skin preparation before their application for sensory NCSs. Unlike the arrangement in motor studies, sensory recording electrodes are generally placed at a fixed relative distance (usually 3–4 cm apart along the course of the recorded nerve).[15]

There are several relevant physiologic differences between CMAPs and SNAPs. First, whereas CMAPs reflect a unidirectional recording that involves a nerve action potential, neuromuscular transmission, and a muscle action potential, SNAPs reflect only summated nerve action potentials. Therefore, SNAPs may be recorded either proximally or distally from the nerve to the point of stimulation. SNAPs recorded proximal to the point of stimulation are described as orthodromic (in the same direction as native sensory signal transmission), and SNAPs recorded distal to the point of stimulation are termed antidromic (in the opposite direction from native transmission). As a result of this flexibility, sensory conduction studies may be performed with 1 recording site and 2 or more points of stimulation, as with motor studies, or with 1 point of stimulation and multiple sites of recording (see **Fig. 1**).

A second distinguishing feature of SNAPs is their configuration (see **Fig. 2**). Unlike CMAPs, which are recorded at the point of initiation of the underlying compound action potential and show an initial negativity, the component nerve action potentials generated in SNAP approach the recording electrodes along the nerve. Therefore, there is often an initial positivity (downward deflection) at the onset of an SNAP. These differences in configuration necessitate differences in measurement approaches, outlined later.

Compared with motor axons, sensory axons within sensory and mixed nerves are (1) more variable in caliber and (2) more variable in degree of myelination.[12] These factors conspire to create differential conduction velocities within a propagating SNAP, with the practical result being appreciably smaller SNAP recordings with greater distance between stimulating and recording electrodes (phase cancellation of these desynchronized nerve action potentials plays a role as well). This is therefore a third important difference between CMAPs and SNAPs.

A fourth difference between SNAPs and CMAPs is the size of the obtained response. SNAPs are generated by much smaller volumes of tissue (nerves) than CMAPs (muscle), and its amplitudes are recorded on the order of microvolts. As a result of this low amplitude, SNAPs are challenged by a low signal to noise ratio. Careful attention to technique as well as using digital signal averaging (available on most electrodiagnostic platforms) helps mitigate this problem.

The quantitated elements of sensory NCSs are very similar to those of motor NCSs, with some important differences. As discussed earlier, the SNAP onset is often initially positive. Therefore, a peak-to-peak measurement of amplitude may be obtained and is the generally preferred approach. Further, although this onset latency with distal stimulation may itself be measured, the latency to the negative peak is more commonly used and is essentially synonymous with the distal latency of the SNAP. Sensory conduction velocities are measured in a manner similar to motor studies, although with multiple recording sites and a single point of stimulation, the distance between recording sites may be used to calculate the velocity.

F waves

For the various technical and anatomic reasons outlined earlier, most NCSs are performed on distal limb structures. As a result, the health of more proximal nerve segments is only indirectly interrogated by conventional NCS. However, there are some studies that do offer insight into the function of these more proximal nerves.

One such technique is F-wave recording. Initially noted during motor conduction studies recorded from foot muscles (leading to the moniker),[16,17] F waves reflect the depolarization of a small number of anterior horn cells by the proximal-traveling action potential created at the distal point of stimulation (**Fig. 3**).

As outlined earlier, the nerve action potential generated with surface stimulation travels in both directions along the nerve. Although the distal-traveling action potential generates the CMAP, the proximal-traveling action potential enters the anterior horn of the spinal cord via the ventral root and activates a small assortment of motor neurons. This small number of spinally generated action potentials then travels the full length of

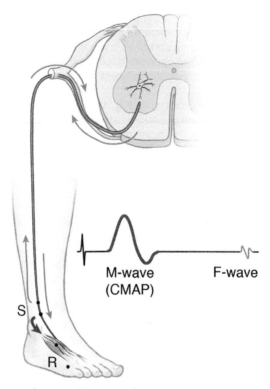

M-wave
(CMAP)   F-wave

Fig. 3. F waves. A normal peroneal F wave is shown, demonstrating how the long latency of the F wave is a reflection of the long proximal course of the action potential pathway. R, recording site; S, stimulation site.

the peripheral nerve and may be recorded in the innervated muscle. In practice, F waves may be reliably recorded from only a select number of distal upper and lower limb nerves and muscles (**Table 5**). F-wave studies are often performed after conventional motor studies of the same nerves and must be performed with supramaximal

Table 5
Studies of proximal nerve segments

Technique	Nerve	Stimulation Site	Recording Site
F wave			
	Median	Wrist (between PL and FCR tendons)	Abductor pollicis brevis
	Ulnar	Wrist (medial to the FCU tendon)	Abductor digiti minimi
	Peroneal	Ankle (lateral to AT tendon)	Extensor digitorum brevis
	Tibial	Ankle (behind the medial malleolus)	Abductor hallucis
H reflex			
	Tibial	Popiteal fossa	Soleus
	Median	Antecubital fossa	FCR or PT

Abbreviations: AT, anterior tibialis; FCR, flexor carpi radialis; FCU, flexor carpi ulnaris; PL, palmaris longus; PT, pronator teres.

stimulation; the anode may be rotated off of the nerve to reduce the risk of anodal block of the orthodromic volley.[18] The specific anterior horn cells that generate the F waves vary from stimulation to stimulation, and, generally speaking, 6 to 12 F-wave recordings are attempted in each study.

As a result of this long excursion, the F waves (which are small but can be distinguished from the CMAP owing to their much longer latency) offer some insight into the speed of conduction and integrity of proximal motor nerve segments. Several features of the F waves may be examined, such as their amplitude, configuration, reproducibility, and duration, but the most reproducible and commonly recorded characteristic is their latency.[19] Of the number of F waves present in a given study, the earliest reproducible latency is recorded.

The normal values for F-wave latencies may be calculated from studies of normal subjects, and, when done so, factors such as age and height should be taken into account. F-wave latencies may also be compared with an F estimate, calculated by the formula

$$F \text{ estimate} = \frac{2 \times F \text{ distance (mm)}}{\text{conduction velocity (m/s)}} + \text{distal latency}$$

where F distance is an approximate measurement of the distance the F-wave volley travels along the proximal nerve (this may be taken from the point of distal stimulation to the xiphoid process for lower limb studies and to the sternal notch for upper limb studies). The conduction velocity and distal latency used are those calculated during the preceding motor study of the same nerve. When there is disproportionate slowing in proximal nerve segments, F-wave latencies will be prolonged beyond the estimate. Conversely, when slowing is primarily distal, the F-wave latency will fall well within the estimate.

H reflexes

Unlike F waves, which reflect a purely motor pathway, the H reflex represents the electrophysiologic analogue of a monosynaptic muscle stretch reflex. With stimulation of a mixed nerve, the action potentials generated in the motor axons in turn generate a CMAP in the innervated muscle. Simultaneously, 1a-afferent proprioceptive sensory fibers innervating muscle spindles are stimulated. The proximal-traveling action potentials in these fibers enter the spinal cord via the dorsal roots and via a monosynaptic reflex excite segmentally corresponding anterior horn cells, generating a recorded response in the same muscle. This is the H reflex (**Fig. 4**).

H reflexes are technically feasible in a very limited number of nerves (see **Table 5**). Tibial H reflexes are by far the most commonly performed, although they may be performed in the upper limb as well.[20] Stimulation uses a low-amplitude, longer-duration current (generally on the order of 5–25 mA for 1 ms). The cathode should be oriented proximally to the nerve, and low rates of stimulation should be ensured. With increasing current, the H reflex becomes apparent and then diminishes in amplitude progressively with the appearance of the much larger M wave (CMAP), likely as a result of central inhibition. Measurements of the H reflex can include the latency (which is similar to that of the F waves) or the amplitude of the response.[21]

H reflexes (named not after a body part but rather Hoffmann, who was the first to describe them[22,23]) are therefore another tool used to assess proximal nerve segments, and they provide one of the few electrophysiologic opportunities to interrogate the dorsal root.

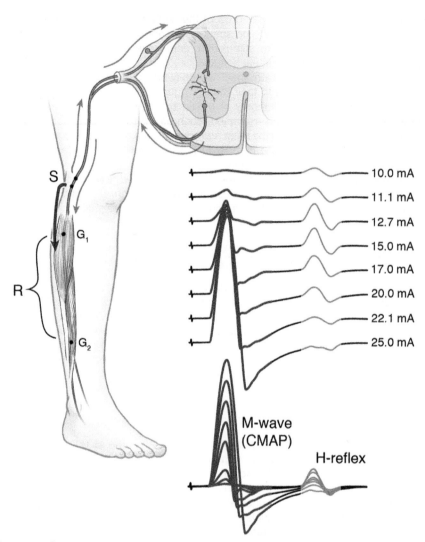

Fig. 4. H reflexes. In contrast to the F wave, the course of the tibial H reflex traverses the dorsal root, creating a monosynaptic reflex and subsequent muscle contraction in the recorded soleus. Note the appearance and subsequent disappearance of the H reflex with increasing levels of current, while the M wave (CMAP) continues to increase in amplitude. R, recording site; S, stimulation site.

TECHNICAL ELEMENTS OF NCSs

Careful adherence to technique is critical for the execution of valid reproducible NCSs. In addition to the general principles outlined in the foregoing sections, some additional factors require mention.

Temperature

For all NCSs, limb temperature must be measured and ideally monitored. With decreasing temperature, changes in membrane channel kinetics result in slowing of conduction velocities and prolongation of distal latencies, and SNAP amplitudes may be increased. Limbs that are too cool (generally <30°C in the lower limb and 32°C in the upper limb, measured with a cutaneous thermistor) should be warmed, ideally with warm water immersion or heat packs. Surface heat lamp warming primarily prevents further cooling and directly warms up the thermistor, leading to false reassurance. Published temperature correction factors for conduction velocity should be avoided. All warming should be performed with the patient's safety in mind (ie, warming patients should be supervised to prevent burns, and many unconventional techniques such as warming damp towels in the microwave are unsafe).

Safety

NCSs may be uncomfortable for the patient but are generally well tolerated with patience and preceding explanation and are overall very safe. There are, however, unusual circumstances in which additional attention to safety is required. The cutaneous impedance inherent in surface stimulation provides a protective current sink that is compromised in patients with indwelling cardiac catheters.[24,25] In these patients, nerve stimulation adjacent to these catheters should be avoided. Several small series have demonstrated that patients with implanted cardiac pacemakers and defibrillators may safely undergo routine NCS of the distal limbs,[26,27] although none have addressed the safety of proximal ipsilateral upper limb nerve stimulation, and therefore these techniques should generally be avoided in these patients absent a compelling need.

Artifacts and Other Sources of Error

In an electrically active world, there are myriad potential sources of electrical interference with NCS. Ubiquitous alternating current artifact (in the United States, this 60-Hz or 60-cycle artifact reflects the alternating rate used in the consumer power grid) can be minimized by effective grounding or ideally in an electrically shielded laboratory. Increasingly, implantable devices are a source of artifact. Poor relaxation of skeletal muscles may be a source of unwanted electrical noise in studies in which higher gains are used, such as sensory NCSs or F waves. Further, there are other more prosaic sources of error, such as measurement errors, anomalous innervation, understimulation, and overstimulation, which are explored in further detail in a later article by Devon Rubin's elsewhere in this issue.

Limitations of NCS

Although NCSs are a very useful tool in neuromuscular diagnosis, there are some limitations inherent in the technique. NCSs selectively assess large, more heavily myelinated fibers and are unhelpful in excluding neuropathies that selectively affect small nerve fibers. For the variety of technical reasons already reviewed, NCSs are generally performed on distal limbs; as a result, although NCS changes may be seen distally with proximal axonal lesions[28] (whose features are discussed in the next section), demyelination or conduction block that occurs only proximally is more difficult to detect (also explored later).[19,29] Conventional NCS cannot detect clinically meaningful processes that primarily or exclusively affect the dorsal root, and alternative techniques such as H reflexes (if at the corresponding level) or somatosensory evoked potentials may be required.

NCS CORRELATES OF NEUROMUSCULAR DISEASE
General Principles

While conventional NCS can provide useful information about all elements of the peripheral nervous system, they provide the richest detail for the neurogenic pathology explored further in this section. Myopathies may demonstrate low-amplitude CMAPs when severe and when they affect the recorded muscle, but this is rather uncommon, and there are other, more useful components of the electrodiagnostic evaluation for the identification and characterization of myopathies (such as the needle electrode examination). Repetitive stimulation is an invaluable tool in the diagnosis of disorders of neuromuscular transmission and is reviewed in further detail in a later article by Vern Juel's elsewhere in this issue. It is very uncommon for NCSs to indicate a central nervous system abnormality.[30]

The design of the electrodiagnostic evaluation, including the choice of NCSs, should be tailored to the clinical diagnostic considerations at hand. This burden is incumbent upon the electrodiagnostician; the referring provider who sees only normal study in the report may not be aware that lower limb studies do not exclude a median neuropathy at the wrist. Although clinical scenarios and individual practice styles vary, a good general rule is to ensure that when possible, motor conduction studies are performed in the distribution of weakness and sensory studies are performed in areas of sensory symptoms or findings.

It is important to recall that electrodiagnostic abnormalities often correlate very well, but not perfectly, with their corresponding pathologic substrates. Therefore, the patterns of NCS changes discussed here are best considered to anticipate, not define, these underlying pathophysiologic processes.

Changes in individual NCSs must be interpreted not only in the patient's clinical context but also in conjunction with other NCS findings. Whereas focal disorders may show abnormalities in only one study, diffuse neuromuscular disorders typically show more widespread derangements. In general, the design of the electrodiagnostic evaluation should presume that abnormalities reflect a diffuse process until its borders are delineated. For example, NCSs performed in only a single lower limb in a patient with a sciatic mononeuropathy may show changes that cannot be electrodiagnostically distinguished from a diffuse length-dependent peripheral neuropathy unless additional evaluation of another limb is pursued. This principle of bracketing the lesion should inform not only the choice of NCS to perform but also how the generated results are interpreted. Bracketing requires flexibility and real-time interpretation of NCS results so the evaluation can be appropriately adjusted as it is performed.

Axonal Loss

As the conducting elements of peripheral nerve, the loss of axons results in characteristic pathologic changes and accompanying electrophysiologic correlates. Regardless of mechanism, axonal loss occurs when axonal continuity is disrupted between anterior horn cells or sensory cell bodies and their distal targets. Therefore, axonal lesions at the level of the peripheral nerve or brachial or lumbosacral plexi may cause corresponding changes on motor or sensory NCS.[31] Conventionally, root-level axonal processes may cause changes on motor studies but spare sensory NCS (most dorsal root ganglia are distal enough to be spared in intraspinal disorders), although less commonly radiculopathies may result in SNAP changes.[32]

For both motor and sensory NCSs, the hallmark of axonal loss is reduction in CMAP or SNAP amplitude (**Fig. 5**).[33,34] Conduction velocities may be mildly slowed and distal latencies mildly prolonged, owing to selective loss of larger-diameter and therefore

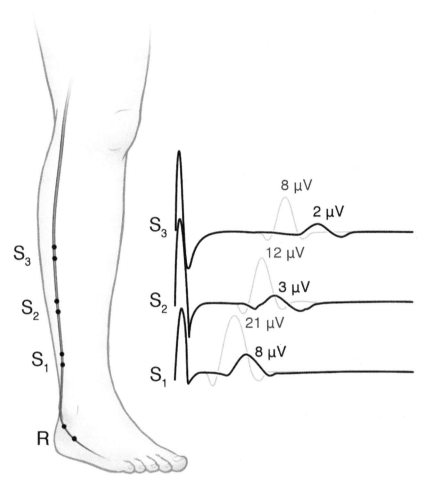

Fig. 5. Axonal loss. A sural SNAP with 3 points of stimulation along the dorsolateral leg in a patient with a length-dependent peripheral neuropathy. The low-amplitude SNAPs are in contrast to the expected normal amplitudes (shaded SNAPs). Note that there is much more reduction in amplitude than there is prolongation of latency, which is characteristic of axonal processes. R, recording site; S, stimulation site.

faster-conducting axons. These secondary changes in the speed of conduction become more prominent with more extensive axonal loss. Following acute axonal lesions, wallerian degeneration takes place on the order of days after the injury, over which time the loss of amplitude develops.[35] For chronic, slowly progressive axonal disorders, reinnervation of denervated muscle fibers through axonal sprouting may result in preservation of CMAP amplitude until advanced stages of axonal loss.[36] For most disorders that result in loss of both sensory and motor axons, SNAP amplitudes are affected earlier and more conspicuously.[33,37] It is also important to recall that severe demyelination may result in secondary axonal loss (**Table 6**).

Demyelination

The saltatory propagation of action potentials along the internodes of myelinated axons allows for high velocity of conduction, and, unsurprisingly, the neurophysiologic

Table 6
Summary of NCS changes seen with axonal loss and demyelination

	Amplitude	Conduction Velocity	Distal Latency
Axonal loss	Decreased	Generally preserved Mild slowing may be seen with prominent axonal loss	Generally preserved Mild prolongation may be seen with prominent axonal loss
Demyelination	Preserved with uniform demyelination May be decreased with temporal dispersion or conduction block	Significant slowing	Significant prolongation

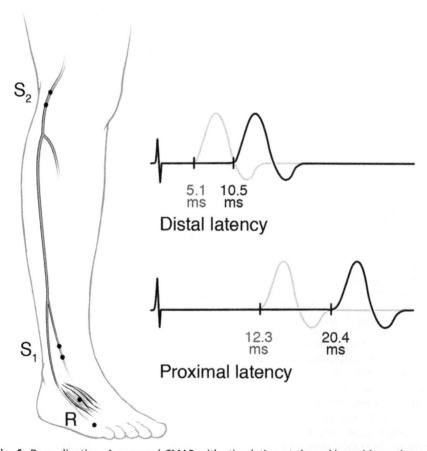

Fig. 6. Demyelination. A peroneal CMAP with stimulation at the ankle and knee demonstrates prolonged distal and proximal latencies compared with a normal waveform (shaded CMAPs). Over a fixed distance, the particularly prolonged proximal latency translates into a slowed conduction velocity. Note the preserved amplitudes, suggesting that the demyelination is uniform within the nerve, a common characteristic of inherited myelinopathies, such as with peripheral myelin protein 22 duplications. R, recording site; S, stimulation site.

hallmark of demyelination is slowing of conduction velocity and prolongation of distal latencies (**Fig. 6**).[38,39] In disorders in which the slowing is uniform among all fascicles of the nerve, CMAP and SNAP amplitudes may be spared (eg, among some inherited demyelinating neuropathies).[40,41] For many acquired primary disorders of myelin, the various fascicles within the nerve may be affected to differing degrees, resulting in temporal dispersion of the CMAP (discussed later).[42]

Because of the degree of slowing that may be seen with axonal loss and the therapeutic import of accurately identifying demyelinating peripheral neuropathies such as chronic inflammatory demyelinating polyradiculoneuropathy, there have been several specific criteria proposed for the definition of demyelination.[38,43] Regardless of the specific criteria used, the primary principle to recall is that the slowing of conduction is out of proportion to any changes noted in amplitude (see **Table 6**).

Demyelination that affects proximal nerve segments may result in prolongation of F-wave or H-reflex latencies (**Fig. 7**).[44] Blink reflexes, performed by stimulation of the supraorbital nerve and recording the ipsilateral and contralateral reflex contraction of the orbicularis oculi, are also a useful tool for characterizing very proximal demyelination or neuropathies that have abolished limb sensory responses. For demyelinating disorders that primarily or exclusively affect proximal neural structures, these may be the only revelatory electrodiagnostic tests.

Temporal Dispersion

As mentioned earlier, it is critically important for the electrodiagnostician to visually inspect NCS waveforms for qualitative abnormalities. One of the changes that

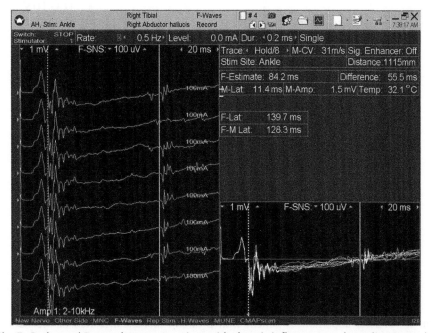

Fig. 7. Prolonged F-wave latency. A patient with chronic inflammatory demyelinating polyradiculoneuropathy demonstrates a very prolonged tibial F-wave latency of 139.7 ms, both in absolute terms and in comparison with the calculated estimate of 84.2 ms. This suggests proximal slowing out of proportion to the clear distal slowing.

may be visually striking but may escape description with automated CMAP measurement is temporal dispersion (**Fig. 8**). Classically reflecting demyelination that differentially affects various fascicles of motor nerves, temporal dispersion essentially represents a desynchronization of the CMAP.[45] As a result, the CMAP amplitude is decreased, the duration is prolonged, and the normally smooth contour of the waveform is replaced by a jagged configuration. Although prominent temporal dispersion usually reflects histopathologic demyelination, very-low-amplitude CMAPs resulting from axonal pathologic condition may have a similar appearance.

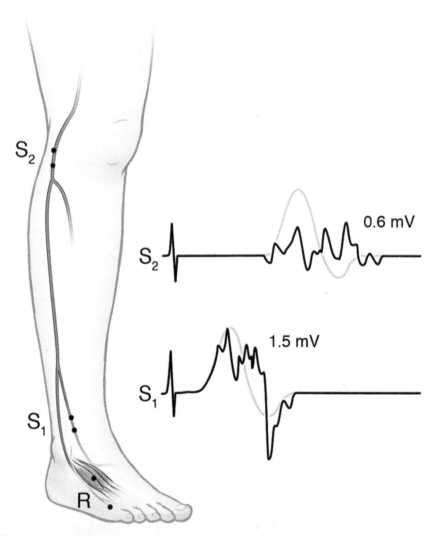

Fig. 8. Temporal dispersion. A patient with a chronic immune-mediated demyelinating peripheral neuropathy demonstrates significant temporal dispersion of the peroneal CMAP (compared with the normally contoured shaded CMAP). This suggests differential degrees of slowing within the various fascicles of the affected nerve. R, recording site; S, stimulation site.

Conduction Block and Focal Slowing

When a focal nerve lesion is of sufficient severity to partially or completely arrest the traversing nerve action potentials, some degree of conduction block is present.[46,47] Electrophysiologically, conduction block is demonstrated by lower-amplitude responses with stimulation across the area of block (**Fig. 9**). Although conduction block may occur in any component of any peripheral nerve, the physiologic decreases in SNAP amplitude with increasingly distant stimulation essentially limits the electrophysiologic characterization of block to motor studies alone.

As discussed earlier, CMAP amplitudes are generally preserved with increasingly proximal stimulation. Observation of conduction block is therefore usually expressed as a percentage decrease in CMAP amplitude or area compared with a more distal preserved CMAP. Criteria may also be applied to formally define conduction block,[47] and qualifying decreases in amplitude generally range from 20% to 50% over long segments of nerve to just 10% over a short segment of nerve. Implied is the need to stimulate across the area of block; when the block affects proximal neural structures, it may only be demonstrated by very proximal nerve stimulation (such as with needle stimulation of spinal nerves) or inferred from absent F waves.

Conduction block represents a focal pathologic process affecting peripheral nerve. However, although conduction block is generally used interchangeably with suspected underlying segmental demyelination, axonal pathology may also create clinically and electrophysiologically observable conduction block.[48,49] For example, acute focal axonal lesions and chronic immune-mediated neuropathies such as multifocal motor neuropathy with conduction block may both be characterized by some

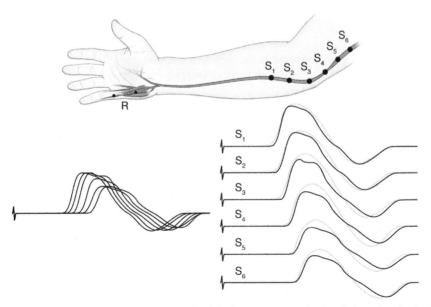

Fig. 9. Conduction block demonstrated with short segmental stimulation (inching). A patient with an ulnar neuropathy at the elbow demonstrates focal block of ulnar motor conduction between stimulus points S_3 and S_5, corresponding to the depicted nerve compression. The degree of block can be measured by the percentage loss of amplitude or area, in this case approximately 40% between the S_3 and S_5 sites. Note the subtle associated focal slowing in the same segment of nerve. R, recording site; S, stimulation site.

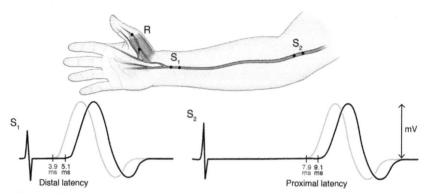

Fig. 10. Focal slowing. A patient with clinical carpal tunnel syndrome demonstrates a prolonged median motor distal latency compared with a normal CMAP (*shaded*). The proximal latency shows a similar degree of change, anticipating a normal conduction velocity. R, recording site; S, stimulation site.

degree of axonally mediated conduction block.[35,47] Typically, once wallerian degeneration has occurred, the block in conduction is replaced by low-amplitude CMAPs at all points of stimulation along the nerve, as would be conventionally suspected in an axonal process. Therefore, the identification of conduction block not only has diagnostic and therapeutic value but also demonstrates the presence of preserved but at-risk axons caused by the disorder at hand.

Frequently, a focal process affecting the nerve may be insufficient to cause frank conduction block but may cause focal slowing (**Fig. 10**). This is usually attributed to focal dysmyelination. When assessed over long interstimulation distances, areas of focal slowing may be missed via an averaging effect with more plentiful segments of unaffected rapidly conducting nerve. Therefore, focal slowing is usually apparent with stimulation over shorter distances (such as a focally prolonged distal latency or with short segmental stimulation, or inching, techniques).[50] Isolation of focal conduction block or slowing with short segmental stimulation is one of the most powerful localizing tools in clinical neurophysiology and, in the setting of compressive pathology, can lead directly to definitive interventional management.

SUMMARY

NCSs are a useful tool in the evaluation of patients with suspected neuromuscular disorders and provide a valuable complement to other elements of the electrodiagnostic evaluation. The quantitative information obtained with NCS allows for precise determination of the presence or absence of many neuromuscular diseases. With careful attention to technique, NCS can be performed safely, reliably, and reproducibly, although its results should always be interpreted in the patient's broader clinical context.

ACKNOWLEDGMENTS

The author would like to thank Veneliza Salcedo and Bob Morreale for assistance with the illustrations.

REFERENCES

1. Lambert E. Diagnostic value of electrical stimulation of motor nerves. In: Pinelli P, editor. Progress in electromyography. Amsterdam: Elsevier; 1962. p. 9–16.

2. Kimura J. Kugelberg lecture. Principles and pitfalls of nerve conduction studies. Electroencephalogr Clin Neurophysiol Suppl 1999;50:12–5.
3. Isaacson W. Benjamin Franklin: an American life. New York: Simon and Schuster; 2003.
4. Barkhaus PE, Periquet MI, Nandedkar SD. Influence of the surface EMG electrode on the compound muscle action potential. Electromyogr Clin Neurophysiol 2006;46(4):235–9.
5. Falck B, Stalberg E. Motor nerve conduction studies: measurement principles and interpretation of findings. J Clin Neurophysiol 1995;12(3):254–79.
6. Watson JC, Daube JR. Compound muscle action potentials. In: Daube JR, Rubin DI, editors. Clinical neurophysiology. 3rd edition. Oxford: Oxford University Press; 2009. p. 327–67.
7. Sorenson E. Sensory nerve action potentials. In: Daube JR, Rubin DI, editors. Clinical neurophysiology. 3rd edition. Oxford: Oxford University Press; 2009. p. 239–56.
8. Kincaid JC, Brashear A, Markand ON. The influence of the reference electrode on CMAP configuration. Muscle Nerve 1993;16(4):392–6.
9. Dyck PJ, O'Brien PC, Litchy WJ, et al. Use of percentiles and normal deviates to express nerve conduction and other test abnormalities. Muscle Nerve 2001; 24(3):307–10.
10. Wang SH, Robinson LR. Considerations in reference values for nerve conduction studies. Phys Med Rehabil Clin N Am 1998;9(4):907–23, viii.
11. Bromberg MB, Jaros L. Symmetry of normal motor and sensory nerve conduction measurements. Muscle Nerve 1998;21(4):498–503.
12. Wilbourn AJ. Sensory nerve conduction studies. J Clin Neurophysiol 1994;11(6): 584–601.
13. Bastron JA, Lambert EH. The clinical value of electromyography and electric stimulation of nerves. Med Clin North Am 1960;44:1025–36.
14. Buchthal F, Rosenfalck A. Sensory potentials in polyneuropathy. Brain 1971;94(2): 241–62.
15. Wee AS, Ashley RA. Effect of interelectrode recording distance on morphology of the antidromic sensory nerve action potentials at the finger. Electromyogr Clin Neurophysiol 1990;30(2):93–6.
16. Magladery JW, Mc DD Jr, Stoll J. Electrophysiological studies of nerve and reflex activity in normal man. II. The effects of peripheral ischemia. Bull Johns Hopkins Hosp 1950;86(5):291–312.
17. Mayer RF, Feldman RG. Observations on the nature of the F wave in man. Neurology 1967;17(2):147–56.
18. Young MS, Triggs WJ. Effect of stimulator orientation on F-wave persistence. Muscle Nerve 1998;21(10):1324–6.
19. Weber F. The diagnostic sensitivity of different F wave parameters. J Neurol Neurosurg Psychiatry 1998;65(4):535–40.
20. Jabre JF. Surface recording of the H-reflex of the flexor carpi radialis. Muscle Nerve 1981;4(5):435–8.
21. Misiaszek JE. The H-reflex as a tool in neurophysiology: its limitations and uses in understanding nervous system function. Muscle Nerve 2003;28(2): 144–60.
22. Hoffmann P. Uber die beziehungen der schnenreflexe zur willkurlichen bewegun und zum tonus. Zeitschrift fur Biologie 1918;68:351–70 [in German].
23. Laughlin RS. H-reflexes. In: Daube JR, Rubin DI, editors. Clinical neurophysiology. 3rd edition. Oxford: Oxford University Press; 2009. p. 519–27.

24. Lagerlund TD. Electrical safety in the laboratory and hospital. In: Rubin DI, Daube JR, editors. Clinical neurophysiology. 3rd edition. Oxford: Oxford University Press; 2009. p. 21–32.
25. Mellion ML, Buxton AE, Iyer V, et al. Safety of nerve conduction studies in patients with peripheral intravenous lines. Muscle Nerve 2010;42(2):189–91.
26. Derejko M, Derejko P, Przybylski A, et al. Safety of nerve conduction studies in patients with implantable cardioverter-defibrillators. Clin Neurophysiol 2011. [Epub ahead of print].
27. Schoeck AP, Mellion ML, Gilchrist JM, et al. Safety of nerve conduction studies in patients with implanted cardiac devices. Muscle Nerve 2007;35(4):521–4.
28. Wilbourn AJ, Aminoff MJ. AAEM minimonograph 32: the electrodiagnostic examination in patients with radiculopathies. American Association of Electrodiagnostic Medicine. Muscle Nerve 1998;21(12):1612–31.
29. Rivner MH. The contemporary role of F-wave studies. F-wave studies: limitations. Muscle Nerve 1998;21(8):1101–4 [discussion: 1104–5].
30. Goodman BP, Smith BE, Ross MA. Electromyographic findings in central nervous system disorders: case series and literature review. J Clin Neurophysiol 2008; 25(4):222–4.
31. Chaudhry V, Glass JD, Griffin JW. Wallerian degeneration in peripheral nerve disease. Neurol Clin 1992;10(3):613–27.
32. Levin KH. L5 radiculopathy with reduced superficial peroneal sensory responses: intraspinal and extraspinal causes. Muscle Nerve 1998;21(1):3–7.
33. Albers JW. Clinical neurophysiology of generalized polyneuropathy. J Clin Neurophysiol 1993;10(2):149–66.
34. Dyck PJ, Karnes JL, O'Brien PC, et al. The Rochester Diabetic Neuropathy Study: reassessment of tests and criteria for diagnosis and staged severity. Neurology 1992;42(6):1164–70.
35. Robinson LR. Traumatic injury to peripheral nerves. Muscle Nerve 2000;23(6): 863–73.
36. Mulder DW, Lambert EH, Bastron JA, et al. The neuropathies associated with diabetes mellitus. A clinical and electromyographic study of 103 unselected diabetic patients. Neurology 1961;11(4 Pt 1):275–84.
37. Gilliatt RW, Sears TA. Sensory nerve action potentials in patients with peripheral nerve lesions. J Neurol Neurosurg Psychiatry 1958;21(2):109–18.
38. Research criteria for diagnosis of chronic inflammatory demyelinating polyneuropathy (CIDP). Report from an Ad Hoc Subcommittee of the American Academy of Neurology AIDS Task Force. Neurology 1991;41(5):617–8.
39. Donofrio PD, Albers JW. AAEM minimonograph #34: polyneuropathy: classification by nerve conduction studies and electromyography. Muscle Nerve 1990; 13(10):889–903.
40. Lewis RA, Sumner AJ. The electrodiagnostic distinctions between chronic familial and acquired demyelinative neuropathies. Neurology 1982;32(6):592–6.
41. Lewis RA, Sumner AJ, Shy ME. Electrophysiological features of inherited demyelinating neuropathies: a reappraisal in the era of molecular diagnosis. Muscle Nerve 2000;23(10):1472–87.
42. Gutmann L, Fakadej A, Riggs JE. Evolution of nerve conduction abnormalities in children with dominant hypertrophic neuropathy of the Charcot-Marie-Tooth type. Muscle Nerve 1983;6(7):515–9.
43. Saperstein DS, Katz JS, Amato AA, et al. Clinical spectrum of chronic acquired demyelinating polyneuropathies. Muscle Nerve 2001;24(3):311–24.

44. Albers JW, Donofrio PD, McGonagle TK. Sequential electrodiagnostic abnormalities in acute inflammatory demyelinating polyradiculoneuropathy. Muscle Nerve 1985;8(6):528–39.
45. Schulte-Mattler WJ, Jakob M, Zierz S. Assessment of temporal dispersion in motor nerves with normal conduction velocity. Clin Neurophysiol 1999;110(4): 740–7.
46. Cornblath DR, Sumner AJ, Daube J, et al. Conduction block in clinical practice. Muscle Nerve 1991;14(9):869–71 [discussion: 867–8].
47. Olney RK, Lewis RA, Putnam TD, et al. Consensus criteria for the diagnosis of multifocal motor neuropathy. Muscle Nerve 2003;27(1):117–21.
48. Jamieson PW, Giuliani MJ, Martinez AJ. Necrotizing angiopathy presenting with multifocal conduction blocks. Neurology 1991;41(3):442–4.
49. Parry GJ, Linn DJ. Conduction block without demyelination following acute nerve infarction. J Neurol Sci 1988;84(2-3):265–73.
50. Campbell WW. The value of inching techniques in the diagnosis of focal nerve lesions. Inching is a useful technique. Muscle Nerve 1998;21(11):1554–6 [discussion: 1561].

Needle Electromyography: Basic Concepts and Patterns of Abnormalities

Devon I. Rubin, MD

KEYWORDS

- Needle electromyography • Spontaneous • Motor unit potential
- Fibrillation potential • Myotonic discharge
- Complex repetitive discharge • Recruitment

 Videos of needle electromyography accompany this article at www.neurologic. theclinics.com.

Needle electromyography (EMG) is a major component of a standard electrodiagnostic examination. Through recording the electrical signals generated from muscle fibers, needle EMG can provide complementary information to nerve conduction studies to help localize a disorder and characterize the underlying pathologic changes that are occurring in motor units within muscles. Different types and patterns of abnormal spontaneously firing electrical signals and changes in motor unit potentials (MUPs) occur with disorders of anterior horn cells or peripheral nerves, neuromuscular junction, and muscle. The performance of reliable EMG studies depends on the technical skills of the physician in inserting, moving, and recording with a needle electrode; assessing clinical neuromuscular problems; and analyzing electric signals recorded from muscle using auditory pattern recognition and semiquantitation. This article reviews basic concepts related to the technique of needle EMG and the types and significance of EMG waveforms recorded.

TECHNIQUE OF NEEDLE EXAMINATION

Needle EMG involves recording the electrical signals that are generated from muscle fibers. Although these signals can sometimes be recorded from the skin surface overlying a muscle using surface recording electrodes, this method is insensitive at recording very small amplitude potentials, such as fibrillation potentials, and does not allow for accurate assessment of subtle changes in an individual MUP.[1] Therefore,

Department of Neurology, Mayo Clinic, 4500 San Pablo Road, Jacksonville, FL 32224, USA
E-mail address: Rubin.Devon@mayo.edu

Neurol Clin 30 (2012) 429–456
doi:10.1016/j.ncl.2011.12.009
0733-8619/12/$ – see front matter © 2012 Elsevier Inc. All rights reserved.

standard EMG studies involve inserting a recording electrode into a muscle, slowly moving the needle through different regions of muscle, and recording the electrical signals that are occurring at rest, initiated by the needle movement, and during voluntary muscle contraction. Several technical factors can affect the collection and interpretation of the signals.

Needle Electrode Types

There are several different types of needle electrodes used during routine clinical EMG to record the electric activity within a muscle (**Fig. 1**). For most routine studies, concentric or monopolar electrodes are used.[2]

Concentric-needle electrode

The concentric-needle electrode consists of a 24- to 26-gauge hollow needle with a fine wire down the center and beveled at the tip to produce an active, oval recording surface of 125 μm × 580 μm. The electrode is referenced to the shaft of the needle; thereby canceling activity from distant, surrounding muscle. This electrode type has several advantages over the monopolar electrode (**Table 1**).

Monopolar needle electrode

The monopolar electrode consists of a Teflon-coated 22- to 30-gauge stainless steel needle electrode with a bare tip of approximately 500 μm in diameter. The active recording tip is referenced to a separate surface electrode applied on the skin of the limb being examined. Although the monopolar electrode records essentially the same activity as the standard concentric electrode, the configuration and reference difference results in the recorded MUPs being slightly longer in duration and higher in amplitude than those recorded with the concentric-needle electrode.[3]

Single fiber electrode

The single fiber needle electrode is a specialized electrode specifically used for the technique of single fiber EMG (SFEMG). This electrode has a small (25 μm) recording surface allowing for the recording of only a single or few muscle fibers in the immediate

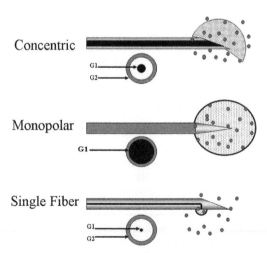

Fig. 1. Types of needle electrodes used in recording EMG signals. The conceptual recording areas of each electrode type are shown by the hashed regions. G1, active recording site; G2, reference site.

Table 1 Differences among needle electrode types			
	Concentric	**Monopolar**	**Single Fiber**
Noise or interference from surrounding muscles	Less	More	Much less
Separate reference electrode	No	Yes	No
Recording area	Smaller	Larger	Very small
MUP duration or amplitude	Shorter or lower	Longer or higher	Very short (single fiber) and low
Defined quantitative values	Yes	Less well defined	Yes
Cost	More	Less	Very expensive

vicinity of the electrode. SFEMG is used primarily to study disorders of neuromuscular transmission, such as myasthenia gravis, because it can detect variation in a motor unit ("jitter") more readily than with other needle electrodes. SFEMG can also be used to quantify the density of muscle fibers in a motor unit (fiber density). Because single fiber electrodes are very expensive, the electrodes are reusable following appropriate sterilization. Due to increasing concerns about the performance of studies using reusable needle electrodes in patients with transmissible disorders, many laboratories have eliminated the use of single fiber needle electrodes and perform SFEMG with concentric-needle electrodes. Normative data have been developed for concentric-needle SFEMG.[4,5]

Conducting the Needle Examination

The ability to efficiently and effectively record the electric activity from muscle depends considerably on an electromyographer's skills of patient interaction and needle electrode handling. Special attention to several steps of the study helps to ensure a more reliable study.

Preparing the patient
Educating the patient about the test and explaining that a needle will be inserted into several muscles, which may cause some minor discomfort, may help reduce anxiety during the study and allow for better muscle relaxation and more efficient recording of the electrical signals.

Muscle selection
The muscles to be tested are selected initially based on the clinical problem. Certain algorithms or protocols can help guide the approach to an individual patient; however, adjustments from the algorithms are frequently necessary depending on the findings obtained during the studies.[6] In evaluating certain diseases, the distribution of findings will often vary among muscles as well as in different regions of the same muscle. For example, in many myopathies, abnormalities are more commonly seen in proximal muscles; in some myopathies, such as dermatomyositis, the superficial layers of the muscle may show more prominent changes than deeper portions. In a patient with suspected amyotrophic lateral sclerosis (ALS), multiple distal and proximal limb muscles supplied by different roots and nerves may be necessary to examine to demonstrate a widespread disease of motor neurons. In a patient with a suspected single root radiculopathy or mononeuropathy, the needle examination will be more focused on muscles in a single limb.

Needle movement

During the examination, three types of activity are recorded: (1) the activity that occurs with or following each needle movement at rest (insertional activity), (2) spontaneously firing activity at rest, and (3) activity during voluntary muscle contraction (voluntary activity). Because the needle electrode primarily records activity from a small area in a muscle, the electrode must be moved to record the activity in multiple different regions of the muscle to obtain a more complete assessment of the underlying changes that may have occurred in the motor units or muscle fibers. The movement of the needle through the muscle is the predominant generator of the discomfort experienced during the examination. To reduce this discomfort, the muscle should be examined by moving the needle along a straight line through the muscle in short steps (0.5–1 mm).[7] Complete assessment of a muscle usually requires 2 to 4 different passes through the muscle.

Examining a resting muscle

Examination of the muscle at rest is performed to assess for abnormal spontaneous discharges that may be indicators of an underlying disease. Several types of electrical signals normally occur in a resting muscle. Insertional activity is the electric response of the muscle to the mechanical damage by a small movement of the needle. Evaluation of insertional activity requires a pause of 0.5 to 1 second or more following cessation of needle movement to observe any repetitive or slowly firing potentials, such as infrequent fibrillation potentials or fasciculation potentials. Insertional activity may be increased, decreased, or elicit specific waveforms, such as myotonic discharges.

Examining a contracting muscle

The contracting muscle is best examined at a low level of contraction that activates only a few motor units. Measurements of MUPs are typically made by one of two methods: (1) isolation and measurement of a single MUP (semiquantitative or quantitative EMG) or (2) interference pattern analysis. Quantitative EMG is the classic method of measuring MUP parameters by isolating and recording at least 20 MUPs in different areas of the muscle at low-to-moderate levels of muscle contraction. Assessment of the mean of the parameters of all MUPs recorded can then be compared with normative data from the same muscle in normal subjects of the same age. This method provides no quantitative assessment of recruitment or stability, although these parameters can be assessed semiquantitatively with this technique. Variants of quantitative EMG analysis using computer algorithmic template matching, such as decomposition quantitative EMG, have and are being developed to allow for more rapid assessment of three to five individual MUPs firing at one time.

Details of individual characteristics of MUPs cannot be measured reliably during a strong voluntary contraction, which normally produces a dense pattern of multiple superimposed potentials called an interference pattern. Interference pattern analysis summates the effect of recruitment with the duration and amplitude of the MUPs and records the number of turns and total amplitude of the electric activity during a fixed time with an automatic counting device.[8,9] With examination at stronger levels of contraction, less dense patterns may occur if there is a loss of motor units, poor effort, or an upper motor lesion or if the muscle is powerful. The latter three conditions can be distinguished from a loss of motor units only by estimates of firing rates. This method varies with patient effort, which must be accounted for in measurements.

EMG WAVEFORM RECOGNITION

Interpreting the variety of waveforms that may be encountered during an EMG examination requires specialized skills that must be learned, mastered, and continually practiced by electromyographers. The main skill required for accurate waveform identification is auditory pattern recognition. Each of the different EMG waveforms fire in one of six distinct patterns, defined by the pattern of change of the interpotential interval of successive potentials. Because the configuration of different waveforms may be identical and a specific type of waveform (eg, fibrillation potential) can have different configurations, only by recognizing the pattern of firing can a potential be accurately identified. The six different characteristic firing patterns of EMG waveforms are listed in **Table 2** and shown in **Fig. 2**. A second skill used is auditory semiquantitation, which allows the electromyographer to rapidly recognize various MUP parameters to determine the presence and temporal course of a neuromuscular disease. Once mastered, this skill allows for accurate assessment of parameters such as firing frequency, rise time, MUP size, and number of turns or phases.

ELECTROMYOGRAPHIC POTENTIALS

A variety of normal and abnormal EMG waveforms may be recorded from the muscle. The generators of all EMG potentials are the action potentials of the muscle fibers that are firing singly or in groups, spontaneously or under voluntary control, near the recording electrode (**Fig. 3**; **Table 3**).[10] Neuromuscular diseases may result in abnormal spontaneous discharges, abnormal voluntary MUPs, or both. The electromyographer must be able to recognize specific discharges, understand their significance, and know with which disease processes they are associated. In most cases, a specific discharge may be associated with several different diseases. The following discussion reviews the types of abnormal EMG waveforms.

Table 2
Patterns of firing of EMG waveforms

Pattern	Spike Recurrence	Examples
Regular with no change	Precisely defined intervals that do not change on a moment-to-moment basis	Complex repetitive discharge
Regular with linear change	Precisely defined intervals that change linearly	Fibrillation potential
Regular with exponential change	Precisely defined intervals that change slowly or rapidly in an exponential manner	Myotonic discharge
Irregular	Random intervals with no definable intervals.	End plate spike Fasciculation potential
Semirhythmic	Orderly, but not precise, intervals. The variation in the change of interpotential interval is approximately 10%.	Voluntary MUP
Burst	Groups of single or few spikes firing repetitively in a burst, with the bursts recurring at intervals that may be regular, irregular, or semirhythmic	Myokymic discharge Hemifacial spasm Tremor

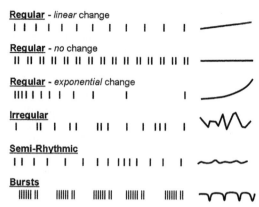

Regular - *linear* change

Regular - *no* change

Regular - *exponential* change

Irregular

Semi-Rhythmic

Bursts

Fig. 2. Firing patterns of EMG potentials.

SPONTANEOUS EMG WAVEFORMS

Spontaneous EMG waveforms are those that occur while the muscle is in a resting, noncontracting state. Some spontaneous activity may be induced by needle irritation of the muscle fibers and other occur independent of any stimulation of the fibers. Several spontaneous waveforms are normal phenomena, although the presence of most is indicative of an underlying pathologic condition.

Insertional Activity

Insertional activity is the electrical activity that occurs because of mechanical depolarization of the muscle fibers due to needle insertion and movement through the muscle. Insertional activity is generated by single muscle fiber action potentials and is composed of combinations of positive and negative spikes. The length of the insertional activity reflects the number of muscle fibers that depolarize because of mechanical

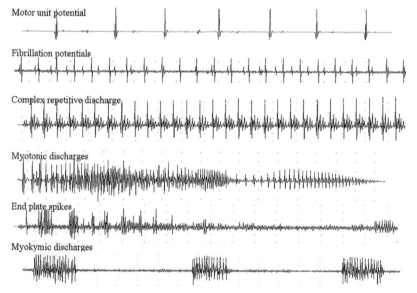

Motor unit potential

Fibrillation potentials

Complex repetitive discharge

Myotonic discharges

End plate spikes

Myokymic discharges

Fig. 3. Examples of EMG waveforms.

Table 3
Generators of EMG waveforms

	Single Muscle Fibers	Groups of Adjacent Muscle Fibers (Different Motor Units)	MUP (Same Motor Unit)
Spontaneous	Fibrillation potentials Myotonic discharges End plate spikes	Complex repetitive discharges Insertional activity	Fasciculation potentials Myokymic discharges Neuromyotonic discharges Hemifacial spasm Tremor Dystonia
Voluntary	(Severely short duration or nascent MUP)	—	Voluntary MUP Synkinesis

irritation. With larger needle movements the length is longer and with smaller needle movements the length is shorter (Video 1; please go to www.neurologic.theclinics. com to view video). In a normal muscle, the activity ceases immediately following cessation of needle movement.

Abnormal insertional activity may be increased or decreased. Increased insertional activity may occur as two types of normal variants, as a result of denervated muscle, or associated with myotonic discharges. The normal variants are recognized by their widespread distribution, most often occurring in younger, muscular persons. One normal variant is composed of short trains of regularly firing positive waves.[11] Some patients with this type of diffuse increased insertional activity have been found to have mutations in the CLCN1 gene associated with myotonia congenita.[12] The second type is characterized by short recurrent bursts of irregularly firing potentials, sometimes referred to as "snap, crackle, pop." Increased insertional activity may also be the initial early sign (usually within the first 2–3 weeks) of denervation following an acute neurogenic disorder, such as an early radiculopathy or mononeuropathy (**Fig. 4**). Increased insertional activity typically occurs before the development of more sustained fibrillation potentials (Video 2). In addition, because needle movement often leads to the generation of fibrillation potentials in denervated muscle, most muscles that demonstrate fibrillation potentials have increased insertional activity.

Decreased insertional activity may occur in conditions in which muscle fibers are unable to produce action potentials in response to membrane irritation. This most commonly occurs in end-stage neurogenic or myopathic disorders in which the muscle is completely atrophic or has been replaced by fibrous connective tissue. Additionally, disorders such as periodic paralysis (during paralysis) or myophosphorylase deficiency myopathy (McArdle disease) (during a contracture) may demonstrate decreased insertional activity or electrical silence during needle movement through the muscle.

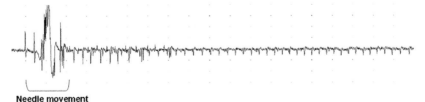

Needle movement

Fig. 4. Increased insertional activity.

End plate Activity

Normal muscle fibers show no spontaneous electric activity at rest outside of the end plate region. In the end plate region, miniature end plate potentials (MEPPs) are recorded owing to random spontaneous release of individual quanta of acetylcholine. These MEPPs are recorded as monophasic, low amplitude (<10 μV), short duration (<1–3 milliseconds) negative waves called end plate noise. Individual potentials occur irregularly but usually cannot be distinguished. This activity has a typical "seashell sound" (**Fig. 5**; Video 3). The action potentials of some individual muscle fibers caused by mechanical depolarization of a nerve terminal may be recorded in the end plate region as end plate spikes.[13] These have a rapid irregular firing pattern, often with interspike intervals of less than 50 milliseconds. Although usually initially negative, end plate spikes may be triphasic or even as irregularly firing positive waves. End plate spikes sound like "sputtering fat in a frying pan." End plate activity is normal and has no clinical significance. However, because recording from the end plate region is usually uncomfortable, recording end plate activity should prompt repositioning of the needle electrode.

Fasciculation Potentials

Fasciculation potentials are spontaneously and randomly discharging MUPs that may be generated anywhere along the lower motor neuron from the anterior horn cell to the nerve terminal (Video 4). Fasciculation potentials may be of any size and shape, depending on the characteristics of the motor unit from which they arise and their relation to the recording electrode; they may have the appearance of normal or abnormal MUPs. The firing rates may vary from a few per second to fewer than 1 per minute. They are identified by their irregular firing pattern and may sound like "popcorn kernels just beginning to pop." Fasciculation potentials occur in normal persons as well as in many diseases. They are especially common in chronic neurogenic disorders but have been found in all neuromuscular disorders (**Table 4**). Needle EMG cannot reliably distinguish between benign fasciculations and those associated with specific diseases and the presence of fasciculations alone, without fibrillation potentials or

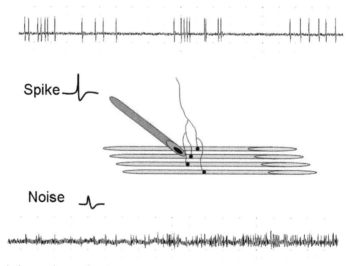

Fig. 5. End plate spikes and noise.

Table 4	
Disorders associated with fasciculation potentials	
Type of Disease	**Examples**
No disease	Benign fasciculation syndrome
	Postexercise
Peripheral nerve hyperexcitability syndrome	Cramp fasciculation syndrome
	Isaacs syndrome
Neurogenic disorders	Anterior horn cell diseases (eg, ALS, Kennedy disease, spinal muscular atrophy)
	Peripheral neuropathies, axonal
	Radiculopathies
Metabolic disorders	Hyperthyroidism
Medications	Anticholinesterase agents

changes in voluntary MUPs, is not sufficient to make a diagnosis of progressive motor neuron disease, such as ALS. In normal persons, fasciculations occur more rapidly, on average, and are more stable.[14]

Fibrillation Potentials

Fibrillation potentials are the action potentials of single muscle fibers that fire spontaneously in the absence of innervation. These potentials typically fire in a regular pattern at rates of 0.5 to 15 Hz and take one of two forms, a spike or a positive wave (**Fig. 6**). The morphologic differences in the two forms reflect the site of the initiation of the fibrillation potential along the muscle fiber relative to the site of the needle electrode. The amplitude of a fibrillation potential is variable and is proportional to the muscle fiber diameter; they may be low in diseases with muscle fiber atrophy and high in hypertrophic muscle fibers.[15] Because there is a wide range of sizes of and configurations of fibrillation potentials, recognition relies on identifying the slow, regular firing pattern, which sounds like the "ticking or tocking of a clock."

Fibrillation potentials occur in neurogenic or myopathic processes, and occasionally in neuromuscular junction disorders (**Table 5**). They may occur in muscle fibers that (1) have lost their innervation, (2) have been sectioned transversely or divided longitudinally, (3) are regenerating, or (4) have never been innervated. In neurogenic disorders, such as radiculopathies, mononeuropathies, or motor neuron disease, loss or

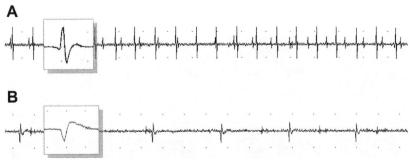

Fig. 6. Fibrillation potentials. (*A*) Spike form. (*B*) Positive waveform.

Table 5
Diseases associated with fibrillation potentials

Type of Disease	Examples
Neurogenic disorders	Anterior horn cell diseases (eg, ALS, spinal muscular atrophy, acute poliomyelitis, West Nile virus)
	Axonal polyradiculopathies
	Radiculopathies
	Plexopathies
	Peripheral neuropathies, axonal
	Mononeuropathies
Neuromuscular junction diseases	Myasthenia gravis, severe
	Lambert-Eaton myasthenic syndrome, severe
	Botulinum toxin administration (iatrogenic)
	Botulism
Myopathies	Inflammatory (eg, polymyositis, dermatomyositis, inclusion body myositis)
	Infiltrative (eg, sarcoidosis, amyloid)
	Muscular dystrophies (eg, Duchenne, Becker, limb-girdle)
	Myotonic dystrophy
	Toxic myopathies (eg, lipid-lowering agents, chloroquine)
	Metabolic myopathies (eg, acid maltase)
	Congenital myopathies (eg, myotubular, late-onset rod myopathy)
	Infectious myopathy (eg, viral myositis)

degeneration of axons leads to denervated muscle fibers. In myopathies characterized by muscle fiber necrosis or splitting, functional denervation of individual or segments of muscle fibers occurs as the fiber becomes separated from the end plate zone. In myopathies, fibrillation potentials are often of low amplitude and have a slow firing rate (eg, 0.5 Hz). The density of fibrillation potentials is a rough estimate of the number of denervated muscle fibers and is commonly graded from 1+ (few fibrillation potentials in most areas of the muscle) to 4+ (profuse fibrillations filling the baseline in all areas) (Videos 5 and 6).

Myotonic Discharges

Myotonic discharges are single muscle fibers firing spontaneously and repetitively with a pattern that waxes and wanes in amplitude and frequency because of an abnormality in the membrane of the muscle fiber. Myotonic discharges are induced by needle movement or voluntary contraction and fire with a pattern of exponentially changing frequency, usually between 40 and 100 Hz (**Fig. 7**; Video 7). It has been

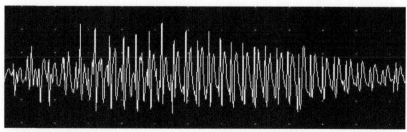

Fig. 7. Myotonic discharge.

suggested the degree of waxing and waning differs between different forms of myotonic disorders. In myotonic dystrophy type 1 (DM1), myotonic discharges has been reported to mostly wax and wane (increase and then decrease in firing rate), whereas in myotonic dystrophy type 2 (DM2) the discharges more often wane in frequency.[16] However, a study comparing the abundance of myotonic discharges in patients with sodium and chloride channelopathies, including myotonia congenita, paramyotonia congenita, and hyperkalemic periodic paralysis found no difference in the degree of myotonic discharges among the diseases.[17] Therefore, a diagnosis of a specific myotonic disorder cannot usually be made solely based on the characteristics of the myotonic discharge.[18] Slowly firing myotonic discharges that bear some resemblance to fibrillation potentials, but demonstrate a more rapid rate of change in firing frequency and amplitude, may also occur in myopathic and some neurogenic disorders.[19] Myotonic discharges may occur in disorders with or without associated clinical myotonia (**Table 6**). When prominent and diffuse, myotonic dystrophy type 1 and 2 (DM1 and DM2) or myotonia congenita should be considered.

Complex Repetitive Discharges

Complex repetitive discharge (CRD) are the action potentials of groups of individual muscle fibers arising from several different neighboring motor units firing spontaneously in near synchrony in a regular, repetitive fashion. A CRD occurs as a single muscle fiber action potential ephaptically spreads to and depolarizes a neighboring muscle fiber. Subsequently, a group of 3 to 10 or more neighboring muscle fibers may be depolarized in sequence until the "circuit" is complete, causing the initial muscle fiber to discharge again. CRDs fire in a regular pattern, characteristically with an abrupt onset and cessation, at rates ranging from 3 to 40 Hz (Video 8). During the discharge, there may be a sudden change in the configuration or firing rate of the CRD (**Fig. 8**). CRDs sound like "a motor boat" or a "jackhammer."

CRDs are nonspecific in significance but occur in neurogenic and myopathic disorders that are chronic or longstanding in nature, such as old or chronic radiculopathies, peripheral neuropathies, or slowly progressive myopathies (**Table 7**). In rare cases of patients with chronic S1 radiculopathies associated with pain and calf hypertrophy, CRDs are seen in the gastrocnemius in approximately 50%, raising the possibility that CRDs may contribute to neurogenic hypertrophy in these cases.[20] Rarely, CRDs occur in otherwise normal muscles, such as the iliopsoas or biceps.

Table 6 Diseases associated with myotonic discharges	
Type of Disease	**Examples**
Myopathies (with clinical myotonia)	Myotonic dystrophy type 1 and 2 (DM1, DM2) Myotonia congenita Paramyotonia congenita
Myopathies (without clinical myotonia)	Hyperkalemic periodic paralysis Polymyositis Dermatomyositis Acid maltase deficiency Cholesterol lowering agent myopathy Toxic myopathies (eg, colchicine myopathy)
Neurogenic disorders	Severe axonal disorders (eg, peripheral neuropathies, radiculopathies)

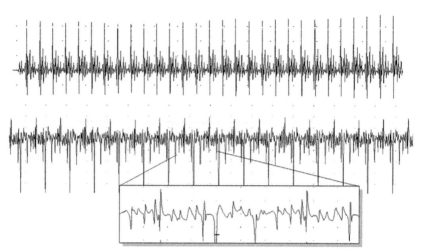

Fig. 8. Complex repetitive discharge.

Myokymic Discharges

Myokymic discharges are spontaneously firing MUPs that fire repetitively in a burst pattern. The individual potentials within each burst often have the appearance of normal MUPs, although they may also be long duration or polyphasic. Each burst may be composed of one or a few MUPs, and the MUPs may fire a few or many times within the burst. The rate of firing of potentials within each burst is typically 40 to 60 Hz. Each burst fires with a regular or semirhythmic pattern at intervals of 0.1 to 10 seconds (**Fig. 9**). The firing pattern or rate is unaffected by voluntary activity and simultaneously occurring myokymic discharges may have different burst durations or firing rates. Some myokymic discharges sound similar to "marching soldiers" (Video 9).

Myokymic discharges may or may not be associated with clinical myokymia, which appears as undulation or quivering of the muscle. Although myokymic discharges are more commonly found in limb muscles, clinical myokymia is more often observed in facial muscles, probably due to less subcutaneous tissue than in limb muscles. Diseases associated with myokymic discharges are listed in **Table 8**. Most commonly, myokymic discharges occur with radiation-induced nerve injury, chronic compressive neuropathies, or polyradiculopathies. The myokymic discharges seen in chronic compressive neuropathies, such as carpal tunnel syndrome, are often composed of a single or few potentials.

Table 7
Disorders associated with CRDs

Type of Disease	Examples
Neurogenic disorders	Chronic anterior horn cell diseases (eg, ALS, spinal muscular atrophy, polio) Chronic radiculopathies Chronic axonal neuropathies
Myopathies	Chronic inflammatory myopathies (eg, inclusion body myositis) Muscular dystrophies Hypothyroid myopathy

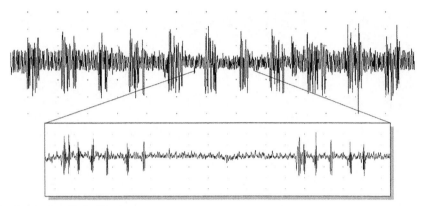

Fig. 9. Myokymic discharge.

Neuromyotonic Discharges

Neuromyotonic discharges, or neuromyotonia, are rare, spontaneously firing MUPs that fire at very high frequencies (100–300 Hz) (**Fig. 10**). These potentials may decrease in amplitude because of the inability of muscle fibers to maintain discharges at rates greater than 100 Hz. The discharges may be continuous for long intervals or recur in short bursts (Video 10). Neuromyotonic discharges are seen in disorders of peripheral nerve hyperexcitability, such as Isaacs syndrome, and may occur because of a defect in potassium channels in the nerve membrane (**Table 9**).[21] Some forms of syndromes of peripheral nerve hyperexcitability are also associated with bursts of doublet, triplet, or multiplet discharges, with intraburst frequencies often ranging from 40 to 350 Hz, which may appear similar to myokymic discharges.[21,22] Neuromyotonia may also occur with tetany, Morvan syndrome, or following radiation.[23,24]

A form of neuromyotonic discharges, called "neurotonic discharges" occur intraoperatively with the mechanical irritation of cranial or peripheral nerves. These discharges are brief bursts of MUPs discharging at very high rates, similar to the rates of spontaneously occurring neuromyotonic discharges. The identification of neurotonic discharges intraoperatively is valuable in alerting surgeons to possible nerve damage.

Table 8
Disorders associated with myokymic discharges

Location	Associated Conditions
Facial muscles	Radiation to head and neck Multiple sclerosis Brainstem neoplasms Polyradiculopathy (eg, AIDP) Facial neuropathy (eg, Bell palsy) ALS
Extremity muscles	Radiation (plexopathy, mononeuropathy) Chronic nerve compression (eg, chronic carpal tunnel syndrome) Syndrome of peripheral nerve hyperexcitability (Isaacs syndrome) Morvan syndrome

Abbreviation: AIDP, acute inflammatory demyelinating polyradiculopathy.

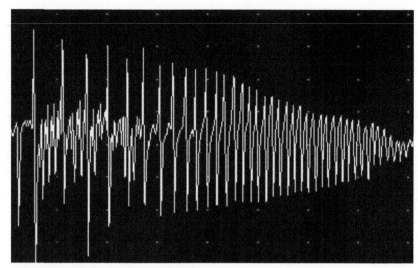

Fig. 10. Neuromyotonic discharge. Spike fires at rates of up to 300 Hz.

Cramp Potentials (Cramp Discharge)

Cramps are painful, involuntary contractions of muscle. The discharges associated with a muscle cramp (cramp discharges) are composed of MUPs that fire in a unique firing pattern, which distinguishes them from other spontaneous activity and normal strong voluntary activation. The configuration of the individual potentials resemble MUPs. However, in contrast to the pattern of activation that occurs with voluntary contraction, potentials in cramp discharges usually have an abrupt onset, rapid buildup and addition of subsequent potentials, and a rapid or "sputtering" cessation. The potentials fire rapidly (40–60 Hz) and may fire in an irregular pattern, especially just before termination. Cramps are a common phenomenon in normal persons, usually when a muscle is activated strongly in a shortened position. In addition, cramps may occur with chronic neurogenic disorders, in metabolic or electrolyte disorders, or in disorders of peripheral nerve hyperexcitability (such as cramp fasciculation syndrome) (**Table 10**).

Synkinesis

The aberrant regeneration of axons after nerve injury may occasionally result in two different muscles being innervated by the same axon (synkinesis).When this happens,

Table 9	
Disorders associated with neuromyotonic discharges	
Type of Disorder	**Examples**
Hyperexcitable nerve syndromes	Isaacs syndrome
	Voltage-gated potassium channel antibody syndromes
	Morvan syndrome
Neurogenic disorders	Chronic spinal muscular atrophy
	Hereditary motor neuropathy
	Postradiation

Table 10 Disorders associated with cramp discharges	
Type of Disorder	**Examples**
Neurogenic disorders	Chronic radiculopathies
	Peripheral neuropathy
	Motor neuron disorders
Metabolic or electrolyte disorders	Salt depletion
	Pregnancy
	Hypothyroidism
	Chronic renal failure (dialysis)
Peripheral nerve hyperexcitability disorders	Cramp fasciculation syndrome
Other	Benign nocturnal cramps

MUPs in one muscle fire in response to voluntary activation of a different distant muscle. Sometimes the MUPs fire in bursts, such as when groups of MUPs are activated in the orbicularis oris during blink in facial synkinesis following reinnervation from facial neuropathy (eg, Bell palsy). With synkinesis, MUPs may have normal or long duration (due to reinnervation from a neurogenic lesion). Synkinesis is most common in facial muscles or in the arm ("arm-diaphragm synkinesis" or "the breathing arm or hand") in which potentials in shoulder girdle or hand muscles fire in association with respiration because of aberrant regeneration of the phrenic nerve following brachial plexus injuries.[25-27]

Hemifacial Spasm

Hemifacial spasm is an involuntary, peripherally generated movement disorder manifest as intermittent, unilateral, or bilateral irregular contractions of one or several facial muscles. Hemifacial spasm occurs because of chronic, intermittent compression of the facial nerve, usually by an aberrant artery, causing demyelination of the proximal facial nerve or remodeling of the facial nerve nucleus within the brainstem. As a result, spontaneously generated action potentials are initiated in the facial nerve and ephaptically spread to adjacent axons. The responses are recorded as bursts of several MUPs firing at very rapid rates (often over 100 Hz). The bursts may be long or short duration and fire with irregular intervals.

Tremor

Tremor is a centrally driven pattern of motor unit firing in which MUPs fire in groups in a burst pattern. Each burst is composed different and a variable number of MUPs and each burst changes slightly in morphology. Recognition of tremor is based on the rhythmic (often regular) firing pattern and changing appearance of each burst. Although the electrical discharge in tremor is often associated with a visible tremor, subtle tremor discharges can be recognized without clinical tremor. Minimal activation, with slightly increasing and decreasing effort, often allows a single MUP to be identified. Tremor discharges may be confused with polyphasic MUPs or myokymic discharges, but have distinct differences that should be readily distinguishable. In tremor, the potentials of these motor units are superimposed and may resemble polyphasic, complex, or long-duration MUPs. In contrast to tremor, myokymic discharges are composed of the same MUPs firing repetitively within a burst, so the morphology of each burst changes minimally or not at all (**Fig. 11**; Video 11). Tremor can occur because of a variety of disorders and the

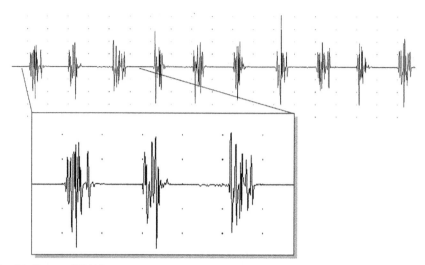

Fig. 11. Tremor (10 Hz).

firing frequency of the tremor burst can sometimes be useful to help distinguish among different types of tremor (eg, 4–6 Hz in Parkinson disease, 8–10 Hz in essential tremor).

Dystonia, Rigidity, Spasticity, and Stiff-Man Syndrome

MUP firing patterns and morphology in dystonia, rigidity, spasticity, and stiff-man syndrome are normal. However, voluntary control of firing of MUPs is lost and, therefore, continuously firing MUPs may occur even with attempted complete relaxation. The MUP findings in these conditions may be identical to that of persistent voluntary activation. In patients with upper motor neuron weakness (such as following a stroke or spinal cord injury), patients cannot maintain motor unit firing or recruit a large number of motor units. The MUP morphology is normal, but only a few MUPs may be activated at attempted strong contraction (poor activation).

VOLUNTARY MUPs

MUPs are the electrical responses recorded from motor units within the muscle and consist of a group of muscle fibers innervated by a single anterior horn cell that are located within the recording area of the needle electrode. By assessing the various features of each of many different MUPs, information about the presence or absence of a neuromuscular disorder can be obtained. Several factors contribute to the characteristics of the recorded MUPs, including the number of motor units within the muscle, the number and diameter of muscle fibers, the arrangement and density of the fibers within the motor unit, and the synchrony of firing of each of the muscle fibers. MUPs are recognized by the distinct semirhythmic pattern of firing (Video 12).

The appearance, including duration, amplitude, number of turns, and rise time, is assessed for each MUP (**Fig. 12**). Each of these characteristics is affected by technical, physiologic, and pathologic factors. Technical factors that have a major influence on the appearance of MUPs include the type of needle electrode used to record the potentials, the filter settings, and the proximity of the recording needle to the muscle fibers being recorded. Physiologic variables that affect the appearance of MUPs include the subject's age, the muscle being studied, temperature, and the

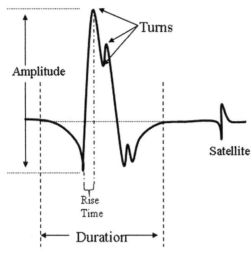

Fig. 12. An MUP showing characteristics that can be measured.

strength of activation.[28] The appearance of an MUP from one motor unit also varies with electrode position because only a small proportion of the fibers in a motor unit are near the electrode and those at a distance contribute little to the recorded MUPs (**Fig. 13**). If the technical and physiologic factors are controlled, the normal

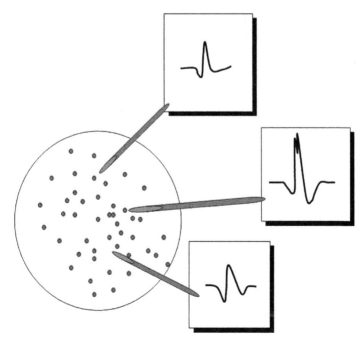

Fig. 13. Variation of MUP morphology with electrode position. Each recorded potential is derived from the same motor unit.

anatomic and histologic features of the motor unit, including the innervation ratio (number of muscle fibers in the motor unit) and fiber density (number of muscle fibers per given cross-sectional area), and any pathologic changes that may affect these features will determine the characteristics of the MUPs.

Assessment of each of the different MUP parameters (recruitment, stability, phases, and duration or amplitude) is necessary to determine whether a neuromuscular disorder is present. Because a single MUP may not be fully representative of all of the MUPs within a muscle, appropriate assessment of a muscle relies on recording multiple MUPs from different sites within the muscle.

Recruitment

Recruitment refers to the relationship between the number of MUPs activated and the firing rates of the activated MUPs at time relative to force of muscle contraction. Recruitment is assessed by comparing the rate of firing of a single MUP with the total number of MUPs that are firing. In most normal muscles, as contraction is initiated at a low level of force, a single or a few MUPs begin to fire at rates of approximately 5 to 8 Hz. With increasing force, the firing rates steadily increase up to 20 to 40 Hz while, at the same time, the threshold of firing of additional motor units is reached and additional MUPs are "recruited."

Normal recruitment

Recruitment can be judged by two methods during routine EMG: assessing recruitment frequency or the recruitment ratio. The recruitment frequency is measured as the rate of firing of an initially activated MUP when a second MUP is recruited (**Fig. 14**). Recruitment frequencies vary in different muscles. A normal recruitment frequency for the second MUP is between 7 and 10 Hz in most limb muscles and up to 16 Hz for motor units in cranial muscle.[29] The recruitment ratio is defined by the ratio of the rate of firing of an individual MUP to the number of MUPs that are active. For most normal limb muscles, this ratio is five or less. For example, if an MUP is firing at 10 Hz there should be two MUPs firing near the recording electrode;

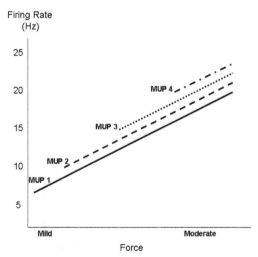

Fig. 14. Graph demonstrating the normal relationship between force of contraction, MUP firing rate, and number of MUPs (recruitment frequency) in normal muscles.

if an MUP is firing at 15 Hz, three MUPs should be present; and four MUPs should be firing at rates of 20 Hz.

Reduced recruitment

In the presence of neurogenic disorders in which there is either a loss of motor units or a block of conduction along some of the axons, fewer MUPs are activated with increasing force of contraction. As a result, the recruitment frequency and the recruitment ratio increase as MUPs fire more rapidly before additional MUPs are recruited (**Fig. 15**; Video 13). If the ratio is greater than five (for example, two MUPs firing at 16 Hz for a recruitment ratio of eight), there is virtually always some decrease in the number of motor units. This higher recruitment frequency or recruitment ratio is termed reduced recruitment (also termed "poor recruitment"). Reduced recruitment is characteristic of neurogenic disorders but can occasionally be seen in patients with severe or end-stage myopathic disorders, due to the loss of all muscle fibers within a motor unit.

Poor activation

In patients in whom relatively few MUPs fire because of pain, upper motor neuron lesions, or poor cooperation, the term "poor activation" is used. In these situations, few MUPs are activated with attempted strong effort. In contrast to reduced recruitment, in which a few MUPs fire at rapid rates, with poor activation the MUPs fire slowly with a normal rate of recruitment (eg, recruitment ratio <5).

Rapid recruitment

Rapid recruitment refers to an increased number of motor units relative to the force of contraction. With this type of recruitment, a large number of MUPs fire with normal recruitment frequencies but with minimal patient effort. Rapid recruitment can only be identified when the force exerted by the patient is known because the recruitment frequencies are entirely normal. Rapid recruitment is characteristic of myopathies.

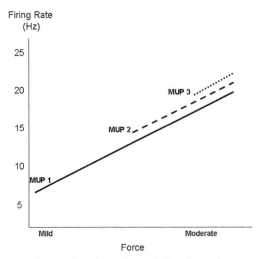

Fig. 15. Graph demonstrating reduced recruitment. The firing frequency in increased relative to the number of MUP firing with increasing force.

Duration and Amplitude

The duration of the MUPs is measured as the time from the initial deflection away from baseline to the final return to baseline (see **Fig. 12**). It varies with the muscle and increases slightly with cool muscle temperature and older age. The duration reflects the area of the muscle fibers in a motor unit. The size of MUPs is also dependent on the level of activation, with larger MUPs becoming active at a stronger force. The amplitude of the potential is the maximal peak-to-peak amplitude of the main spike and consists of the action potentials of only a few muscle fibers closest to the tip of the needle electrode. Although amplitude changes typically correlate with duration changes in neuromuscular diseases, amplitude may be normal in situations in which the MUP duration is abnormally short or long. Therefore, assessing amplitude alone does not fully assess whether an MUP is normal or abnormal. The normal MUP duration in most limb muscles is 8 to 12 millseconds.[30]

Phases

A phase is defined as the number of times the potential crosses the baseline plus one (see **Fig. 12**). An MUP may be biphasic, triphasic, or it may have multiple phases. The configuration depends on the synchrony of firing of the muscle fibers in the region of the electrode. Usually, only a small proportion (<15%) of MUPs in a muscle have more than four phases (polyphasic). A turn is a change in direction of a spike that does not cross the baseline and has the same significance and physiologic generator as a phase. A late spike, distinct from the main potential that is time locked to the main potential, is called a satellite potential (see **Fig. 12**). The satellite potential is generated by a muscle fiber in a motor unit that has a long nerve terminal, narrow diameter, or distant end plate region.

Stability

Normally, MUPs are stable and appear identical each time they fire. Variability, or instability, of an MUP is any change in its configuration, amplitude, or both as the motor unit fires repetitively, in the absence of movement of the recording electrode. Abnormal MUP variation occurs in disorders affecting neuromuscular transmission, including neuromuscular junction disorders or reinnervating motor units in neurogenic disorders. Assessing stability requires recording MUPs at low levels of steady contraction. MUP stability can be quantified with SFEMG.

ABNORMAL MUPs: CHANGES IN DISEASE

Alterations in MUP parameters occur in different types of neuromuscular diseases. The types of these alterations, in conjunction with the presence of spontaneous discharges, help to identify the underlying type, temporal course, and severity of a neuromuscular disorder.

Neurogenic Disorders

In neurogenic disorders, such as radiculopathies, mononeuropathies, peripheral neuropathies, or motor neuron disorders, the MUP changes occur in a temporal continuum and the findings reflect the time of the study in relation to the onset of the disease or nerve injury as well as the extent of reinnervation that has occurred (**Table 11**).

Table 11
Typical evolution of needle EMG findings following acute neurogenic disorder

Time from Injury	Spontaneous Activity or Fibrillations	Recruitment	Stability	Turns or Phases	Duration
1–10 days	Normal	Reduced	Stable	Normal	Normal
11–15 days	Increased	Reduced	Stable	Normal	Normal
16 days–1 month	Fibrillations	Reduced	Stable	Turns	Mildly long
1–2 months	Fibrillations	Reduced	Unstable	Polyphasic	Long
2–6 months	Normal (fibrillations if incomplete reinnervation)	Reduced	Stable or unstable	Polyphasic	Long
>6 months	Normal (fibrillations if incomplete reinnervation)	Reduced	Stable	Normal or polyphasic	Long

Reduced recruitment

The first change that occurs on needle EMG in neurogenic disorders in which there is loss of axons or block of conduction is reduced recruitment. Reduced recruitment may be the earliest finding in an acute axonal lesion (radiculopathy or mononeuropathy) when fibrillation potentials or other MUP changes have not yet developed. It may be the only finding in a neurapraxic lesion in which the sole abnormality is a focal conduction block. Although a hallmark of neurogenic disorders, reduced recruitment may also be seen in severe or end-stage myopathies in which entire motor units are lost owing to primary muscle fiber degeneration, such as in end-stage muscular dystrophies.

Unstable MUPs

As reinnervation from collateral sprouting begins following an acute nerve injury, the nerve terminals of the newly formed collateral nerve sprouts are immature and neuromuscular transmission is not fully effective. Therefore, each time a motor unit fires, a different number of muscle fiber action potentials are depolarized resulting in a changing morphology and variability of the amplitude and/or number of turns of the MUP. This variation, recorded with a concentric or monopolar needle electrode, is termed jiggle (Video 14). Unstable MUPs are commonly seen in chronic or progressive neurogenic processes, such as a recovering radiculopathy or ALS.

Polyphasic MUPs

Polyphasic MUPs ($\geq$5 phases) in neurogenic disorders occur because of collateral sprouting, reinnervation, and an increase in fiber density. Polyphasic MUPs occur at a stage of ongoing reinnervation in neurogenic disorders, usually beginning approximately 1 month following an acute neurogenic lesion. Polyphasic MUPs in reinnervating neurogenic processes may be of any duration: normal, long, or short. In most cases, the duration is normal or slightly increased, but with continued reinnervation MUP duration increases. In nerve injuries producing severe axonal loss, early reinnervation to only a few muscle fibers in a motor unit produces nascent MUPs, in which the MUP duration is short, amplitude low, and recruitment is severely reduced (**Fig. 16**).

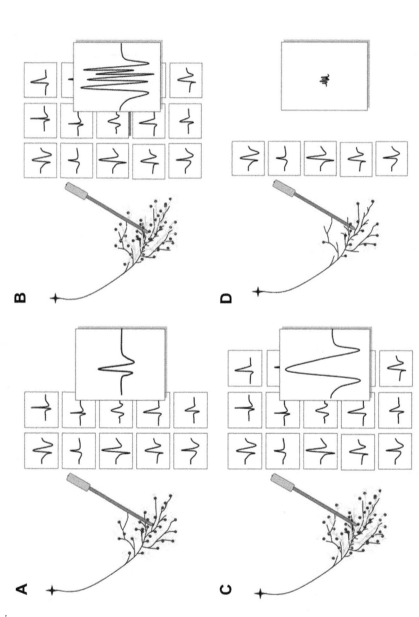

Fig. 16. Summation of muscle fiber action potentials in a motor unit that generate (*A*) a normal MUP, (*B*) a polyphasic MUP during reinnervation from a neurogenic disorder, (*C*) a long-duration MUP in a longstanding neurogenic disorder, and (*D*) a short-duration, low-amplitude, polyphasic MUP in a myopathy.

Long-duration MUPs

MUP duration reflects the density, area, and synchrony of firing of fibers of a motor unit (see **Fig. 16**; Video 15). Long-duration MUPs occur in diseases in which there is increased fiber density or number of fibers or loss of synchronous firing of fibers in a motor unit, typically due to collateral sprouting and reinnervation. Long-duration MUPs generally have high amplitude and show reduced recruitment, but the amplitude may be normal. Long-duration MUPs typically occur in chronic neurogenic disorders and develop several weeks to months following an acute nerve injury (**Table 12**). Once reinnervation is complete, the long-duration MUP persist indefinitely.

Myopathies

Rapid recruitment

The characteristic recruitment pattern in myopathies is rapid recruitment. In myopathies, loss of individual muscle fibers within individual motor unit results in a lower force generation relative to effort. As a result, more MUPs are activated relative to force. Although, in many cases, abnormalities in MUP configuration will also be present, rapid recruitment may be the only abnormality identified on needle examination, particularly in early or mild myopathies (Video 16).

Short-duration and polyphasic MUPs

Short-duration MUPs are characteristic of many types of myopathies and occur in diseases in which there is either physiologic or anatomic loss of muscle fibers from the motor unit or atrophy of component muscle fibers. In these disorders, the number of innervated muscle fibers within the recording region of the electrode is decreased, thereby leading to a decrease in the area of that motor unit. Commonly, these potentials also have low amplitude and show rapid recruitment with minimal effort, but they may have normal or reduced recruitment and normal amplitudes. Some short-duration MUPs may be as short as 1 to 3 milliseconds if only a single muscle fiber is in the recording area. Short-duration MUPs are most characteristic of primary muscle diseases in which loss of muscle fibers from necrosis or degeneration occurs (**Table 13**). Some myopathies, such as metabolic and endocrine disorders, demonstrate only minimal or no reduction in MUP duration. Short-duration MUPs may also occur in severe neuromuscular junction disorders or in newly reinnervated motor units (nascent MUPs) following severe nerve injury. Polyphasic MUPs are also common in myopathies and result from asynchrony of firing of those remaining fibers in the recording area of the needle electrode (see **Fig. 16**). Occasionally, patients with

Table 12 Disorders associated with long duration MUP	
Type of Disorder	**Examples**
Neurogenic disorders	Motor neuron diseases (eg, ALS, poliomyelitis, spinal muscular atrophy)
	Chronic axonal neuropathies (eg, hereditary motor sensory neuropathy type 2)
	Chronic radiculopathies or the residua of an old radiculopathy
	Chronic mononeuropathies or the residua of an old mononeuropathy
Myopathies	Chronic myopathies (eg, inclusion body myositis)

Table 13
Disorders associated with short duration MUP

Type of Disorder	Examples
Myopathies	Muscular dystrophies Inflammatory myopathies (eg, polymyositis, inclusion body myositis) Infiltrative myopathies (eg, sarcoidosis, amyloid) Toxic myopathies (eg, lipid-lowering agents, chloroquine) Congenital myopathies Endocrine myopathies (eg, hypothyroid)
Neuromuscular junction disorders	Myasthenia gravis Lambert-Eaton myasthenic syndrome Botulinum intoxication
Neurogenic disorders	Early reinnervation after nerve damage (nascent MUP)
Disorders of muscle membrane	Periodic paralysis

chronic myopathies, such as inclusion body myositis, have a combination of short-duration and long-duration MUPs.

Neuromuscular Junction Disorders

Varying (unstable) MUPs

When MUPs fire repetitively under voluntary control, they normally have the same amplitude, duration, and configuration each time they fire. Fluctuation of any of these variables (varying or unstable MUPs) is indicative of dysfunction of neuro-muscular transmission. Moment-to-moment variation of MUPs is caused by block-ing of the discharge of action potentials of one or a few of the individual muscle fibers composing the motor unit. The disorders in which varying MUPs occur are listed in **Table 14**. Varying MUPs are characteristic of disorders of neuromuscular transmission, such as myasthenia gravis or Lambert-Eaton myasthenic syndrome, in which impairment of the presynaptic or postsynaptic neuromuscular junction affects the stability of the recorded potentials. Varying MUPs are also commonly seeing in reinnervating neurogenic disorders and occasionally in myopathies (**Fig. 17**).

Table 14
Disorders associated with varying (unstable) MUP

Type of Disorder	Examples
Neuromuscular junction disorders	Myasthenia gravis Lambert-Eaton myasthenic syndrome Botulism Congenital myasthenic syndromes
Neurogenic disorders	Reinnervation after nerve injury Progressing neurogenic disorders (eg, ALS)
Myopathies	Inflammatory myopathies

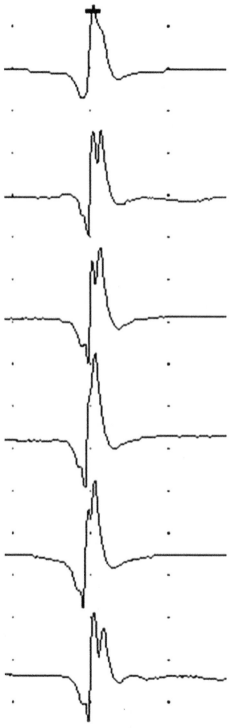

Fig. 17. A varying MUP. Six sequential firings of a single MUP shown in raster mode. The recording is made without movement of the needle electrode and demonstrates MUP instability. Note the slightly different morphologies of the MUP each time it fires.

Table 15
Patterns of MUP abnormalities in different diseases

Recruitment	MUP Configuration	MUP Variation	Example
Normal	Normal	No	Normal
			Some myopathies (metabolic, endocrine, steroid)
			Central nervous system or upper motor neuron disorders
		Yes	Neuromuscular junction disorders (eg, myasthenia gravis, Lambert-Eaton myasthenic syndrome)
	Short duration, polyphasic	No	Myopathies
		Yes	Severe neuromuscular junction disorders (eg, MG, Lambert-Eaton myasthenic syndrome, botulism)
			Myopathies (occasionally)
	Mixed short and long duration	No or yes	Chronic myopathies (eg, inclusion body myositis)
Reduced	Normal	No	Acute neurogenic lesion
		Yes	Subacute neurogenic lesion
	Long duration, polyphasic	No	Chronic neurogenic lesion
		Yes	Chronic, progressing neurogenic lesion
	Short duration, polyphasic	No	Severe or end-stage myopathy
			End-stage neurogenic disorder
		Yes	Early reinnervation after severe nerve damage (nascent MUPs)
			Severe, reinnervating neurogenic disorders
	Mixed short and long duration	No or yes	Rapidly progressing neurogenic disorders (eg, ALS)
Rapid	Normal	No	Mild myopathies
		Yes	—
	Short duration	No	Myopathies
		Yes	Myopathies
	Long duration	No	Chronic myopathies
		Yes	Chronic myopathies (occasionally)

Abbreviation: MG, myasthenia gravis.

SUMMARY

Each of the MUP variables may change separately or in combination with one or more of the others in different neuromuscular disorders. The overall findings on needle EMG should be interpreted in the context of known pathophysiologic mechanisms that occur in diseases. The pattern of changes in MUP recruitment, stability, and configuration can assist in determining the underlying pathologic process affecting the muscle (**Table 15**). Each pattern of abnormality changes with the severity and duration of the disease.

SUPPLEMENTARY DATA

Supplementary data related to this article can be found online at doi:10.1016/j.ncl. 2011.12.009.

REFERENCES

1. Meekin GD, So Y, Quan D. American Association of Neuromuscular & Electrodiagnostic Medicine evidence-based review: use of surface electromyography in the diagnosis and study of neuromuscular disorders. Muscle Nerve 2008;38: 1219–24.
2. Dumitru D, King JC, Nandedkar SD. Motor unit action potential duration recorded by monopolar and concentric needle electrodes. Physiologic implications. Am J Phys Med Rehabil 1997;76:488–93.
3. Chan RC, Hsu TC. Quantitative comparison of motor unit potential parameters between monopolar and concentric needles. Muscle Nerve 1991;14:1028–32.
4. Kouyoumdjian JA, Stalberg EV. Reference jitter values for concentric needle electrodes in voluntarily activated extensor digitorum communis and orbicularis oculi muscles. Muscle Nerve 2008;37:694–9.
5. Stalberg EV, Sanders DB. Jitter recordings with concentric needle electrodes. Muscle Nerve 2009;40:331–9.
6. Rubin DI, Daube JR. Application of clinical neurophysiology: assessing peripheral neuromuscular symptom complexes. In: Daube JR, Rubin DI, editors. Clinical neurophysiology. New York: Oxford University Press; 2009. p. 801–37.
7. Strommen JA, Daube JR. Determinants of pain in needle electromyography. Clin Neurophysiol 2001;112:1414–8.
8. Fuglsang-Frederiksen A, Ronager J. EMG power spectrum, turns-amplitude analysis and motor unit potential duration in neuromuscular disorders. J Neurol Sci 1990;97:81–91.
9. Pfeiffer G, Kunze K. Turn and phase counts of individual motor unit potentials: correlation and reliability. Electroencephalogr Clin Neurophysiol 1992;85:161–5.
10. Stålberg E, Karlsson L. Simulation of the normal concentric needle electromyogram by using a muscle model. Clin Neurophysiol 2001;112:464–71.
11. Weichers DO, Johnson EW. Diffuse abnormal electromyographic insertional activity: a preliminary report. Arch Phys Med Rehabil 1979;60:419–22.
12. Mitchell CW, Bertorini TE. Diffusely increased insertional activity: "EMG Disease" or asymptomatic myotonia congenita? A report of 2 cases. Arch Phys Med Rehabil 2007;88:1212–3.
13. Brown WF, Varkey GP. The origin of spontaneous electrical activity at the endplate zone. Ann Neurol 1981;10:557–60.
14. de Carvalho M, Swash M. Fasciculation potentials: a study of amyotrophic lateral sclerosis and other neurogenic disorders. Muscle Nerve 1998;21:336–44.

15. Kraft GH. Fibrillation potential amplitude and muscle atrophy following peripheral nerve injury. Muscle Nerve 1990;13:814–21.
16. Logigian EL, Ciafaloni E, Quinn C, et al. Severity, type, and distribution of myotonic discharges are different in type 1 and type 2 myotonic dystrophy. Muscle Nerve 2007;35:479–85.
17. Fournier E, Arzel M, Sternberg D, et al. Electromyography guides toward subgroups of mutations in muscle channelopathies. Ann Neurol 2004;56:650–61.
18. Massey R, Daube J. Characteristics of myotonic discharges in neurogenic disorders. Muscle Nerve 2010;42:688–9.
19. Barkhaus PE, Nandedkar SD. "Slow" myotonic discharges. Muscle Nerve 2006; 34:799–800.
20. Costa J, Graca P, Evangelista T, et al. Pain and calf hypertrophy associated with spontaneous repetitive discharges treated with botulinum toxin. Clin Neurophysiol 2005;116:2847–52.
21. Hart IK. Acquired neuromyotonia: a new autoantibody-mediated neuronal potassium channelopathy. Am J Med Sci 2000;319:209–16.
22. Maddison P, Mills KR, Newsom-Davis J. Clinical electrophysiological characterization of the acquired neuromyotonia phenotype of autoimmune peripheral nerve hyperexcitability. Muscle Nerve 2006;33:801–8.
23. Loscher WN, Wanschitz J, Reiners K, et al. Morvan's syndrome: clinical, laboratory, and in vitro electrophysiological studies. Muscle Nerve 2004;30:157–63.
24. Weiss N, Behin A, Psimaras D, et al. Postirradiation neuromyotonia of spinal accessory nerves. Neurology 2011;76:1188–9.
25. Friedenberg SM, Hermann RC. The breathing hand: obstetric brachial plexopathy reinnervation from thoracic roots? J Neurol Neurosurg Psychiatry 2004;75: 158–60.
26. Swift TR. The breathing arm. Muscle Nerve 1994;17:125–9.
27. Swift TR, Leshner RT, Gross JA. Arm-diaphragm synkinesis: electrodiagnostic studies of aberrant regeneration of phrenic motor neurons. Neurology 1980;30: 339–44.
28. Bischoff C, Machetanz J, Conrad B. Is there an age-dependent continuous increase in the duration of the motor unit action potential? Electroencephalogr Clin Neurophysiol 1991;81:304–11.
29. Gunreben G, Schulte-Mattler W. Evaluation of motor unit firing rates by standard concentric needle electromyography. Electromyogr Clin Neurophysiol 1992;32: 103–11.
30. Buchthal F, Rosenfalck P. Action potential parameters in different human muscles. Acta psychiatrica et neurologica Scandinavica 1955;30:125–31.

The Electrodiagnostic Approach to Carpal Tunnel Syndrome

James C. Watson, MD

KEYWORDS

- Carpal tunnel syndrome • Electrodiagnosis • Electromyogram
- Nerve conduction studies • Median neuropathy at the wrist

Carpal tunnel syndrome (CTS) is caused by compression of the median nerve as it passes under the transverse carpal ligament and between the tubercles of the scaphoid and trapezium radially and the pisiform and hook of the hamate carpal bones medially. It is the most common entrapment neuropathy seen in the electrodiagnostic laboratory[1] and was responsible for 0.2% of all US ambulatory care visits in 2007.[2] The incidence of CTS is 376 per 100,000 person years and affects women twice as often as men.[3] Notably, in this epidemiology study from Rochester, Minnesota, the incidence of CTS increased by 164% between the beginning (1981–1985) and the end of the study period (2000–2005; incidence increased from 258 to 424 per 100,000). Since the 1990s, the greatest increase in incidence has been in elderly people.[3] It is estimated that the lifetime risk of CTS is just under 10%.[4] In 2006, 577,000 carpal tunnel releases were performed nationally.[5] Mirroring incidence trends, the greatest increase in surgical release rates has been in elderly patients.[3]

THE GOLD STANDARD QUESTION AND THE ROLE OF ELECTRODIAGNOSTICS

The gold standard for the diagnosis of CTS has been debated. CTS is a clinically defined constellation of symptoms caused by a median neuropathy at the wrist (**Box 1**).[6] Clinical examination signs, such as the Tinel and Phalen signs, are not included in the proposed criteria, as they are limited in specificity. A Tinel or Phalen sign has been reported in 20% or more of healthy subjects.[7–9] Similarly, there can be misdiagnoses (false-positives) with the clinical symptoms alone.[10] Electrodiagnostics have several important roles in suspected CTS (**Box 2**), including confirming the clinically suspected diagnosis by identifying a median neuropathy at the wrist.

Patient-reported symptoms can show significant variability among patients with CTS and may suggest alternative diagnoses (cervical radiculopathy, other mononeuropathy, or peripheral neuropathy). Patients may report involvement of only some, but

Disclosures: no pertinent disclosures.
Department of Neurology, Mayo Clinic, 200 First Street SW, Rochester, MN 55905, USA
E-mail address: watson.james@mayo.edu

Neurol Clin 30 (2012) 457–478
doi:10.1016/j.ncl.2011.12.001
0733-8619/12/$ – see front matter
neurologic.theclinics.com

Box 1

Clinical diagnosis of carpal tunnel syndrome

- Sensory symptoms for 1 month
  - Involving at least 2 digits of digits 1 to 4
  - Intermittent or, if constant, were previously intermittent
  - May have accompanying pain, but not pain alone
- Aggravating precipitants (1 of):
  - Sleep
  - Sustained hand or arm positioning
  - Repetitive hand actions
- Sensory symptoms improved by (1 of):
  - Change in hand position
  - Shaking hand out
  - Use of wrist splints
- If pain present, it involves the hand and fingers > proximal arm/forearm and neck
- No history or examination findings suggestive of an alternative diagnosis

Data from Jablecki CK, Andary MT, Floeter MK, et al. Second AAEM literature review of the usefullness of nerve conduction studies and needle electromyography for the evaluation of patients with carpal tunnel syndrome. Muscle Nerve 2002;(Suppl X):S924–78. Available at: http://www.aanem.org/Practice/Practice-Management/Practice-Guidelines.aspx.

---

not other, median innervated fingers or report a sense of involvement of nonmedian innervated fingers or parts of the hand or arm.[11] Pain above the level of the wrist raises concerns of an alternative diagnosis, such as cervical radiculopathy, but is common (20%–40%) in CTS cases without any identifiable proximal pathology.[11–13] Electrodiagnostics are effective at excluding alternative neurogenic processes mimicking CTS. A series evaluating patients referred for electromyography (EMG)/nerve conduction studies (NCS) with upper extremity nerve complaints with a suspected clinical diagnosis (CTS or other), found that electrodiagnostics changed the final diagnosis 42% of the time.[14]

Electrodiagnostics used alone are not the answer to defining CTS, however, as they are limited in sensitivity and specificity for the clinical syndrome and need to be interpreted in the clinical context. Specificity is high in clinically suspected cases of CTS[6];

Box 2

Role of electrodiagnostic studies in the diagnosis of CTS

- Confirm the diagnosis
  - Localize the median nerve abnormalities to the carpal tunnel
- Exclude alternative diagnoses mimicking CTS
- Diagnose superimposed disorder(s) contributing to symptoms that may cause ongoing symptoms after treatment of CTS (cervical radiculopathy, peripheral neuropathy)
- Define severity of the neurogenic injury
- Baseline before surgery

---

however, in cohorts of clinically asymptomatic workers incidentally found to have electrophysiologically defined median neuropathies at the wrist, up to 75% of them did not develop symptoms of CTS during follow-up of 7 to 11 years.[15–17] On the flip side, it is estimated that 10% to 15% of clinically defined CTS cases will have no electrodiagnostic abnormalities.[17] As such, an unremarkable study does not exclude CTS, but it does exclude significant axonal loss or conduction block, which should push toward conservative treatment options as an initial treatment strategy. Similarly, severe electrodiagnostic abnormalities indicating advanced neurogenic injury could influence a provider to consider more invasive treatment options earlier. Defining the extent of neurogenic impairment in cases of CTS will often influence treatment decisions.

Several consensus statements from multidisciplinary groups have concluded that for clinical practice and particularly before invasive treatment considerations, the combination of clinical symptoms and electrodiagnostic abnormalities are preferable to clinical signs and symptoms or to electrodiagnostics alone in defining CTS.[10,18–20] It has been proposed that the constellation of clinical symptoms alone define cases of probable CTS, but that a classification of definite CTS should be reserved for patients with clinical and concordant electrodiagnostic abnormalities.[18] A recent proposal of quality measures for the electrodiagnosis in suspected CTS recommended that preoperative EMG/NCS should be completed in all work-related CTS cases. This part of the proposal has proved controversial.[20]

In relation to this article's focus on the electrodiagnostic evaluation of CTS, it should be noted that the reported sensitivities and specificities of NCS are in relation to clinically defined cases of CTS, as they must be compared against a CTS diagnosis that was made independent of the electrodiagnostic results.

THE ELECTRODIAGNOSTIC EVALUATION FOR CTS

A practice parameter for electrodiagnostic studies in carpal tunnel syndrome was published in 2002 after being endorsed by the American Association of Neuromuscular and Electrodiagnostic Medicine (AANEM), the American Academy of Neurology (AAN), and the American Academy of Physical Medicine and Rehabilitation (AAPMR),[18,21] with its full details and annotated bibliography published in a supplement.[6] This still serves as an excellent review and the pooled sensitivities and specificities for CTS of older NCS reported here are from this source. This article includes but emphasizes advances and new data since that review.

Sensory fibers are more sensitive to compression in CTS than motor fibers and, as such, sensory NCS (SNCS) are diagnostically more sensitive for CTS than motor NCS (MNCS). There are multiple reasons for this discrepancy. Sensory fibers are more susceptible to ischemic change, given a larger proportion of large myelinated fibers and higher energy requirements than motor fascicles and hence show damage from compression earlier.[17] SNCS are also low-amplitude responses (microvolts) with a low signal-to–background noise ratio and, as such, SNCS are sensitive to smaller changes in the signal (a reduced safety margin for detecting a response). In addition, when there is damage to a motor axon, there are compensatory mechanisms to preserve function, including collateral sprouting from unaffected axons to reinnervate denervated myofibers. There is no such compensatory mechanism when sensory fascicles are damaged.

The goal of the electrodiagnostic evaluation in clinically suspected CTS is to use the most sensitive tests available to confirm CTS in an efficient and technically reliable way, while also being comprehensive enough to exclude mimickers or superimposed neurogenic processes.

SENSORY NERVE CONDUCTION STUDIES
Median Antidromic SNCS Recording Over Digit 2

Technique
Recording ring electrodes are placed over the second digit (pointer finger) with G1 over the proximal phalanx and G2 over the distal part of middle phalanx.[22] The median nerve is stimulated 13 cm proximal to the G1 electrode just above the wrist where it runs between the easily palpated flexor carpi radialis tendon radially and the palmaris longus tendon medially. More proximal stimulation can be performed over the median nerve in the antecubital fossa, medial to the biceps tendon overlying the brachial artery to calculate a conduction velocity over the forearm.

Normal values
Normal values are distal latency less than 3.6 ms, amplitude greater than 15 μV, conduction velocity greater than 56 m/s.[6,22]

Role in CTS
Antidromic SNCS are quick and easy to perform and have good inter-rater and intra-rater reliability. They usually have well-defined responses that are higher in amplitude than traditional orthodromic sensory responses. As the median nerve is stimulated at the level of the wrist, motor fascicles are also stimulated and median muscles in the thenar eminence contract. This produces a volume-conducted motor response that can contaminate the sensory nerve action potential (SNAP) recording distally over the finger. This motor response usually occurs late with a slow rise time and long duration. The SNAP can be distinguished from this motor response, if necessary, by moving the recording electrode distally (the SNAP latency will increase, the motor response will not).[22]

In CTS, a median neuropathy at the wrist would be confirmed with prolongation of the distal latency (>3.6 ms). It should be noted for all SNCS that amplitude is more variable and a low SNCS amplitude without evidence of slowing across the carpal tunnel (ie, prolonged distal latency) should be interpreted with caution and is generally not an indication of CTS. Other median SNCS could be considered in that situation.

The digit 2 median antidromic SNCS is a routine, and in many laboratories default, upper limb median SNCS. Its sensitivity in cases of suspected CTS is limited, however, with a pooled sensitivity of 65%, but with a high specificity (98%) when applied to a patient population with a clinical suspicion for CTS.[6] Despite this, the AANEM/AAN/AAPMR practice parameter recognizes this SNCS as being widely used and a reasonable first study in the CTS electrodiagnostic evaluation. If there is no distal latency prolongation, however, a more sensitive SNCS needs to be performed in suspected CTS cases. In the practice parameter, median motor NCS are lower in priority and performed later.[21]

This methodology may lead to unnecessary studies. As such, in Mayo Clinic EMG laboratories, a practical approach is used where the median motor NCS (which is known to be less sensitive for CTS) is performed first for clinically suspected cases of CTS. If it shows a prolonged distal latency (suggesting a median neuropathy at the wrist), the sensory fascicles would also be expected to be affected and the SNCS of choice is the digit 2 median antidromic sensory response, given its ease of use. If the median MNCS does not show an abnormality, a more sensitive SNCS is used and the digit 2 median antidromic SNCS is not performed.

Other considerations
The median antidromic SNCS has also been well studied recording over the third digit.[23–25] There is no difference in sensitivity of detecting CTS between recording

over the second or third digit.[26] Appropriate normal values need to used for the method chosen.[27] After 2 older studies, there has been a renewed interest in whether provocative maneuvers increase the sensitivity of median SNCS.[28,29] A recent study in patients with clinically defined CTS but normal NCS found that 5 minutes of wrist flexion increased the sensitivity of the median antidromic SNCS in detecting CTS, without a significant change in median motor or control group distal latencies.[30]

Orthodromic Palmar Studies

Technique
When performed, both the median and ulnar orthodromic palmar studies should be performed in the same limb.[22] The median G1 recording electrode is placed proximal to the wrist crease and 8 cm proximal to the stimulator cathode. It should overlie the median nerve between the flexor carpi radialis and palmaris longus tendons. The ulnar G1 electrode is placed proximal to the wrist crease just medial of the flexor carpi ulnaris tendon and 8 cm proximal to the cathode stimulation site. The G2 electrodes are placed 3.5 to 4.0 cm proximal to G1 for each nerve. In addition, recording electrodes can be placed over the median nerve in the antecubital fossa at the elbow and over the ulnar nerve about 5 cm proximal to the medial epicondyle to calculate the conduction velocity along each nerve. For median stimulation, the cathode is placed on the thenar crease overlying the second metacarpal. For ulnar stimulation, the cathode is placed on the palmar crease between the fourth and fifth metacarpals. For each, the anode begins distal to this but usually needs to be rotated (without moving the cathode) to decrease shock artifact.

Normal value
The median normal values are distal latency less than 2.3 ms, amplitude greater than 50 μV, conduction velocity greater than 56 m/s. The ulnar normal values are distal latency less than 2.3 ms, amplitude greater than 15 μV, conduction velocity greater than 55 m/s. The difference between median and ulnar latency is 0.3 ms or less.[6,22]

Technical considerations
Palmar stimulation is a mixed NCS, as both sensory and motor (innervating the median lumbricals or ulnar dorsal interosseous) fascicles are stimulated. The recorded response at the wrist is primarily sensory, however.[1] Therefore, these studies are billed as SNCS.

The distance between the stimulator and G1 is short (8 cm) and shock artifact often makes it difficult to mark a well-defined SNAP onset. Sliding the stimulator when a response is initially obtained (but not supramaximal) to maximize position over the nerve of interest will reduce the stimulation necessary for a supramaximal response. Rotating the anode and using a smaller stimulating head also help to reduce shock artifact. Amplitudes show higher levels of variability than antidromic studies and an isolated low-amplitude palmar response should be interpreted with caution and other SNCS considered. As with all SNCS, a low-amplitude response without evidence of slowing across the carpal tunnel (distal latency prolongation) is not diagnostic of CTS.

Role in suspected CTS
Median palmar distal latencies can be examined for an absolute prolongation relative to normal values and for a relative prolongation in comparison with the ulnar palmar distal latency over the same distance. Palmar studies are the preferred method for diagnosing CTS in the Mayo Clinic EMG laboratories and are an appropriate choice for a "sensitive SNCS" in the AANEM/AAN/AAPMR practice parameter.[21]

Absolute prolongation of the median palmar distal latency (>2.3 ms for patients 60 years old and younger, and >2.4 for those older than 60) is more sensitive for the diagnosis of CTS than the traditional median antidromic SNCS (digit 2). The pooled sensitivity is 74%, with a specificity of 97% in cohorts of patients with suspected CTS.[6] Sensitivity is improved over median antidromic studies by excluding the normally conducting segments of the median nerve from the palm to the finger that dilutes the slowing across the carpal tunnel.[1,17]

In addition, the median palmar distal latency can be compared with the ulnar palmar distal latency to see if there is a significant "relative" prolongation of the median latency (**Fig. 1**). This difference has been called the "palmdiff." The pooled sensitivity

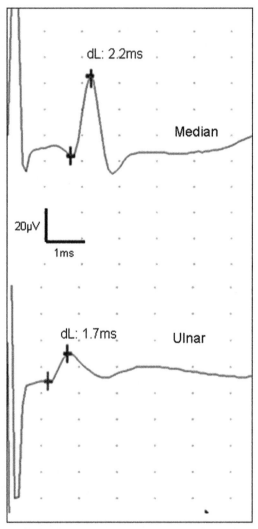

Fig. 1. Median (*upper tracing*) and ulnar (*lower tracing*) palmar studies. The absolute peak (distal) latencies for both are within normal limits (<2.3 ms); however, there is a relative prolongation of the median palmar latency (0.5 ms in this case) compared with the ulnar palmar latency when tested over the same distance (8 cm). Given a similar caliber, degree of myelination, and temperature of the nerves in the tested segment, the primary difference in their course and conduction is the carpal tunnel and the relative prolonged median latency can be rationally attributed to median slowing through the carpal tunnel.

for this technique alone is 71% with 97% specificity.[6] In combination with assessment of the absolute palmar latency, however, this appears to add additional sensitivity.[31] The median and ulnar nerves at the wrist and through the palm are similar in caliber and myelination. In addition, they course at similar depths and therefore are at similar temperatures. All of these factors suggest that the median and ulnar nerves over these segments would be anticipated to conduct at a similar velocity and, therefore, if examined over the same stimulator-to-G1 distance, have similar distal latencies. If the median palmar latency is significantly prolonged (>0.3 ms if younger than 60 years, >0.4 ms if older than 60) relative to the ulnar palmar latency over the same distance (even if still within normal limits for the absolute palmar distal latency), this can rationally be attributed to being secondary to compression of the median nerve at the carpal tunnel, as passing through the carpal tunnel is the only significant difference in the nerves' course. The most important technical consideration is ensuring the median and ulnar palmar studies were examined over the same distance.

Median-Ulnar Ring Finger Antidromic Sensory Latencies Difference (Ringdiff)

Technique
Ring electrodes are placed over digit 4 (ring finger). The median and ulnar nerves are stimulated above the wrist at a distance of 14 cm proximal to the proximal ring electrode (G1) (**Fig. 2**).[22] The distances must be identical.

Normal value
A prolongation of the median distal latency relative to the ulnar distal latency over the same distance of 0.4 ms or more is considered significant (some have recommended ≥0.5 ms). This has been called the "ringdiff."[31-35]

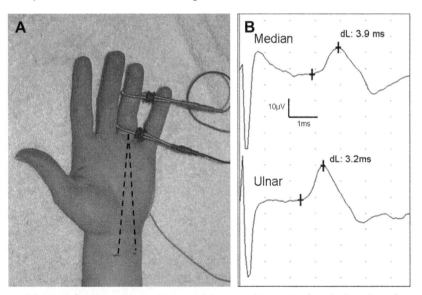

Fig. 2. (A) Setup for the median–ulnar antidromic studies to the fourth digit (ring finger). Ring electrodes are placed over the ring finger with the proximal electrode being G1. The distance from G1 to the median and to the ulnar stimulation sites is 14 cm. The distances must be identical. (B) Tracings from median (*upper*) and ulnar (*lower*) antidromic SNCS recording over the ring finger showing a "ringdiff" (the latency difference between the median and the ulnar studies) of 0.7 ms (abnormal ≥0.4 ms). This confirms relative slowing of the median nerve through the carpal tunnel.

Role in CTS

The premise behind being able to compare the median and ulnar nerve latencies is the same as for palmar studies. This study has the advantages of other antidromic SNCS (quick and easy to perform with well-defined, reproducible responses). It has a high pooled sensitivity of 85% and specificity of 97%.[21] It has several potential roles in CTS. The AANEM/AAN/AAPMR practice parameter considers palmar studies and median versus ulnar antidromic SNCS to be "high-sensitivity" SNCS for CTS and the sensory studies of choice when there is a high clinical suspicion of CTS. As such, it is reasonable to use as the SNCS of choice when evaluating suspected CTS. At Mayo Clinic EMG laboratories, palmar studies have remained our preferred SNCS primarily secondary to experience with it. Although the published pooled sensitivities in the practice parameter seem to favor the ringdiff measurement compared with the palmar studies, there is overlap in the confidence intervals of reported sensitivities for the 2 techniques. The Mayo Clinic practice is to perform the ringdiff evaluation when there is a high clinical suspicion of CTS but normal palmar studies and clinical symptoms more predominant in or toward the ring finger (note that the literature supports the sensitivity of these studies regardless of which fingers show the predominance of symptoms).

Median–Radial Thumb Antidromic Sensory Latency Difference (Thumbdiff)

Technique

Ring electrodes are placed over digit one (thumb). The median and radial nerves are stimulated above the wrist at a distance of 10 cm proximal to the proximal ring electrode (G1) (**Fig. 3**).[22] The distances must be identical.

Normal value

A prolongation of the median distal latency relative to the radial distal latency over the same distance of 0.5 ms or more is considered significant compared with normal values.[35,36]

Role in CTS

The pooled sensitivity for the thumbdiff is 65% with a 99% specificity.[21] Its role is primarily in patients whose symptom complex is suggestive of CTS but predominately affects the thumb and whose other SNCS are unrevealing. It could also be considered in patients who have a known ulnar neuropathy affecting the ulnar SNCS, which negates the usefulness of median–ulnar comparison studies.

The Combined Sensory Index

The combined sensory index (CSI) was proposed as a way to decrease the chance of random error in a single NCS causing a false-positive or false-negative result (ie, improved sensitivity and specificity) and as a way to magnify slight differences from normal, but still within normal limits in an individual study, to confirm the diagnosis of CTS in very mild cases.[35] It is a summation of the latency differences between the median-ulnar palmar, median-ulnar fourth digit, and median-radial thumb studies (palmdiff + ringdiff + thumbdiff). A CSI of 1.0 ms or greater is considered abnormal and was suggested to have greater sensitivity (83%) than the individual studies with excellent specificity.[35] Further study, however, demonstrated that if there was an abnormality in any 1 of the 3 SNCS components of the CSI (palmdiff $\geq$0.4 ms, ringdiff $\geq$0.5 ms, thumbdiff >0.7 ms), it was highly predictive of an abnormal CSI, negating the utility of the CSI.[37] If those thresholds were not met, it was proposed to complete the full CSI in patients with a high clinical suspicion. A recent retrospective study found that CSI correlated with surgical outcomes in patients, particularly if there was a high CSI (2.5–4.6).[38]

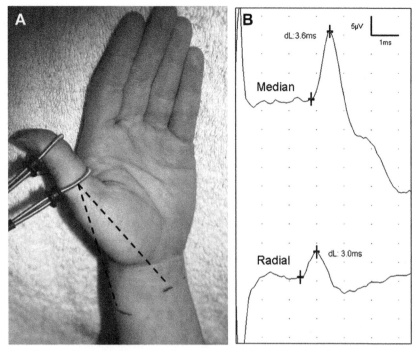

Fig. 3. (*A*) Setup for the median–radial antidromic studies to the thumb. Ring electrodes are placed over the thumb with the proximal electrode being G1. The distance from G1 to the median and radial stimulation sites is 10 cm. The distances must be identical. (*B*) Tracing from median (*upper*) and radial (*lower*) antidromic SNCS recording over the thumb showing a "thumbdiff" (the latency difference between the median and the radial studies) of 0.6 ms (abnormal ≥0.5 ms). This confirms relative slowing of the median nerve through the carpal tunnel.

The Mayo Clinic practice is to perform one of the other SNCS if the clinical symptoms are suggestive of CTS and the more standard antidromic or palmar studies are normal (ie, thumbdiff performed if the patient has a predominance of symptoms toward the thumb and palmar studies are normal). The CSI is occasionally, but not routinely, performed. It should be noted that in these situations, it is electrophysiologically very mild cases of CTS that are being identified with the CSI and if the syndrome has already been defined clinically this may not alter management. It may be worthwhile, however, if there is a diagnostic dilemma.

MOTOR NERVE CONDUCTION STUDIES
Median MNCS Recording Over the Abductor Pollicis Brevis

Technique
The G1 recording electrode is placed at the midpoint of the abductor pollicis brevis (ABP) muscles on the thenar eminence one-third the distance between the major creases at the metacarpal-carpal and metacarpal-phalangeal joints of the thumb.[22] G2 sits just distal to the metacarpal-phalangeal joint on the lateral side of the thumb. The stimulator cathode is placed 7 cm proximal to G1 over the median nerve between the flexor carpi radialis and palmaris longus tendons.

Normal values

Normal values are distal latency less than 4.5 ms, amplitude greater than 4.0 mV, and conduction velocity greater than 48 m/s.[6,22]

Role in CTS

The median MNCS recording over the APB is a routine upper limb MNCS for most patients undergoing electrodiagnostic evaluation for upper limb symptoms. Although the SNCS are more sensitive for CTS and can confirm the diagnosis alone, it is still worthwhile to perform the median MNCS to assess the involvement of the motor fascicles that help to define electrophysiologic severity of CTS (later section) and influence management. The practice parameter's pooled sensitivity of a prolonged median MNCS (recording over the APB) distal latency to confirm CTS is 63% with a high specificity.[21] Several studies have suggested a much lower sensitivity. In a cohort of patients with CTS in Rochester, Minnesota, only 38% had prolonged median motor distal latencies (>4.5 ms) and 2% had no responses.[39] This is in keeping with other more recent studies of the median motor distal latency showing sensitivities of 44% to 55%.[25,40]

The median motor distal latency (recording APB) can be compared with the ulnar MNCS recording over the abductor digiti minimi (ADM), the routine ulnar MNCS. Unlike SNCS comparison studies, however, the distance and nerve parameters (size, myelination, depth) are not directly comparable. Mayo laboratories use a conservative difference of 1.8 ms or more as a significant abnormality[1,41]; however, others have suggested a lower cutoff (as low as a 1.2-ms difference being significant).[42,43]

The median motor distal latency can also be compared with the opposite side and a difference of 1.0 ms or more considered significant. However, CTS occurs bilaterally almost 60% of the time, making this comparison less useful.[1] If the median motor latency relative to the opposite side or to the ulnar motor latency to the ADM is considered in addition to absolute prolongation of the median motor distal latency, the sensitivity of the median motor study improved from almost 40% to 51% in the previously cited study.[39]

Similar to sensory studies, an isolated abnormality of the median MNCS amplitude without significant distal latency prolongation should not be interpreted as evidence of a median neuropathy at the wrist. Conduction block of the motor fascicles is possible and can be evaluated by inching the stimulator across the carpal tunnel from above the wrist in 1-cm increments. In practice, this is difficult (and therefore not commonly performed), given the course of the recurrent median motor branch to the thenar eminence and the proximity of the thenar eminence and risk of direct muscle stimulation when stimulating below the wrist crease.[6] In addition, a prolonged median motor distal latency without any median sensory latency prolongation is rare in CTS. In a study of 2700 hands with typical signs and symptoms of CTS, Repaci and colleagues[44] reported only 0.6% of their series had abnormal median motor latencies without latency abnormalities in high-sensitivity SNCS. In an older study, 1.1% of a CTS cohort showed this motor-only pattern, but it was acknowledged that early cases in that series may not have had more sensitive SNCS performed.[39] Although fascicular involvement of only the motor fascicles of the median nerve could explain this phenomenon, it is rare enough that the electromyographer should extend the electrodiagnostic study to exclude alternative etiologies, such as a disorder of the C8/T1 anterior horn cell, motor root (cervical radiculopathy), or of a motor neuropathy.[39]

Proximal Conduction Velocity Slowing in CTS

In approximately 10% of patients with CTS, there will be mild slowing of the median motor conduction velocity in the forearm. The cause of this has been debated and may be caused by retrograde degeneration, axonal atrophy, or conduction block of large rapidly conducting nerve fibers in the carpal tunnel.[45–50] It is important to recognize this phenomenon, as it alone does not suggest a more proximal median neuropathy (pronator syndrome or ligament of Struthers syndrome).

Median-to-Ulnar Crossover

Median-to-ulnar crossover (the Martin Gruber anastomosis) is an autosomally dominant inherited, common (present in 15%–30% of the healthy population and bilateral in 70%), normal anatomic variant, whereby median nerve fascicles pass over to the ulnar nerve in the proximal one-third of the forearm. These fascicles then travel with the ulnar nerve to the hand and innervate ulnar muscles in the thenar region (first dorsal interosseous, flexor pollicis brevis, and/or adductor pollicis) or hypothenar eminence or both.[51–55] A crossover innervating the thenar eminence is the least common form.[56] Crossovers are of no clinical significance, but can confound the interpretation of the nerve conduction studies if not well understood.

The key to recognizing a median-to-ulnar crossover innervating the thenar eminence is recognizing that the proximal median MNCS amplitude is higher than the distal median MNCS amplitude. This never occurs from disease. If this occurs, one must first exclude overstimulation of the proximal median motor site with current spread directly to the ulnar nerve and understimulation (ie, not supramaximal) at the distal median stimulation site. If these have been excluded, a median-to-ulnar crossover should be confirmed. This can usually be accomplished by stimulating the ulnar nerve at the wrist and at sites above the elbow with the recording electrodes still overlying the abductor pollicis brevis (the usual median MNCS setup). Because the crossover fibers are not present at the ulnar nerve above the elbow, it would be theorized that stimulation there would yield no response; however, because there are true ulnar innervated muscles (first dorsal interosseous, adductor pollicis, flexor pollicis brevis) in the region of the recording electrodes over the thenar eminence, stimulation of the ulnar nerve at the elbow will usually produce a volume-conducted response from these ulnar muscles, even in the absence of a crossover. This volume-conduction ulnar response usually is of low amplitude and always has a large positive wave preceding it. The positivity before the response indicates that the recording electrode over the APB is not over the endplate of the contracting muscle. Without moving the recording electrodes, the ulnar nerve is then stimulated at the wrist. Similar to the elbow, a volume-conducted response will be recorded over the thenar eminence; however, in the presence of a crossover, the response recorded with ulnar/wrist stimulation will sometimes have an initial negative (upward) deflection and be much higher in amplitude than the response with ulnar/elbow stimulation. The amplitude difference between the ulnar wrist and above-elbow sites represents the contribution of the crossover fibers and should equal (roughly) the difference between the median proximal and distal stimulation site amplitudes (**Fig. 4**).

Another phenomenon unique to a crossover in the setting of CTS is that the proximal median motor response, in addition to being of higher amplitude than the distal response, may have a large positivity preceding it. These are present in cases of more severe CTS where the median fibers contributing to the CMAP response are slowed significantly through the carpal tunnel, but the crossover fibers bypass this slowing and arrive at the thenar eminence before the median fibers through the carpal tunnel. Because these crossover fibers may activate thenar myofibers not directly under the APB G1 recording electrode, they appear as a large positivity preceding the median CMAP. When this proximal median simulation positivity is seen in the setting of CTS, a crossover should be presumed and confirmed (see **Fig. 4**).

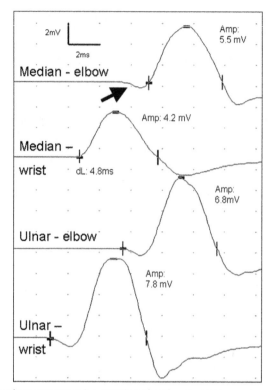

Fig. 4. Median-to-ulnar crossover innervating the thenar eminence in a patient with CTS. The recording electrodes are overlying the abductor pollicis brevis (APB) for all studies. Top 2 tracings: Median nerve stimulation demonstrates a higher CMAP at the elbow than the wrist with an initial positivity at the elbow. The arrow in the top tracing indicates the crossover fibers that are arriving at the thenar eminence sooner than the median fibers, which are slowed passing through the carpal tunnel (the following large CMAP response). This finding is indicative of a crossover in the setting of CTS. Bottom 2 tracings: Ulnar stimulation at the elbow and wrist shows responses with initial positivity at both sites owing to volume-conducted responses from ulnar innervated muscles. The difference between the ulnar elbow and wrist CMAP amplitudes approximates the crossover fibers.

Median–Ulnar Lumbrical versus Interosseous Study

Technique
The G1 recording electrode is placed in the midpalm on the distal thenar crease between the second and third metacarpals.[22] G2 is placed over the proximal index finger or in the web space between the second and third digits. In this position, the active recording electrode (G1) is immediately over the median innervated second lumbrical and deep to that (ie, dorsally) sits the ulnar innervated second palmar and interosseous muscle. Stimulation of the median and ulnar nerves is then performed proximal to the wrist crease at a distance of 9 to 10 cm from G1 (**Fig. 5**).

Normal value
A prolongation of the medial distal latency to the second lumbrical compared with the ulnar latency to the second interosseous of 0.5 ms or more is considered significant for median slowing across the carpal tunnel.[57–60]

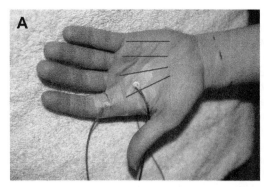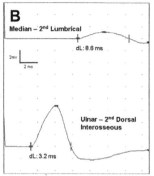

Fig. 5. (*A*) Setup for median–ulnar lumbrical versus second dorsal interosseous motor study. Lines indicate metacarpals. G1 is placed between the second and third metacarpal. G2 is over the proximal index finger. The stimulation sites are 10 cm proximally over the median and ulnar nerves. (*B*) Tracings in a case of very severe CTS where all routine median MNCS and SNCS were absent. There is a marked prolongation of the median latency recording over the second lumbrical (*top tracing*) compared with the ulnar latency to the second dorsal interosseous (abnormal ≥0.5 ms).

Role in CTS

In mild CTS cases, with median stimulation there is a recordable small sensory nerve action potential that precedes the large, broad compound muscle action potential over the second lumbrical. This premotor response represents a traveling wave of median digital sensory fibers. A distal (peak) latency of greater than 2.7 ms of this SNAP is considered abnormal with a sensitivity of 77% for CTS.[61] It has been used as part of the routine electrodiagnostic evaluation of CTS,[57,60,62] but it is unclear how much value is added compared with more routine and sensitive sensory studies. More commonly, these studies are used in very severe CTS where routine MNCS and SNCS are absent. The median innervated lumbricals are relatively spared compared with the median innervated fibers in the thenar eminence and the lumbrical response is usually still obtainable. This allows demonstration of slowing across the carpal tunnel with a prolonged median motor distal latency.[63,64] In these situations, the premotor sensory potential is no longer elicitable. Finally, the lumbrical–interosseous studies are useful in the setting of generalized peripheral neuropathy (discussed later in this article).

THE ROLE OF ELECTROMYOGRAPHY—THE NEEDLE EXAMINATION

The role of the needle examination in CTS has been debated in the literature.[65,66] On one side, it is argued that if the clinical suspicion was for CTS and the NCS confirmed that diagnosis, the needle EMG adds little except discomfort and cost. The counter argument is that confirming the diagnosis is only one of the roles of electrodiagnostic studies in CTS. It is just as important to exclude mimickers and processes that, if present (cervical radiculopathy or peripheral neuropathy), may cause continued signs and symptoms even if the identified CTS was treated. One small review found that 7.4% of the CTS cases in their laboratory had a superimposed cervical radiculopathy ("double crush").[65] Needle EMG easily accomplishes this goal. Further, if the patient ends up having CTS alone, a screening needle examination of the affected limb takes very little time with limited discomfort in an experienced electromyographer's hands. Obviously, this benefit ratio may become unfavorable if a patient has a significant coagulopathy or significant anxiety, but in the author's EMG laboratory, a screening needle examination is routinely performed. The needle examination is listed as an option in the AANEM/AAN/AAPMR practice parameter.[21]

A reasonable screening needle examination should include 1, and ideally 2, muscles from each cervical root to the upper extremity, passing through different parts of the brachial plexus and different peripheral nerves. A reasonable screening needle examination might include the deltoid (C5/6 root, upper trunk, posterior cord, axillary nerve), biceps (C5/6 root, upper trunk, lateral cord, musculocutaneous nerve), triceps (C6/7/8 roots, all trunks, posterior cord, radial nerve), pronator teres (C6/7 roots, upper/middle trunk, lateral cord, proximal median nerve), first dorsal interosseous (C8/T1 roots, lower trunk, medial cord, ulnar nerve), and abductor pollicis brevis (C8/T1 roots, lower trunk, medial cord, median nerve). All roots, parts of the brachial plexus (trunks and cords), and all of the major peripheral nerves in the upper extremity are quickly covered. The screening examination should be modified to fit a patient's symptoms.

The needle examination of the median innervated muscles in the thenar eminence (abductor pollicis brevis, opponens pollicis) is uncomfortable. Of patients with CTS, 40% to 60% may have no definable motor fascicle involvement on MNCS[6,39] and, as such, needle EMG changes in the median innervated muscles of the thenar eminence would not be expected in many patients. Some have suggested the needle examination of these muscles offers nothing additional to the median MNCS and should not be performed routinely.[67] A survey suggested that 74% of electromyographers do a needle examination of a median thenar muscle in CTS cases.[68] Performing needle EMG of the thenar median innervated muscles only if the median MNCS amplitude was less than 7 mV was found to detect 95% of all cases with denervation and would spare 52% of patients from needle examination of these uncomfortable muscles.[69] A recent proposal of quality measures for the electrodiagnosis in suspected CTS recommends that CTS should be classified as severe only if the median MNCS is low amplitude or absent, or if there are changes on the needle examination of the median thenar muscles.[20]

It would seem reasonable to include needle examination of the thenar median innervated muscles only in cases with a reduced (<7 mV) median compound muscle action potential amplitude. If the thenar eminence is deferred and a screening upper limb needle examination is performed, it is reasonable to include another median innervated C8/T1 muscle that is better tolerated, such as the flexor pollicis brevis.

SPECIAL SITUATIONS
Peripheral Neuropathy

Identifying CTS in patients with superimposed peripheral neuropathies can be challenging both clinically and electrophysiologically. It can be difficult to determine if the median NCS distal latency prolongation is disproportionate to the changes seen in other NCS. A comparison latency study would seem most appropriate for this determination, as the peripheral neuropathy would be expected to affect both the median and ulnar nerves similarly. The lumbrical–interossei motor studies have been shown to be effective discriminators of CTS on a background peripheral neuropathy and superior to palmar studies and median–ulnar antidromics recording over the ring finger.[70] A greater than 0.8 ms (or in another study 1.0 ms) prolongation of the median-to–second lumbrical latency compared with that of the ulnar-to–second dorsal interosseous latency was found to optimize sensitivity and specificity.[70,71]

Ulnar Nerve Conduction Abnormalities in CTS

There has been recent attention brought to a reasonable frequency of abnormalities of the ulnar sensory nerve conduction studies in patients with CTS. It is reported that ulnar SNCS abnormalities can occur with CTS of all severities, although the degree of ulnar SNCS abnormalities increases with increasing electrophysiologic severity of CTS.[72–74] The mechanism is presumed to be transmitted forces from the increased pressure in the carpal tunnel to the ulnar nerve as it passes through the Guyon canal. Following carpal tunnel release there is a decrease in the pressure in the Guyon canal[75] and an improvement in ulnar SNCS.[76] Further support for this theory was provided by a recent ultrasound study that showed an increase in ulnar nerve cross-sectional area at the Guyon canal following carpal tunnel release, which corresponded with improvement in ulnar SNCS. Notably, the bulk of this literature comes from a single group and others have questioned this association, suggesting that further study is needed.[77]

Grading the Severity of CTS

There has been debate as to the appropriateness of grading the severity of CTS based on electrodiagnostic findings.[78–81] The primary issue is that the patient's clinical and electrophysiologic severity often do not correlate.[82] There is some evidence that there is a correlation, however, albeit imperfect, between electrodiagnostic severity and surgical outcome.[83] In the Mayo EMG laboratories, CTS cases are graded as to their electrophysiologic severity with a scale proposed by Stevens (**Box 3**).[1] A slight variation has been proposed by others,[17,40] and a more complicated grading scheme has been proposed by Bland.[84] When using an electrophysiologic grading scale, it is important to recognize that it is the severity of the median neuropathy at the wrist that is being graded and that the severity of the clinical syndrome is separate and based on patient report. Both are important for the treating physician and can influence treatment recommendations. For example, a physician may have a lower threshold for considering carpal tunnel release to prevent progressive neurologic

---

Box 3
Electrophysiologic severity of a median neuropathy at the wrist

- Mild CTS
  - Prolonged sensory or mixed (palmar) distal latency ± amplitude reduction
- Moderate CTS
  - Above, PLUS
  - Prolonged median motor distal latency
- Severe CTS
  - Absent sensory response OR
  - Low amplitude motor response
- Very Severe CTS
  - Absent routine sensory and thenar motor responses
  - Lumbrical response may still be present with prolonged latency

Data from Stevens JC. AAEM minimonograph #26: the electrodiagnosis of carpal tunnel syndrome. American Association of Electrodiagnostic Medicine. Muscle Nerve 1997;20(12):1477–86.

decline in a patient with NCS evidence of significant sensory and motor axonal loss, even if symptoms are reported only as mild. Conversely, if NCS show little evidence of neurogenic injury, a physician may be more comfortable giving a longer trial of conservative management. Finally, a patient with very mild or even normal NCS, with a compelling history for CTS, which is clinically severe despite conservative management, could still deserve consideration for carpal tunnel release. No concrete recommendations can be made based on the NCS grading alone. They must be considered in the clinical context, but do provide useful information on the extent of neurogenic injury.

Recurrent CTS After Carpal Tunnel Release

Reevaluating patients with residual or recurrent symptoms of CTS after surgical carpal tunnel release (CTR) is challenging. Following CTR, corresponding with clinical improvement, there is improvement in the median NCS. The maximum improvement in NCS occurs in the first 6 weeks after surgery,[85] but the exact timing is unknown and the degree of improvement variable and often incomplete (ie, median latencies do not return to normal).[86–91] Of median sensory distal latencies, 79% remained abnormal at up to the 1 year follow-up in one study.[92] Postoperative repeat electrodiagnostic studies are not routine. As such, when patients are evaluated for residual or recurrent symptoms of CTS, it is usually unknown how things improved after the CTR, and repeat electrodiagnostic evaluation is often limited in its conclusions, even if pre-CTR NCS are available for comparison. In these situations, if repeat electrodiagnostic studies again confirm CTS and exclude mimickers, imaging (magnetic resonance imaging or ultrasound) may be reasonable to exclude treatable etiologies (operative bed scar, incomplete resection of the transverse carpal ligament).[93,94]

Box 4
Recommended electrodiagnostic approach to CTS

1. Median MNCS: recording over the abductor pollicis brevis

2. Median SNCS

   a. If median MNCS abnormal, do median antidromic SNCS recording over digit 2 or 3.

   b. If median MNCS normal, do more sensitive median SNCS:

      i. Median–ulnar palmar studies (palmdiff) OR

      ii. Median–ulnar antidromic SNCS to ring finger (ringdiff)

   c. If high clinical suspicion, unremarkable studies above, and ongoing diagnostic dilemma, consider other comparator studies based on distribution of clinical symptoms or the combined sensory index

3. MNCS and SNCS of another nerve in the affected limb, if not already performed.

4. If routine median MNCS and SNCS are absent, perform median–ulnar lumbrical versus second dorsal interosseous study to confirm slowing over carpal tunnel.

5. If evidence of a superimposed peripheral neuropathy, perform median–ulnar lumbrical versus second dorsal interosseous study.

6. Needle examination

   a. Examine the abductor pollicis brevis or opponens pollicis if median MNCS amplitude <7 mV.

   b. Strongly consider screening needle examination of affected extremity to exclude superimposed neurogenic process.

PUTTING IT ALL TOGETHER—A TREATMENT ALGORITHM

Box 4 presents a suggested algorithm for the electrodiagnostic approach to the patient with suspected CTS. It incorporates the AANEM/AAN/AAPMR practice parameter guidelines and quality recommendations.[20,21]

SUMMARY

CTS is a clinically defined syndrome; however, there is value added by an evidence-based electrodiagnostic approach to (1) efficiently confirm the diagnosis (particularly before invasive interventions), (2) to identify neurogenic mimickers or superimposed processes that may influence the response to treatment, and (3) to stratify the degree of neurogenic injury to help the clinician make management decisions in conjunction with the severity of the clinical symptoms.

Take-Home Points:
1. CTS is a clinically defined syndrome associated with a median neuropathy at the wrist.
2. Electrodiagnostic studies are useful to confirm the diagnosis of CTS, exclude mimickers, and to define the extent of neurogenic injury.
3. Sensory fascicles are more sensitive to compression than motor fascicles and SNCS are more sensitive than MNCS for CTS.
4. Median-to-ulnar latency sensory comparison studies (palmars and antidromics to the ring finger) are the most sensitive electrodiagnostic studies for confirming CTS.
5. MNCS are abnormal in only 40% to 60% of CTS cases.
6. Median-ulnar latency comparison studies recording over the second lumbrical and dorsal interossei muscles are useful to confirm slowing across the carpal tunnel when traditional MNCS and SNCS are absent and in the setting of a peripheral neuropathy.
7. The electrodiagnostic severity of CTS may not correlate with the clinical severity. Both are useful in directing treatment recommendations for CTS.

ACKNOWLEDGMENTS

I acknowledge Dr J. Clarke Stevens, a Mayo Clinic professor of neurology, electrophysiologist, and respected expert in CTS, whose mentorship and knowledge were instrumental in developing my CTS curriculum, which served as the basis for this article.

REFERENCES

1. Stevens JC. AAEM minimonograph #26: the electrodiagnosis of carpal tunnel syndrome. American Association of Electrodiagnostic Medicine. Muscle Nerve 1997;20(12):1477–86.
2. Schappert SM, Rechtsteiner EA. Ambulatory medical care utilization estimates for 2007. Vital Health Stat 13 2011;(169):1–38.
3. Gelfman R, Melton LJ 3rd, Yawn BP, et al. Long-term trends in carpal tunnel syndrome. Neurology 2009;72(1):33–41.
4. Atroshi I, Gummesson C, Johnsson R, et al. Prevalence of carpal tunnel syndrome in a general population. JAMA 1999;282(2):153–8.
5. Cullen KA, Hall MJ, Golosinskiy A. Ambulatory surgery in the United States, 2006. Natl Health Stat Report 2009;(11):1–25.

6. Jablecki CK, Andary MT, Floeter MK, et al. Second AAEM literature review of the usefullness of nerve conduction studies and needle electromyography for the evaluation of patients with carpal tunnel syndrome. Muscle Nerve 2002;(Suppl X): S924–78. Available at: http://www.aanem.org/Practice/Practice-Management/ Practice-Guidelines.aspx.

7. Stewart JD, Eisen A. Tinel's sign and the carpal tunnel syndrome. Br Med J 1978; 2(6145):1125–6.

8. Seror P. Tinel's sign in the diagnosis of carpal tunnel syndrome. J Hand Surg Br 1987;12(3):364–5.

9. Seror P. Phalen's test in the diagnosis of carpal tunnel syndrome. J Hand Surg Br 1988;13(4):383–5.

10. Rempel D, Evanoff B, Amadio PC, et al. Consensus criteria for the classification of carpal tunnel syndrome in epidemiologic studies. Am J Public Health 1998; 88(10):1447–51.

11. Stevens JC, Smith BE, Weaver AL, et al. Symptoms of 100 patients with electromyographically verified carpal tunnel syndrome. Muscle Nerve 1999;22(10): 1448–56.

12. Nora DB, Becker J, Ehlers JA, et al. Clinical features of 1039 patients with neurophysiological diagnosis of carpal tunnel syndrome. Clin Neurol Neurosurg 2004; 107(1):64–9.

13. Zanette G, Marani S, Tamburin S. Proximal pain in patients with carpal tunnel syndrome: a clinical-neurophysiological study. J Peripher Nerv Syst 2007;12(2):91–7.

14. Haig AJ, Tzeng HM, LeBreck DB. The value of electrodiagnostic consultation for patients with upper extremity nerve complaints: a prospective comparison with the history and physical examination. Arch Phys Med Rehabil 1999;80(10): 1273–81.

15. Nathan PA, Keniston RC, Myers LD, et al. Natural history of median nerve sensory conduction in industry: relationship to symptoms and carpal tunnel syndrome in 558 hands over 11 years. Muscle Nerve 1998;21(6):711–21.

16. Werner RA, Gell N, Franzblau A, et al. Prolonged median sensory latency as a predictor of future carpal tunnel syndrome. Muscle Nerve 2001;24(11):1462–7.

17. Werner RA, Andary M. Electrodiagnostic evaluation of carpal tunnel syndrome. Muscle Nerve 2011;44(4):597–607.

18. Jablecki CK, Andary MT, Floeter MK, et al. Practice parameter: electrodiagnostic studies in carpal tunnel syndrome. Report of the American Association of Electrodiagnostic Medicine, American Academy of Neurology, and the American Academy of Physical Medicine and Rehabilitation. Neurology 2002;58(11):1589–92.

19. Keith MW, Masear V, Chung KC, et al. American Academy of Orthopaedic Surgeons Clinical Practice Guideline on diagnosis of carpal tunnel syndrome. J Bone Joint Surg Am 2009;91(10):2478–9.

20. Sandin KJ, Asch SM, Jablecki CK, et al. Clinical quality measures for electrodiagnosis in suspected carpal tunnel syndrome. Muscle Nerve 2010;41(4):444–52.

21. American Association of Electrodiagnostic Medicine, American Academy of Neurology, and American Academy of Physical Medicine and Rehabilitation. Practice parameter for electrodiagnostic studies in carpal tunnel syndrome: summary statement. Muscle Nerve 2002;25(6):918–22.

22. Daube JR, Rubin DI. Clinical neurophysiology—companion CD. 3rd edition. New York: Oxford University Press; 2009.

23. Casey EB, Le Quesne PM. Digital nerve action potentials in healthy subjects, and in carpal tunnel and diabetic patients. J Neurol Neurosurg Psychiatry 1972;35(5): 612–23.

24. Kuntzer T. Carpal tunnel syndrome in 100 patients: sensitivity, specificity of multi-neurophysiological procedures and estimation of axonal loss of motor, sensory and sympathetic median nerve fibers. J Neurol Sci 1994;127(2):221–9.

25. Padua L, Lo Monaco M, Valente EM, et al. A useful electrophysiologic parameter for diagnosis of carpal tunnel syndrome. Muscle Nerve 1996;19(1):48–53.

26. Wee AS, Abernathy SD. Carpal tunnel syndrome: comparison of the median sensory nerve conduction findings from the index and middle fingers. Electromyogr Clin Neurophysiol 2003;43(4):251–3.

27. Buschbacher RM. Median 14-cm and 7-cm antidromic sensory studies to digits two and three. Am J Phys Med Rehabil 1999;78(Suppl 6):S53–62.

28. Marin EL, Vernick S, Friedmann LW. Carpal tunnel syndrome: median nerve stress test. Arch Phys Med Rehabil 1983;64(5):206–8.

29. Schwartz MS, Gordon JA, Swash M. Slowed nerve conduction with wrist flexion in carpal tunnel syndrome. Ann Neurol 1980;8(1):69–71.

30. Emad MR, Najafi SH, Sepehrian MH. The effect of provocative tests on electrodiagnosis criteria in clinical carpal tunnel syndrome. Electromyogr Clin Neurophysiol 2010;50(6):265–8.

31. Jackson DA, Clifford JC. Electrodiagnosis of mild carpal tunnel syndrome. Arch Phys Med Rehabil 1989;70(3):199–204.

32. Johnson EW, Kukla RD, Wongsam PE, et al. Sensory latencies to the ring finger: normal values and relation to carpal tunnel syndrome. Arch Phys Med Rehabil 1981;62(5):206–8.

33. Cioni R, Passero S, Paradiso C, et al. Diagnostic specificity of sensory and motor nerve conduction variables in early detection of carpal tunnel syndrome. J Neurol 1989;236(4):208–13.

34. Seror P. Sensitivity of the various tests for the diagnosis of carpal tunnel syndrome. J Hand Surg Br 1994;19(6):725–8.

35. Robinson LR, Micklesen PJ, Wang L. Strategies for analyzing nerve conduction data: superiority of a summary index over single tests. Muscle Nerve 1998;21(9):1166–71.

36. Pease WS, Cannell CD, Johnson EW. Median to radial latency difference test in mild carpal tunnel syndrome. Muscle Nerve 1989;12(11):905–9.

37. Robinson LR, Micklesen PJ, Wang L. Optimizing the number of tests for carpal tunnel syndrome. Muscle Nerve 2000;23(12):1880–2.

38. Malladi N, Micklesen PJ, Hou J, et al. Correlation between the combined sensory index and clinical outcome after carpal tunnel decompression: a retrospective review. Muscle Nerve 2010;41(4):453–7.

39. Stevens JC. AAEE minimonograph #26: the electrodiagnosis of carpal tunnel syndrome. Muscle Nerve 1987;10(2):99–113.

40. Padua L, LoMonaco M, Gregori B, et al. Neurophysiological classification and sensitivity in 500 carpal tunnel syndrome hands. Acta Neurol Scand 1997;96(4):211–7.

41. Thomas JE, Lambert EH, Cseuz KA. Electrodiagnostic aspects of the carpal tunnel syndrome. Arch Neurol 1967;16(6):635–41.

42. Sander HW, Quinto C, Saadeh PB, et al. Sensitive median-ulnar motor comparative techniques in carpal tunnel syndrome. Muscle Nerve 1999;22(1):88–98.

43. Melvin JL, Schuchmann JA, Lanese RR. Diagnostic specificity of motor and sensory nerve conduction variables in the carpal tunnel syndrome. Arch Phys Med Rehabil 1973;54(2):69–74.

44. Repaci M, Torrieri F, Di Blasio F, et al. Exclusive electrophysiological motor involvement in carpal tunnel syndrome. Clin Neurophysiol 1999;110(8):1471–4.

45. Wilson JR. Median mixed nerve conduction studies in the forearm: evidence against retrograde demyelination in carpal tunnel syndrome. J Clin Neurophysiol 1998;15(6):541–6.

46. Chang MH, Chiang HT, Ger LP, et al. The cause of slowed forearm median conduction velocity in carpal tunnel syndrome. Clin Neurophysiol 2000;111(6): 1039–44.

47. Chang MH, Lee YC, Hsieh PF. The real role of forearm mixed nerve conduction velocity in the assessment of proximal forearm conduction slowing in carpal tunnel syndrome. J Clin Neurophysiol 2008;25(6):373–7.

48. Chang MH, Liao KK, Chang SP, et al. Proximal slowing in carpal tunnel syndrome resulting from either conduction block or retrograde degeneration. J Neurol 1993; 240(5):287–90.

49. Chang MH, Liu LH, Lee YC, et al. Alteration of proximal conduction velocity at distal nerve injury in carpal tunnel syndrome: demyelinating versus axonal change. J Clin Neurophysiol 2008;25(3):161–6.

50. Chang MH, Wei SJ, Chen LW. The reason for forearm conduction slowing in carpal tunnel syndrome: an electrophysiological follow-up study after surgery. Clin Neurophysiol 2003;114(6):1091–5.

51. Gutmann L. AAEM minimonograph #2: important anomalous innervations of the extremities. Muscle Nerve 1993;16(4):339–47.

52. Budak F, Gonenc Z. Innervation anomalies in upper and lower extremities (an electrophysiological study). Electromyogr Clin Neurophysiol 1999;39(4):231–4.

53. Kimura J, Murphy MJ, Varda DJ. Electrophysiological study of anomalous innervation of intrinsic hand muscles. Arch Neurol 1976;33(12):842–4.

54. Amoiridis G. Median–ulnar nerve communications and anomalous innervation of the intrinsic hand muscles: an electrophysiological study. Muscle Nerve 1992; 15(5):576–9.

55. Crutchfield CA, Gutmann L. Hereditary aspects of median-ulnar nerve communications. J Neurol Neurosurg Psychiatry 1980;43(1):53–5.

56. Amoiridis G, Vlachonikolis IG. Verification of the median-to-ulnar and ulnar-to-median nerve motor fiber anastomosis in the forearm: an electrophysiological study. Clin Neurophysiol 2003;114(1):94–8.

57. Preston DC, Logigian EL. Lumbrical and interossei recording in carpal tunnel syndrome. Muscle Nerve 1992;15(11):1253–7.

58. Uncini A, Di Muzio A, Awad J, et al. Sensitivity of three median-to-ulnar comparative tests in diagnosis of mild carpal tunnel syndrome. Muscle Nerve 1993; 16(12):1366–73.

59. Preston DC, Ross MH, Kothari MJ, et al. The median-ulnar latency difference studies are comparable in mild carpal tunnel syndrome. Muscle Nerve 1994; 17(12):1469–71.

60. Sheean GL, Houser MK, Murray NM. Lumbrical-interosseous latency comparison in the diagnosis of carpal tunnel syndrome. Electroencephalogr Clin Neurophysiol 1995;97(6):285–9.

61. Therimadasamy AK, Li E, Wilder-Smith EP. Can studies of the second lumbrical interossei and its premotor potential reduce the number of tests for carpal tunnel syndrome? Muscle Nerve 2007;36(4):491–6.

62. Resende LA, Adamo AS, Bononi AP, et al. Test of a new technique for the diagnosis of carpal tunnel syndrome. J Electromyogr Kinesiol 2000;10(2):127–33.

63. Logigian EL, Busis NA, Berger AR, et al. Lumbrical sparing in carpal tunnel syndrome: anatomic, physiologic, and diagnostic implications. Neurology 1987; 37(9):1499–505.

64. Trojaborg W, Grewal RP, Weimer LH, et al. Value of latency measurements to the small palm muscles compared to other conduction parameters in the carpal tunnel syndrome. Muscle Nerve 1996;19(2):243–5.
65. Conway RR. The role of needle electromyography in the evaluation of patients with carpal tunnel syndrome: needle EMG is often unnecessary. Muscle Nerve 1999;22(2):284–5.
66. Balbierz JM, Cottrell AC, Cottrell WD. Is needle examination always necessary in evaluation of carpal tunnel syndrome? Arch Phys Med Rehabil 1998;79(5): 514–6.
67. Wee AS. Needle electromyography in carpal tunnel syndrome. Electromyogr Clin Neurophysiol 2002;42(4):253–6.
68. Gnatz SM. The role of needle electromyography in the evaluation of patients with carpal tunnel syndrome: needle EMG is important. Muscle Nerve 1999;22(2): 282–3.
69. Vennix MJ, Hirsh DD, Chiou-Tan FY, et al. Predicting acute denervation in carpal tunnel syndrome. Arch Phys Med Rehabil 1998;79(3):306–12.
70. Ubogu EE, Benatar M. Electrodiagnostic criteria for carpal tunnel syndrome in axonal polyneuropathy. Muscle Nerve 2006;33(6):747–52.
71. Vogt T, Mika A, Thomke F, et al. Evaluation of carpal tunnel syndrome in patients with polyneuropathy. Muscle Nerve 1997;20(2):153–7.
72. Ginanneschi F, Dominici F, Milani P, et al. Evidence of altered motor axon properties of the ulnar nerve in carpal tunnel syndrome. Clin Neurophysiol 2007;118(7): 1569–76.
73. Ginanneschi F, Milani P, Mondelli M, et al. Ulnar sensory nerve impairment at the wrist in carpal tunnel syndrome. Muscle Nerve 2008;37(2):183–9.
74. Ginanneschi F, Milani P, Rossi A. Anomalies of ulnar nerve conduction in different carpal tunnel syndrome stages. Muscle Nerve 2008;38(3):1155–60.
75. Ablove RH, Moy OJ, Peimer CA, et al. Pressure changes in Guyon's canal after carpal tunnel release. J Hand Surg Br 1996;21(5):664–5.
76. Mondelli M, Ginanneschi F, Rossi A. Evidence of improvement in distal conduction of ulnar nerve sensory fibers after carpal tunnel release. Neurosurgery 2009;65(4):696–700 [discussion: 701].
77. Moghtaderi A, Ghafarpoor M. The dilemma of ulnar nerve entrapment at wrist in carpal tunnel syndrome. Clin Neurol Neurosurg 2009;111(2):151–5.
78. Robinson L, Kliot M. Stop using arbitrary grading schemes in carpal tunnel syndrome. Muscle Nerve 2008;37(6):804.
79. Sucher BM. Stop using arbitrary grading schemes in carpal tunnel syndrome. Muscle Nerve 2008;38(5):1526 [author reply: 1527–8].
80. Bland JD. Stop using arbitrary grading schemes in carpal tunnel syndrome. Muscle Nerve 2008;38(5):1527 [author reply: 1527–8].
81. Johnson EW. Stop using arbitrary grading schemes in carpal tunnel syndrome. Muscle Nerve 2008;38(5):1526 [author reply: 1527–8].
82. Chan L, Turner JA, Comstock BA, et al. The relationship between electrodiagnostic findings and patient symptoms and function in carpal tunnel syndrome. Arch Phys Med Rehabil 2007;88(1):19–24.
83. Bland JD. Do nerve conduction studies predict the outcome of carpal tunnel decompression? Muscle Nerve 2001;24(7):935–40.
84. Bland JD. A neurophysiological grading scale for carpal tunnel syndrome. Muscle Nerve 2000;23(8):1280–3.
85. Pascoe MK, Pascoe RD, Tarrant E, et al. Changes in palmar sensory latencies in response to carpal tunnel release. Muscle Nerve 1994;17(12):1475–6.

86. Melvin JL, Johnson EW, Duran R. Electrodiagnosis after surgery for the carpal tunnel syndrome. Arch Phys Med Rehabil 1968;49(9):502–7.
87. Rotman MB, Enkvetchakul BV, Megerian JT, et al. Time course and predictors of median nerve conduction after carpal tunnel release. J Hand Surg Am 2004; 29(3):367–72.
88. Naidu SH, Fisher J, Heistand M, et al. Median nerve function in patients undergoing carpal tunnel release: pre- and post-op nerve conductions. Electromyogr Clin Neurophysiol 2003;43(7):393–7.
89. Borisch N, Haussmann P. Neurophysiological recovery after open carpal tunnel decompression: comparison of simple decompression and decompression with epineurotomy. J Hand Surg Br 2003;28(5):450–4.
90. Goodwill CJ. The carpal tunnel syndrome. long-term follow-up showing relation of latency measurements to response to treatment. Ann Phys Med 1965;8:12–21.
91. Hongell A, Mattsson HS. Neurographic studies before, after, and during operation for median nerve compression in the carpal tunnel. Scand J Plast Reconstr Surg 1971;5(2):103–9.
92. Prick JJ, Blaauw G, Vredeveld JW, et al. Results of carpal tunnel release. Eur J Neurol 2003;10(6):733–6.
93. Campagna R, Pessis E, Feydy A, et al. MRI assessment of recurrent carpal tunnel syndrome after open surgical release of the median nerve. AJR Am J Roentgenol 2009;193(3):644–50.
94. Cudlip SA, Howe FA, Clifton A, et al. Magnetic resonance neurography studies of the median nerve before and after carpal tunnel decompression. J Neurosurg 2002;96(6):1046–51.

Electrodiagnostic Evaluation of Ulnar Neuropathy and Other Upper Extremity Mononeuropathies

Elliot L. Dimberg, MD

KEYWORDS

- Mononeuropathy • Ulnar • Radial • Axillary
- Musculocutaneous • Suprascapular • Long thoracic
- Electromyography

Upper extremity mononeuropathies are common in clinical practice and in the electrodiagnostic (EDX) laboratory. Clinicians and electrodiagnosticians must understand the anatomy and function of peripheral nerves potentially involved, features of the history and physical examination that narrow the differential diagnosis, and EDX findings to arrive at a diagnosis. EDX studies serve to localize a lesion, confirm a suspected diagnosis, exclude alternate possibilities, discover unsuspected conditions, determine the functional involvement and pathophysiology of the lesion, and assess severity, timeframe, and prognosis of the lesion.

Most clinicians and electromyographers have already used their clinical assessment to narrow the differential diagnosis of a possible mononeuropathy to a few most likely localizations before the performance of EDX testing. This article assumes that an appropriate clinical examination has occurred as the first step in the EDX testing and that the suspected nerve localization has been defined. Therefore, the article focuses on the EDX approach to confirming a clinically suspected mononeuropathy using both nerve conduction studies (NCS) and needle examination (NEX), according to each specific mononeuropathy: ulnar, median in the forearm (median neuropathy at the wrist is discussed in a separate article), radial, musculocutaneous, axillary, suprascapular, and long thoracic neuropathy.

The author has no funding support.
The author has nothing to disclose.
Department of Neurology, Mayo Clinic, 4500 San Pablo Road, Jacksonville, FL 32224, USA
E-mail address: Dimberg.Elliot@mayo.edu

In general, EDX studies of suspected mononeuropathies should be performed 2 weeks or more after the suspected onset or injury, if known, to allow for the development of more complete EDX findings and specifically to assess the extent of axon loss. In many cases of nontraumatic mononeuropathies, however, the time of onset of symptoms is not known or the symptoms develop gradually. In either circumstance, most mononeuropathies are characterized by axon loss, whereas focal demyelination may occur but is less common. In lesions characterized by axon loss, nerve conduction studies reveal low-amplitude compound muscle and sensory nerve action potentials. NEX demonstrates fibrillation potentials and reduced recruitment of long duration motor unit potentials, depending on the degree of reinnervation that has occurred. Finally, the electrodiagnosis of a mononeuropathy should be interpreted cautiously when there are only borderline or equivocal findings, especially because there may be surgical implications that result from the findings.

ULNAR NEUROPATHY

The ulnar nerve is derived from the C8 and T1 nerve roots, fibers from which travel through the lower trunk and medial cord of the brachial plexus terminating in the ulnar nerve in the axilla.[1] The ulnar nerve courses in the medial upper arm, through the medial intermuscular septum and its apposed arcade of Struthers, passing behind the medial epicondyle (ME) in the retrocondylar groove (**Figs. 1** and **2**). It then proceeds through the humeroulnar arcade into the cubital tunnel and through the flexor carpi ulnaris (FCU) (**Fig. 3**). As it continues to the wrist it passes through Guyon canal between the pisiform bone and the hook of the hamate before going on through the hand (see **Fig. 1**; **Fig. 4**).

The first branch of the ulnar nerve is the motor branch to the FCU muscle, arising variably above the ME (above elbow [AE]) or below the ME (below elbow [BE]). The next branch to the flexor digitorum profundus (FDP) arises in the forearm. The palmar cutaneous sensory nerve to the medial palm and the dorsal ulnar cutaneous (DUC) nerve to the dorsal medial hand and proximal little and medial ring finger branch next in the forearm. The superficial radial nerve (SRN) may also give rise to the DUC, the importance of which is discussed later.[2]

In the Guyon canal, the nerve separates into the superficial terminal and deep ulnar branches. The superficial terminal branch supplies the palmaris brevis muscle before providing sensory innervation to the palmar aspect and dorsal distal phalanges of the fifth and medial fourth fingers. The deep branch innervates the abductor digiti minimi (ADM) initially before curving around in the hand, supplying the interossei, third and fourth lumbricals, adductor pollicis, and potentially flexor pollicis brevis muscles. The ulnar nerve can be affected at multiple sites along the course of the nerve; however, the most common sites of ulnar neuropathy occur at or around the elbow or at the wrist (see **Figs. 1, 3**, and **4**).

ULNAR NEUROPATHY AT THE ELBOW

Ulnar neuropathy at the elbow (UNE) is the second most common mononeuropathy, behind median neuropathy at the wrist.[3–5] Symptoms include sensory loss in the medial hand, pain or paresthesia in the hand and arm (often subjectively outside of the distribution of the ulnar nerve itself), and weakness and atrophy of ulnar innervated muscles and the ulnar claw with extension of the metacarpophalangeal joints and flexion of the interphalangeal joints of the ring and little fingers. Paresthesias are reported to be the most common symptom and are more common than pain, whereas ulnar distribution sensory loss is more common than weakness.[6] Other conditions that

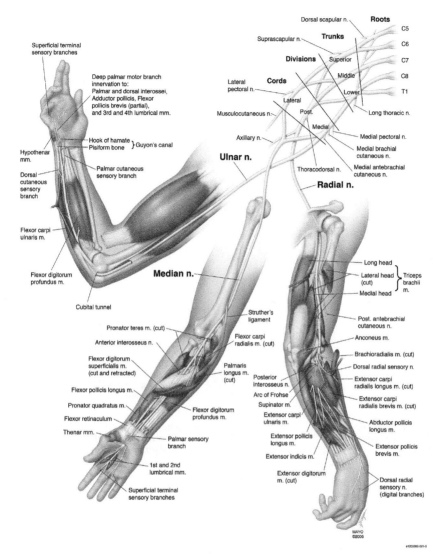

Fig. 1. Courses of the ulnar, median, and radial nerves from origin to termination. Common sites of entrapment are shown for each nerve. Hand positions are those common to associated lesions of the respective nerve. (*From* Neurology board review: an illustrated study guide. Rochester [MN]: Mayo Clinic Scientific Press and Boca Raton: Informa Healthcare USA; 2008. p. 778; used with permission of Mayo Foundation.)

can present with similar clinical features as UNE and are considered in the differential diagnosis include ulnar neuropathy at the wrist (UNE), lower trunk or medial cord brachial plexus neuropathy, C8/T1 radiculopathy, or more widespread motor neuron disease (when sensory findings are absent). There are 4 sites of compression of the ulnar nerve at or near the elbow: the arcade of Struthers (uncommon), the retrocondylar groove (at or a few centimeters AE), the humeroulnar arcade (0–2.5 cm BE),[7,8] and as it exits the FCU (4–7 cm BE, also uncommon).[5,8,9] Although each of these sites may produce clinically identical features, precise localization electrophysiologically can

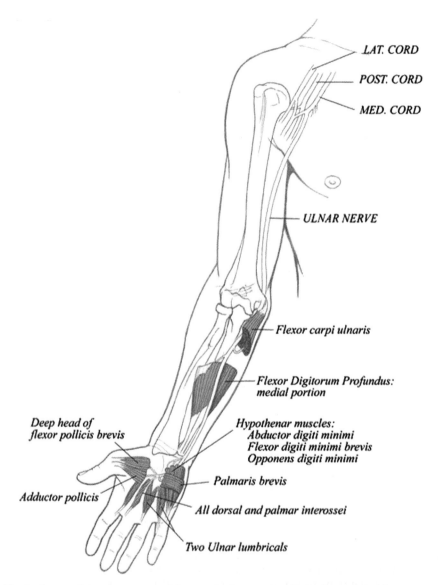

Fig. 2. Course of the ulnar nerve with muscular innervation. (*From* Rosse C, Gaddum-Rosse P. Hollinshead's textbook of anatomy. 5th edition. Philadelphia: Lippincott-Raven; 1997; with permission.)

affect decisions regarding the evaluation for causes and the specific treatments that may be offered, including surgery.

Motor Nerve Conduction Studies

In suspected cases of UNE, an ulnar motor response recording from the ADM is usually obtained first, performed with the elbow flexed to 135° and stimulating AE

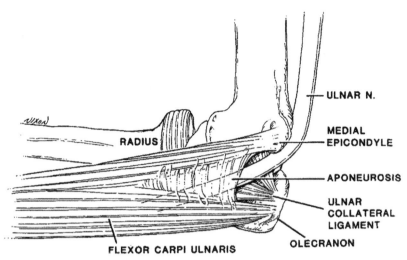

Fig. 3. Medial view of the elbow showing the ulnar nerve passing behind the ME in the retrocondylar groove, through the humeroulnar arcade (aponeurosis), and into the cubital tunnel. (*From* Kincaid JC. AAEE minimonograph #31: the electrodiagnosis of ulnar neuropathy at the elbow. Muscle Nerve 1988;11(10):1006. Copyright 1988 John Wiley & Sons; this material is reproduced with permission of John Wiley & Sons, Inc.)

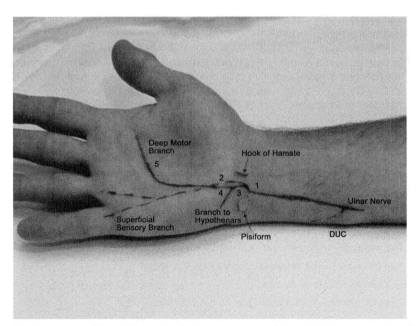

Fig. 4. Volar aspect of the right hand outlining the course of the distal ulnar nerve. Numbers correspond to lesion sites producing the various types of ulnar neuropathies at the wrist: (1) proximal Guyon canal, (2) superficial terminal branch, (3) distal Guyon canal, (4) hook of the hamate, and (5) distal deep ulnar branch (see text and **Table 2**).

and BE with stimulation points 10 cm apart and at the wrist.[10] F waves are also performed to assess for evidence of slowing along the nerve at a site more proximal than the elbow. If NCS are performed with the elbow extended, slack is introduced along the nerve, and the distance measurement made along the course of the skin with the tape measure underestimates the actual length of the nerve, leading to an apparently slow but inaccurate conduction velocity (CV) across the elbow.[11] A median motor response recording from the abductor pollicis brevis (APB) muscle with F waves is performed to identify or exclude other disorders or localizations, such as a C8/T1 radiculopathy or brachial plexopathy.

Ulnar motor conduction studies are generally the most helpful when attempting to determine the precise site of localization of the ulnar neuropathy (**Box 1**). Abnormal, focal slowing across the elbow is indicated when (1) the CV across the elbow segment is less than 50 m/s or (2) when the CV across the elbow segment is greater than 10 m/s slower than the forearm segment.[10,11] A partial conduction block from focal demyelination is indicated by a greater than 20% drop in compound muscle action potential (CMAP) amplitude from BE to AE (**Fig. 5**).[10] Definite partial conduction block is present if there is greater than 50% drop in amplitude or greater than 40% reduction in area with less than 30% increase in duration between the 2 stimulation sites.[12,13] A low-amplitude AE (and BE) ulnar CMAP (<6 mV in our laboratory) is suggestive of an ulnar neuropathy in general but in the absence of focal conduction block or focal slowing is nonlocalizing and can be seen in an ulnar neuropathy with axonal loss at any site along the course of the ulnar nerve or also a C8 radiculopathy, lower trunk or medial cord brachial plexopathy, or motor neuron disease.

In patients in whom the FDI muscle is preferentially weak or in whom there is high suspicion for an ulnar neuropathy but motor studies recording from the ADM are unremarkable, motor studies recording the FDI may be performed. Focal slowing across the elbow can be demonstrated in some patients via this study when the ADM study is normal.[14] In some instances, performing an ulnar motor conduction study using 2-channel recording and recording simultaneously from both the ADM and FDI may be useful. There is possible usefulness of the so-called intranerve ratio, which compares the motor nerve CV recording the FDI with the CV recording the ADM; an FDI:ADM CV ratio of less than or equal to 0.97 has been shown to have a 91% specificity and 68% sensitivity for UNE,[15] but this has yet to be validated.

Box 1
Nerve conduction study criteria for confirming an ulnar neuropathy at the elbow

Conduction velocity

    Ulnar motor CV across the elbow segment <50 m/s

    Ulnar motor CV across the elbow segment >10 m/s slower than forearm segment

CMAP amplitude (ADM or first dorsal interosseous [FDI] recording)

    Reduction of >20% from BE to AE

    Significant change in CMAP configuration between BE and AE

Short segment stimulation

    >10% CMAP amplitude drop across 2-cm segment

    8-ms latency shift or doubling of latency across 2-cm segment

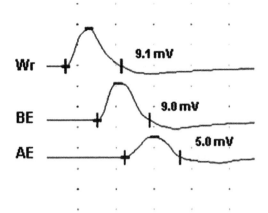

Fig. 5. Ulnar motor NCS with stimulation both above (AE) and below (BE) the elbow demonstrating partial conduction block at the elbow. There is a 45% drop in CMAP amplitude after AE stimulation compared with after BE stimulation. Wr, wrist.

Sensory Nerve Conduction Studies

Sensory nerve conduction studies include both the ulnar and median antidromic sensory responses (recording the fifth and index fingers, respectively) with stimulation at the elbow and wrist. Routine ulnar antidromic sensory studies may show a low-amplitude sensory nerve action potential (SNAP) when axonal loss has occurred in the sensory fibers, but low sensory amplitude is nonlocalizing.[10] Although sensory fibers are often affected first, especially with axon loss, they can also be abnormal in a lower trunk or medial cord brachial plexus neuropathy. Furthermore, because of normal temporal dispersion along sensory fibers with stimulation over longer distances (such as between the wrist and the elbow), it is difficult to demonstrate focal slowing or conduction block on sensory nerve conduction studies.

A particularly problematic scenario in confirming the diagnosis of an ulnar neuropathy occurs when only sensory fibers are affected or when sufficient axon loss has occurred to cause slowing of the motor nerve in the forearm segment as well as across the elbow. In these situations, identifying a focal site of nerve involvement may not be possible. There is some evidence supporting use of sensory or mixed nerve orthodromic studies in this situation specifically.[14,16–18] Mixed nerve studies are performed with the elbow extended, stimulating at the wrist and recording at BE and AE sites. The CV dropoff across the elbow segment compared with the forearm segment should be less than 22 m/s.[16] Recently, comparison of SNAP amplitudes recording the little finger after AE, BE, and wrist stimulation has led to proposed amplitude ratio criteria. A BE:wrist amplitude ratio of less than 0.45 and an AE:BE amplitude ratio of less than 0.65 suggest UNE.[17] Further study is necessary before these criteria are adopted into clinical practice. Mixed and sensory nerve special studies are technically difficult, however, and not commonly performed.

Short Segment (Inching) Motor Studies

When focal changes are not evident on routine motor studies, short segment incremental stimulation (inching) of the motor nerve in quantified segments beginning at the BE stimulation site and continuing across the elbow to the AE stimulation site can demonstrate focal slowing.[8] In our laboratory we use 2-cm segments and consider a latency difference of 8 ms or a doubling of latency difference between 2 sites compared with neighboring sites indicative of focal slowing and a CMAP amplitude reduction of 10% over a 2-cm segment indicative of partial conduction block (**Fig. 6**). Short segment studies allow for precise localization of slowing or partial conduction block.[8,19] Like sensory and mixed nerve stimulation studies, short segment incremental stimulation is more technically difficult and care should be taken to ensure precise measurements.

Dorsal Ulnar Cutaneous Sensory Study

There are times when differentiation between UNE and UNW is not evident after routine studies, such as when there are low CMAP and SNAP amplitudes without focal slowing or conduction block. Bilateral DUC sensory studies are useful in this instance because the DUC leaves the ulnar nerve in the mid-third to distal third of the forearm. A unilaterally low-amplitude (<50% of the amplitude on the unaffected side) or absent

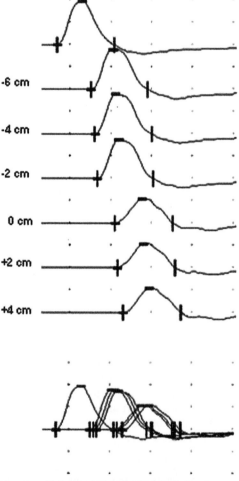

Fig. 6. Short segment incremental stimulation (inching) of the ulnar nerve across the elbow. 0 cm indicates the location of the ME. The first trace is following stimulation at the wrist; other traces are following stimulation across the elbow. Focal slowing and partial conduction block are seen between the ME and 2 cm BE. (*Top*, individual traces rastered; *bottom*, superimposed).

response suggests axonal loss along the DUC from a lesion proximal to the wrist. A normal response should be interpreted with caution, however, because it has been shown that a significant proportion of patients with definite UNE may still have normal DUC sensory response due either to fascicular sparing or to a branch point of the DUC nerve being proximal to the elbow in some patients.[20] Furthermore, if the DUC response is absent, stimulation of the SRN should be performed while recording over the same site as the DUC study because 16% of individuals harbor anomalous innervation of the dorsal ulnar hand by the SRN.[2]

Prognostication of UNE with NCS

Recent studies have demonstrated the prognostic value of NCS findings in ulnar neuropathy. The combination of conduction block in the elbow segment when recording the FDI and a normal CMAP recording the ADM has been shown to be associated with subjective recovery, with 86% of patients achieving full recovery regardless of conservative versus surgical management.[21] Poor rates of recovery (7%) were associated with the absence of conduction block and a low CMAP amplitude recording from the ADM.

Needle Examination

NEX not only can help confirm the localization to the ulnar nerve but also is important to exclude alternate localizations, such as medial cord or lower trunk brachial plexus neuropathy, C8/T1 radiculopathy, and early motor neuron disease. The findings on the NEX help determine the presence of axon loss as well as the temporal profile of the process in UNE. The NEX should include at least the FDI and FDP ulnar head (FDPU) muscles and often the ADM. Distal hand muscles are more commonly affected than proximal muscles, but abnormalities in the FDPU localize the lesion proximal to the wrist. NEX of the FCU and FDP is often normal in UNE, however. Sparing of these muscles may be attributable to branches to these muscles that may arise proximal to the elbow, fascicular sparing of the fibers to these muscles related to nerve fiber location within the nerve, or only mild demyelination in cases in which there is only mild nerve compression.[22] NEX of the APB and extensor indicis proprius (EIP) muscles evaluates for brachial plexus neuropathy and C8/T1 radiculopathy. The author also commonly examines at least one more proximal muscle (such as the pronator teres [PT] or biceps brachii) to exclude a more widespread process. The pattern of findings on NCS and NEX in ulnar neuropathy at the elbow is shown in **Table 1**.

ULNAR NEUROPATHY AT (OR DISTAL TO) THE WRIST

UNW occurs less commonly than UNE but should be considered in patients who have weakness of ulnar innervated hand muscles, with or without sensory deficits in the medial ring and little fingers. Medial dorsal and palmar hand sensation is spared because the palmar branch and DUC originate proximal to the wrist. More common causes of UNW include ganglion cyst, external pressure or repetitive trauma, and neural tumors, such as neuromas. The differential diagnosis for UNW is most commonly that of a UNE but a lower trunk or medial cord brachial plexus neuropathy, C8/T1 radiculopathy, and more widespread motor neuron disease (when sensory findings are absent) are other considerations. There are 5 lesion sites in which the ulnar nerve may be injured at or distal to the wrist (see **Fig. 4**).[23,24]

1. Proximal Guyon canal. At this site, there is involvement of the superficial terminal branch, with sensory loss of the palmar aspect and dorsal distal phalanges of the medial ring and little fingers and the deep motor branch producing weakness

Table 1	
Electrodiagnostic findings in ulnar neuropathy at the elbow	
EDX Study	**Findings in UNE**
Ulnar antidromic sensory	Low amplitude Slow CV
Ulnar motor (ADM or FDI recording)	Low amplitude Slow CV across the elbow Possible conduction block
Inching across the elbow	Focal slowing Possible conduction block
Mixed nerve	Slow CV across the elbow
DUC sensory	Low amplitude (may be normal; check for anomalous innervation from SRN)
NEX FDI, ADM	Abnormal
NEX FDPU, FCU	Abnormal or normal

of all ulnar innervated hand muscles, including the hypothenar muscles. Lesions at this site are most clinically similar to UNE.

2. Superficial terminal branch. There is pure sensory deficit in the distribution of the nerve but no hand weakness.
3. Distal Guyon canal. This causes a pure motor syndrome sparing all sensory function but producing weakness of all ulnar hand muscles (including the hypothenar muscles) other than the palmaris brevis, which is innervated by the superficial terminal branch.
4. Hook of the hamate. This distal deep branch lesion leads to weakness of all ulnar hand muscles other than the palmaris brevis and hypothenar muscles because the branch to the hypothenar muscles originates proximal to the lesion site. There is no sensory loss.
5. Distal deep ulnar branch. This occurs in the hand itself and produces only weakness of the FDI and adductor pollicis brevis muscles.

Nerve Conduction Studies

Similar to UNE, routine ulnar (recording from the ADM) and median motor studies with F waves and ulnar and median antidromic sensory responses are typically obtained as the initial assessment. In addition, an ulnar motor study recording the FDI should be performed because the standard ulnar motor study to the ADM may be spared with more distal wrist lesions. It is often necessary to perform the ulnar motor/FDI study on the unaffected side for comparison.[25] In some cases, UNW may also be determined by use of the lumbrical-interosseous motor study, a study more commonly used in assessment of a median neuropathy at the wrist.[26] With this study, prolongation of the latency to the second palmar interosseus (an ulnar innervated nerve) relative to the first lumbrical (a median innervated nerve) suggests focal slowing in the distal ulnar nerve. Finally, when routine studies are nondiagnostic, short segment incremental stimulation performed across the wrist can demonstrate focal conduction block or segmental slowing at the wrist, but this study is technically challenging and should be interpreted with caution.[27] A DUC sensory study, which should be normal in all UNW localizations, helps confirm that the lesion is distal to its origin and should be performed in all cases of suspected UNW. NCS findings in the 5 types of wrist lesion locations are summarized in **Table 2**.

Table 2
Pattern of electrodiagnostic findings in ulnar neuropathies at or distal to the wrist

Study	Type 1	Type 2	Type 3	Type 4	Type 5
NCS					
Ulnar antidromic sensory	Abnormal[a]	Abnormal[a]	NL	NL	NL
Ulnar motor (ADM)	Abnormal[a]	NL	Abnormal[a]	NL	NL
Ulnar motor (FDI)	Abnormal[a]	NL	Abnormal[a]	Abnormal[a]	Abnormal[a]
Lumbrical-interosseous motor	Abnormal[a]	NL	Abnormal[a]	NL	NL
Inching across the wrist	Possible CB or focal slowing	NL	Possible CB or focal slowing	NL	NL
DUC sensory	NL	NL	NL	NL	NL
NEX					
ADM	Abnormal	NL	Abnormal	NL	NL
FDI	Abnormal	NL	Abnormal	Abnormal	Abnormal
FCU, FDP	NL	NL	NL	NL	NL

Abbreviations: CB, conduction block; NL, normal findings.
 [a] Abnormal indicates low amplitude with prolonged distal latency.

Needle Examination

NEX serves to localize the lesion to the ulnar nerve in general and helps determine specifically which motor branches are involved. The ADM and FDI are abnormal in UNW types 1 and 3, whereas the FDI only is abnormal is types 4 and 5. NEX is normal in type 2. Therefore, NEX should routinely include the ADM and FDI. Examination of the FDPU of FCU should also be performed to assess for UNE. As discussed previously, a normal NEX of these muscles can occur in some patients with UNE and, therefore, does not exclude this site of localization. If these muscles are abnormal, the lesion is proximal to these branches. Examination of the APB and EIP muscles helps exclude a brachial plexus neuropathy and C8/T1 radiculopathy, whereas other non-C8/T1 and ulnar innervated muscles, such as the PT, biceps, or deltoid, help exclude a more diffuse lower motor neuron process.

MEDIAN NEUROPATHY IN THE UPPER ARM AND FOREARM

The median nerve derives from the C5 through T1 nerve roots, all 3 trunks of the brachial plexus, and the medial and lateral cords of the brachial plexus.[28] Sensory fibers primarily course through the C5 and C6 roots, whereas motor fibers arise from the C6 through T1 roots. The median nerve runs in the lateral axilla and through the medial upper arm. At the elbow it courses medial to the biceps tendon under the bicipital aponeurosis (lacertus fibrosus). It commonly passes between the superficial and deep heads of the PT, innervating the PT in the process, but may run deep to both or pierce the superficial head directly. The nerve gives off the anterior interosseous nerve branch and then branches to the flexor digitorum superficialis (FDS) and flexor carpi radialis (FCR) muscles before proceeding under the sublimis bridge, the arch between the two heads of the FDS. The nerve then continues between the FDS and FDP muscles (see **Fig. 1**; **Fig. 7**). After passing through the carpal tunnel, it supplies the APB, opponens pollicis, and first and second lumbrical muscles. The anterior interosseous nerve passes under musculofibrous arches to run between the interosseous membrane and FDP. A pure motor nerve, it supplies the flexor

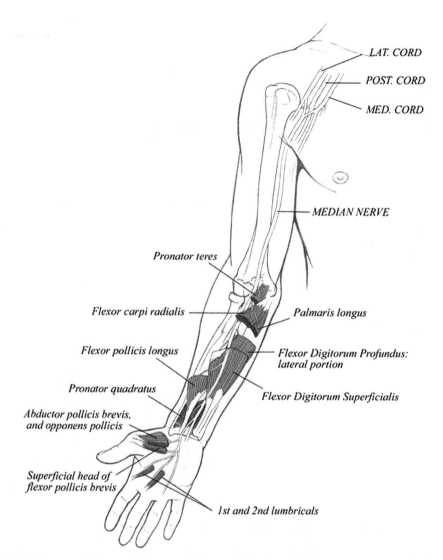

Fig. 7. Course of the median nerve with muscular innervation. (*From* Rosse C, Gaddum-Rosse P. Hollinshead's textbook of anatomy. 5th edition. Philadelphia: Lippincott-Raven; 1997; with permission.)

pollicis longus (FPL), the median head of the FDP (FDPM), and the pronator quadratus (PQ) muscles. The palmar cutaneous branch originates proximal to the carpal tunnel, does not run through it, and provides sensory innervation to the thenar eminence. Digital sensory branches, however, do pass through the carpal tunnel and supply the palmar aspects and distal phalanx of the thumb through lateral ring fingers.

Sites of entrapment of the median nerve proximal to the wrist (carpal tunnel) include the supracondylar spur and ligament of Struthers, the lacertus fibrosus, between the heads of the PT (pronator syndrome), and at the sublimis bridge.[28–32] The median nerve can also rarely be compressed by the brachialis muscle, the accessory head of the FPL, or by a vascular band that can run anterior to the median or anterior interosseous nerve in up to 33% or upper limbs.[32] Symptoms of proximal median neuropathies may be clinically similar at different sites of injury; however, clinical features may also be variable between patients with the same lesion location. Patients with median neuropathies at the ligament of Struthers commonly present with pain in the arm, forearm, or hand and paresthesias and sensory loss in a median nerve distribution, including over the thenar eminence (due to involvement of the palmar cutaneous sensory branch).[30,33] There is typically weakness of all (proximal and distal) median innervated muscles, and some patients may present with only weakness and no sensory loss.[33] Clinical manifestations at the 3 other main proximal sites of entrapment may be similar, although muscle weakness may vary.[29,31,33,34] For example, the PT may be spared in the more distal entrapment sites but the FPL and APB may be involved.[29,31]

Anterior interosseous neuropathy (AION) is characterized by a pure motor syndrome affecting the FPL, FDPM, and PQ muscles in isolation or combination.[31,35–37] There is commonly pain in the forearm but no sensory involvement. Typical sites of compression include the origin of the FDS, an accessory head of the FPL, and the tendinous origin of the deep head of the PT.[31] The anterior interosseous nerve also may be involved in brachial plexus neuropathies, either in isolation or along with involvement of other nerves or sites within the brachial plexus.[35–37]

The differential diagnosis for proximal median neuropathies and AION includes median neuropathy at the wrist, brachial plexus neuropathy, cervical radiculopathy, or motor neuron disease. The pattern of findings on EDX testing can assist in separating among these other disorders.

Nerve Conduction Studies

In proximal median neuropathies, the median motor nerve CV may be slow along the nerve across the site of involvement, either between the wrist and the elbow or between the elbow and upper arm. In some cases where the pathophysiology is focal demyelination, a focal conduction block may be identified.[29–31,33,34] In patients in which there is significant axonal loss, the median CMAP and/or SNAP amplitudes may be low.[31,33] In those cases with low CMAP and SNAP amplitudes without focal conduction block, NCS cannot definitively identify the site of the lesion and NEX may be necessary to help better define the proximal extent of nerve involvement. Ulnar motor and sensory conduction studies are also routinely performed and should be normal.

Because the routine median motor NCS typically records a response from the APB, and because there are no major sensory fibers in the AION muscles, the standard median motor and sensory NCS are normal in AION.[31,33,36] NCS assessing the anterior interosseous branch have been described by stimulating the median nerve at the elbow and recording the PQ via needle electrode or the FPL via surface electrode; however, these studies are technically more difficult and not routinely performed.[36,38,39]

Needle Examination

NEX is highly localizing in proximal median neuropathies and AION.[31,33] The distribution of abnormal muscles helps localize to the AION or proximal median nerve and exclude alternate diagnoses. NEX should include the APB, FPL, FCR, and PT muscles. If abnormalities are seen only in the FPL and AION is suspected, then the PQ should also be studied. To exclude brachial plexus neuropathy, cervical radiculopathy, and motor neuron disease, other nonmedian innervated muscles, such as the first dorsal interosseus, biceps, or triceps brachii muscles, should also be examined.

Furthermore, because brachial plexus neuropathy can present as AION, it is prudent to examine muscles that have been reported as commonly involved in brachial plexus neuropathy (Parsonage-Turner syndrome), such as the infraspinatus, supraspinatus, and serratus anterior muscles.[40] The pattern of findings on NCS and NEX in proximal median neuropathies is shown in **Table 3**.

RADIAL NEUROPATHY

The radial nerve derives its fibers from the C5-C8 and, rarely, T1 nerve roots traveling through all 3 trunks and the posterior cord of the brachial plexus.[41,42] The radial nerve is one of the terminal branches of the posterior cord. It runs in the lateral axilla along the medial humerus where the sensory branch to the posterior upper arm arises (see **Fig. 1**; **Fig. 8**). The proximal portion of the nerve in the upper arm gives off branches that supply the triceps and anconeus as well as the posterior cutaneous sensory nerve of the forearm. The nerve then wraps around the spiral groove to the lateral humerus, where the nerve is most superficial and susceptible to compression. It passes through the lateral intermuscular septum to the anterior arm, giving off motor branches to the brachialis and brachioradialis (BR), extensor carpi radialis longus, and extensor carpi radialis brevis. The nerve then runs between the distal biceps and proximal BR at the elbow and splits into 2 branches: the posterior interosseous nerve (PIN) and the SRN (see **Figs. 2** and **8**). The PIN continues through the arcade of Frohse into the supinator muscle, and innervates the supinator, and the extensor digitorum communis (EDC), extensor carpi ulnaris, extensor pollicis longus and extensor pollicis brevis, abductor pollicis longus (APL), and EIP muscles. The SRN runs deep to the BR then distally along the lateral radius, across the dorsal wrist and over the extensor tendons of the anatomic snuffbox to provide sensation to the dorsolateral hand, thumb, index, middle, and lateral ring fingers.

Clinical Features

Symptoms of radial neuropathies commonly include pain at the lesion site, which may radiate proximally or distally, varying distributions of weakness, and possibly sensory deficit.[43] Clinical examination findings depend on the site of the lesion, most occurring (1) above the spiral groove, (2) at or near the spiral groove, (3) at the arcade of Frohse involving the PIN, or (4) at the SRN.[42,44] The spiral groove is the most common site of entrapment.[45,46] Proximal to the spiral groove, radial neuropathy produces weakness of elbow, wrist, and finger extension (wrist drop); mild weakness of elbow flexion; and sensory abnormalities over the posterior arm, forearm, and dorsolateral hand and

Table 3
Electrodiagnostic findings in proximal median and anterior interosseous neuropathies

	Proximal Median Neuropathy	Anterior Interosseous Neuropathy
Median antidromic sensory	Low amplitude Slow CV	NL
Median motor	Low amplitude Possible partial conduction block Slow CV	NL
NEX APB, FCR, PT	Abnormal	NL
NEX FPL, PQ	Abnormal	Abnormal

Abbreviation: NL, normal findings.

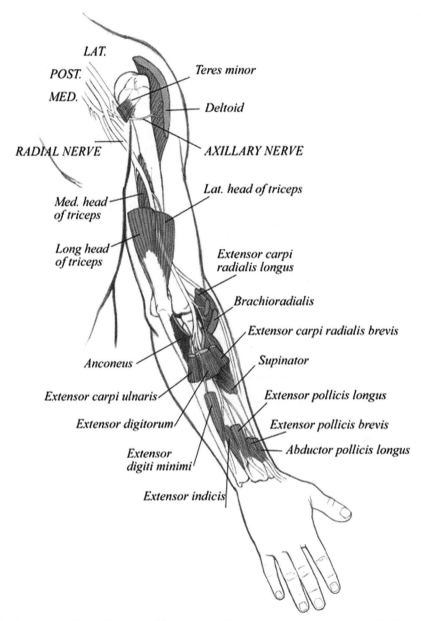

Fig. 8. Course of the radial and axillary nerves with muscular innervation. (*From* Hollinshead WH, Rosse C. Textbook of anatomy. 4th edition. Philadelphia: Harper & Row; 1985; with permission.)

fingers. On examination, the triceps and BR reflexes are diminished or absent. At or near the spiral groove, the triceps (and triceps reflex) is spared as is sensation over the posterior arm and forearm, but the clinical picture is otherwise similar to that of more proximal radial neuropathy. PIN neuropathy displays finger drop and potentially wrist extensor weakness with radial deviation, supination weakness, and thumb abduction weakness, without sensory symptoms or deficits.[44] SRN neuropathies present with sensory deficit in the distribution of the SRN only without motor abnormalities. Common causes of radial neuropathy are listed in **Box 2**.

Sensory Nerve Conduction Studies

The superficial radial sensory NCS is an easily performed study when evaluating patients with suspected radial neuropathies and may demonstrate a low amplitude in lesions of the SRN, in which it may the only EDX finding, or of the proximal radial nerve. The SRN sensory study performed on the affected side should usually be compared with the asymptomatic side, because the response may be preserved but low. Amplitude on the affected side that is less than 50% of the unaffected side is considered abnormal even if the absolute value is greater than the lower limit of normal. The SRN response is normal in PIN neuropathy at the arcade of Frohse but typically abnormal in all other sites of radial neuropathies, unless the underlying pathology of a proximal radial neuropathy is solely focal demyelination (manifest as conduction block).

Motor Nerve Conduction Studies

The radial motor NCS is performed by stimulating at the elbow and spiral groove (at the lateral border of the triceps near the deltoid tendon insertion), recording over the EDC or EIP muscles. With concern for a proximal radial neuropathy at or above the spiral groove, stimulation in the axilla (medial to the triceps muscle) and at the supraclavicular fossa (Erb point) may be performed but is technically more

---

Box 2
Common causes of radial neuropathies according to lesion site

Axilla

  Crutch palsy

  Proximal humeral fracture

  Shoulder dislocation

  Neural tumor

Upper arm

  Midhumeral fracture

  External compression (eg, Saturday night palsy)

  Neural tumor

Posterior interosseous nerve

  Radial fracture

  Compression at the arcade of Frohse

  Compression by supinator muscle

  Neural tumor

Superficial radial sensory nerve

  Compression at the wrist (handcuff, casting, etc.)

  Intravenous placement

  Neural tumor

challenging. Side-to side comparison should be performed to assess for a relative reduction in amplitude. The findings on radial motor NCS in radial neuropathies may be those of focal conduction block with focal demyelination or the response may be absent or low amplitude if significant axonal loss has occurred. Conduction block is common at the spiral groove where it tends to greatly exceed axon loss but less common at other areas along the course of the nerve.[45] Although not as frequently performed, short segment incremental stimulation (inching) studies can be performed around the spiral groove to more precisely localize the site of compression.

Lesions proximal to the spiral groove may manifest as low-amplitude motor (and sensory) responses. Conduction block may also be present if motor nerve stimulation is carried to the axilla or supraclavicular regions. If the lesion is at or near the spiral groove, there may be a low-amplitude SRN response and conduction block is commonly seen on motor studies.

Needle Examination

NEX is useful to assist in localizing the site of the lesion in radial neuropathies and in excluding alternate diagnoses. NEX should include proximal and distal radial inner-vated muscles, and the most proximally affected radial innervated muscle should be identified. A mnemonic that may help in remembering the initial order of the motor branches to the radial nerve is TABES (triceps, anconeus, BR, extensor carpi radialis, supinator). The deltoid and/or teres minor should also be examined to exclude a poste-rior cord brachial plexus neuropathy and other nonradial C6/7 innervated muscles, such as the PT or FCR, are helpful in excluding a C6/7 radiculopathy.

Lesions above the spiral groove produce abnormalities in all radial-innervated muscles. If at or near the spiral groove, the triceps and anconeus are normal but more distal muscles are involved. PIN neuropathy causes abnormalities in the finger and radial wrist extensors. NEX is normal in SRN neuropathy.

There are some data regarding EDX studies and prognosis in traumatic radial neuropathy.[47] In one study, 92% of patients with a recordable radial CMAP from the EIP or full, central, or reduced recruitment from on NEX of the BR muscle had a good recovery (Medical Research Council grade 3 or higher in radial innervated muscles). Of patients with no elicitable CMAP, 65% still had a good outcome. This correlated with those who had discrete recruitment in the BR (67%), whereas only 33% of patients with no voluntary motor unit potentials had a good recovery. EDX studies performed more than 3 months after the trauma were most useful in predicting recovery. The pattern of findings on NCS and NEX in radial neuropathy at the elbow is shown in **Table 4**.

MUSCULOCUTANEOUS NEUROPATHY

The musculocutaneous nerve contains fibers derived mostly from the C5/6 roots (with minor contribution from C7) and upper and middle trunks of the brachial plexus and arises as a branch of the lateral cord.[48,49] It innervates the coracobrachialis muscle, pierces it, and continues through the anterior upper arm to innervate the biceps and brachialis muscles. Its terminal branch is the lateral antebrachial cutaneous (LAC) nerve providing sensory innervation to the lateral volar forearm.

Lesions of the musculocutaneous nerve proper cause weakness of elbow flexion and possibly arm adduction as well as sensory loss over the lateral forearm.[49] More distal lesions at the elbow produce can produce an isolated LAC neuropathy with only sensory abnormalities. Musculocutaneous neuropathies are uncommon and may be clinically mimicked by C5/6 radiculopathy or upper trunk or lateral cord

Table 4
Pattern of electrodiagnostic findings in radial neuropathies

Study	Upper Arm	Spiral Groove	Arcade of Frohse	Posterior Interosseous Nerve	Superficial Radial Sensory Nerve
NCS					
Radial motor	Abnormal	Abnormal[a]	Abnormal[a]	Abnormal[a]	NL
Superficial radial sensory	Abnormal	Abnormal	NL	NL	Abnormal
NEX					
Triceps and anconeus	Abnormal	NL	NL	NL	NL
BR and ECR	Abnormal	Abnormal	NL	NL	NL
Supinator, extensor carpi ulnaris, EDC, EIP	Abnormal	Abnormal	Abnormal	Abnormal	NL

[a] Possible partial conduction block.

brachial plexopathies. Causes to consider include shoulder dislocation, proximal humeral fracture, and external compression.

There are few EDX studies that directly assess the musculocutaneous nerve. In most cases, identifying abnormalities on NEX isolated to muscles innervated by the musculocutaneous nerve is sufficient to make the diagnosis.

Nerve Conduction Studies

The sensory branch of the musculocutaneous nerve can be assessed through the LAC sensory NCS. The LAC amplitudes are often low and, therefore, the response obtained from the affected side should be compared with the unaffected side, with a greater than 50% difference in amplitude considered significant.[50] Because the LAC may also be abnormal in upper trunk brachial plexopathies, assessment of the superficial radial sensory NCS may be useful when the LAC is abnormal to exclude a lesion at this site.

The musculocutaneous motor fibers can be assessed through a motor NCS recording the biceps and stimulating in the axilla and supraclavicular fossa (Erb point).[51–53] In rare cases, a focal conduction block between these sites may be identified, although most lesions produce axon loss, in which an amplitude reduction is seen. Musculocutaneous motor nerve studies are abnormal in musculocutaneous neuropathy but normal in an isolated LAC neuropathy. Also, the musculocutaneous motor NCS may be abnormal in a severe C5/6 radiculopathy or upper trunk or lateral cord plexopathy.

Needle Examination

Because there are few muscles innervated by the musculocutaneous nerve, one of the major roles of the NEX is, in addition to confirming a musculocutaneous neuropathy, excluding other localizations, such as C5/6 radiculopathy and posterior cord or upper trunk brachial plexus neuropathy. NEX of the biceps with or without the brachialis is usually sufficient. In rare situations, the nerve is entrapped in the coracobrachialis; with these lesions, the brachialis and the biceps are involved but the coracobrachialis is spared.[49] Otherwise, there is little to be gained in examining the brachialis, which can have alternate innervation, including by the radial or median nerves.[54] Other non-musculocutaneous innervated muscles that may be useful when trying to exclude other sites of abnormality include the deltoid, supraspinatus, and infraspinatus. NEX is normal in a LAC neuropathy. The pattern of findings on NCS and NEX in usculocutaneous nerve at the elbow is shown in **Table 5**.

AXILLARY NEUROPATHY

The axillary nerve is a terminal branch of the posterior cord, with motor and sensory fibers derived from the C5/6 nerve roots via the upper trunk of the brachial plexus.[48,49] It travels through the quadrilateral space after which it innervates the teres minor. It then separates into its anterior, middle, and posterior branches to supply the deltoid muscle and the upper lateral brachial cutaneous nerve innervating the skin over the deltoid (**Fig. 8**).

Axillary neuropathy causes weakness of arm abduction and possibly mild weakness of shoulder external rotation. Sensory loss may occur over the lateral shoulder. The differential diagnosis includes a posterior cord or upper trunk brachial plexus neuropathy and C5/6 radiculopathy. Although rare, causes include shoulder dislocation, proximal humeral fracture, and external compression.

Nerve Conduction Studies

Although the EDX diagnosis rests primarily on the NEX, motor NCS of the axillary nerve recording over the deltoid should be performed with side-to-side comparison. A 50% or more reduction of amplitude on the affected side is abnormal.[51,53] Routine ulnar and median sensory and motor studies with F waves are also performed to exclude a more widespread disorder. The presence of normal median and superficial radial sensory responses helps exclude posterior cord and upper trunk brachial plexus neuropathies.

Needle Examination

NEX of the deltoid is essential to the diagnosis. The deltoid may be thought of as containing anterior, middle, and posterior regions. If one area is normal on NEX, then other regions should also be studied because abnormalities can be localized to one area of the muscle. The teres minor can also be studied but is more difficult to specifically localize. Examination of the triceps, EDC, or other radial innervated muscles excludes a posterior cord lesion. NEX of the biceps, supraspinatus, and infraspinatus assesses for upper trunk brachial plexus neuropathy and C5/6

Table 5		
Electrodiagnostic findings in musculocutaneous and lateral antebrachial neuropathies		
	Musculocutaneous Neuropathy	**Lateral Antebrachial Cutaneous Neuropathy**
LAC sensory	Abnormal (compare side to side)	Abnormal (compare side to side)
Musculocutaneous motor	Abnormal Possible conduction block	NL
NEX biceps	Abnormal	NL
NEX brachialis	May be normal	NL

Abbreviation: NL, normal findings.

radiculopathy. The pattern of findings on NCS and NEX in axillary neuropathy is shown in **Box 3**.

SUPRASCAPULAR NEUROPATHY

The suprascapular nerve is a branch off the upper trunk of the brachial plexus, therefore has C5/6 root origin. It runs posteriorly through the suprascapular notch to the supraspinous fossa where it innervates the supraspinatus. It then courses around the spinoglenoid notch to innervate the infraspinatus. Either notch can serve as a site of entrapment.[55] Lesions at the suprascapular notch cause pain and weakness of shoulder abduction and external rotation.[49,56,57] Nerve entrapment at the spinoglenoid notch manifests as weakness of external rotation only with or without pain, or pain alone.[58–60] It is commonly involved in idiopathic or hereditary brachial plexus neuropathy.[40] Fractures of the shoulder or proximal humerus and shoulder dislocation are other common causes.

Nerve Conduction Studies

Although the NEX is the most useful component of an EDX for confirming the diagnosis of suprascapular neuropathy, motor NCS of the suprascapular nerve recording over the supraspinatus and infraspinatus can be performed to provide an objective measure of axonal loss within the nerve. From a diagnostic standpoint, a greater than 50% reduction in the CMAP amplitude side-to-side or focal slowing or conduction block at the spinoglenoid notch are abnormal (**Fig. 9**).[53,55] There are no sensory abnormalities in suprascapular neuropathies.

Needle Examination

NEX should include the supraspinatus and infraspinatus, where chronic changes are more common than active denervation.[60] Other, nonsuprascapular innervated muscles, in particular those innervated by the C5/6 roots and upper trunk of the brachial plexus, should be performed. The pattern of findings on NCS and NEX in suprascapular neuropathy is shown in **Box 4**.

LONG THORACIC NEUROPATHY

The long thoracic nerve arises from the C5-7 roots directly, runs beneath the brachial plexus, down the anterior lateral chest to innervate the serratus anterior muscle. It is

---

Box 3
Electrodiagnostic approach to axillary neuropathy

Nerve conduction studies

    Ulnar and median antidromic sensory

    Ulnar and median motor with F-wave responses

    Axillary motor (bilaterally)

    Superficial radial sensory

Needle examination

    Deltoid, teres minor

    Other nonaxillary muscles (eg, supraspinatus, infraspinatus, biceps, triceps, EDC, and cervical paraspinals)

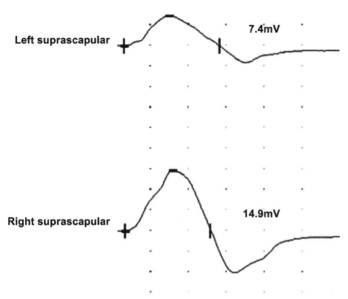

Left suprascapular   7.4mV

Right suprascapular   14.9mV

Fig. 9. NCS in a left suprascapular neuropathy. Left suprascapular CMAP amplitude is less than 50% that of the right.

commonly involved in idiopathic or hereditary brachial plexus neuropathy.[40] Long thoracic neuropathies produce scapular winging with difficulty in shoulder abduction or flexion. Long thoracic neuropathy may occur iatrogenically after various operative procedures, after trauma, or associated with idiopathic or hereditary brachial plexus neuropathy.

Nerve Conduction Studies

Long thoracic NCS have been described stimulating the nerve at Erb point and recording the serratus anterior muscle via needle electrode.[61] In long thoracic neuropathy, the latency is prolonged, but affected patients generally also show abnormalities on NEX, reducing the usefulness of such technically difficult and invasive NCS.

Box 4
Electrodiagnostic approach to suprascapular neuropathy

Nerve conduction studies

    Ulnar and median antidromic sensory

    Ulnar and median motor with F-wave responses

    Suprascapular motor (bilaterally)

    Superficial radial sensory

Needle examination

    Supraspinatus, infraspinatus

    Other non-suprascapular innervated muscles (eg, deltoid, biceps, FDI, serratus anterior, flexor pollicis longus, and cervical paraspinals)

Box 5

Electrodiagnostic approach to long thoracic neuropathy

Nerve conduction studies

    Ulnar and median antidromic sensory

    Ulnar and median motor with F-wave responses

    Superficial radial sensory

Needle examination

    Serratus anterior

    Other nonlong thoracic innervated muscles (eg, infraspinatus, deltoid, biceps, triceps, cervical paraspinals)

Routine ulnar and median sensory and often SRN sensory studies and ulnar and median motor studies with F waves are often performed to exclude a more widespread disorder, particularly a brachial plexus neuropathy.

Needle Examination

NEX should be abnormal only in the serratus anterior muscle, and this should be compared with the unaffected side if only motor unit potential changes are seen. The muscle can be examined with needle insertion lateral to the inferior angle of the scapula or in the midaxillary line, inserting over the upper edge of the inferior rib. The needle should be inserted obliquely, because the major risk during NEX of the serratus anterior is pneumothorax. Other limb muscles should also be examined to exclude C5/6/7 radiculopathy and brachial plexus neuropathy as well as a myopathy, which can also cause scapular winging. The pattern of findings on NCS and NEX in long thoracic neuropathy is shown in **Box 5**.

SUMMARY

Upper extremity mononeuropathies range from the common (ulnar at the elbow and radial) to the uncommon (ulnar at the wrist, proximal median, musculocutaneous, axillary, suprascapular, and long thoracic). Although the history and physical examination are physicians' time-tested tools for localization and diagnosis, EDX studies are an extension of this and aid with assessment of localization, severity, pathophysiology, and prognosis. Appropriately designed studies can confirm the diagnosis and also uncover alternate diagnoses and may direct investigations into possible causes. Serial studies can assess for progression or resolution.

REFERENCES

1. Stewart JD. Ulnar nerve. In: Focal peripheral neuropathies. West Vancouver (Canada): JBJ Publishing; 2010. p. 260–313.
2. Leis AA, Wells KJ. Radial nerve cutaneous innervation to the ulnar dorsum of the hand. Clin Neurophysiol 2008;119(3):662–6.
3. Tackmann W, Vogel P, Kaeser HE, et al. Sensitivity and localizing significance of motor and sensory electroneurographic parameters in the diagnosis of ulnar nerve lesions at the elbow. A reappraisal. J Neurol 1984;231(4):204–11.

4. Merlevede K, Theys P, van Hees J. Diagnosis of ulnar neuropathy: a new approach. Muscle Nerve 2000;23(4):478–81.
5. Campbell WW. Ulnar neuropathy at the elbow. Muscle Nerve 2000;23(4):450–2.
6. Todnem K, Michler RP, Wader TE, et al. The impact of extended electrodiagnostic studies in ulnar neuropathy at the elbow. BMC Neurol 2009;9:52–60.
7. Campbell WW, Pridgeon RM, Riaz G, et al. Variations in anatomy of the ulnar nerve at the cubital tunnel: pitfalls in the diagnosis of ulnar neuropathy at the elbow. Muscle Nerve 1991;14(8):733–8.
8. Campbell WW, Pridgeon RM, Sahni KS. Short segment incremental studies in the evaluation of ulnar neuropathy at the elbow. Muscle Nerve 1992;15(9): 1050–4.
9. Campbell WW, Pridgeon RM, Sahni SK. Entrapment neuropathy of the ulnar nerve at its point of exit from the flexor carpi ulnaris muscle. Muscle Nerve 1988;11(5):467–70.
10. American Association of Electrodiagnostic Medicine, American Academy of Neurology, American Academy of Physical Medicine and Rehabilitation. Practice parameter for electrodiagnostic studies in ulnar neuropathy at the elbow: summary statement. Muscle Nerve 1999;22(3):408–11.
11. Kothari MJ, Preston DC. Comparison of the flexed and extended elbow positions in localizing ulnar neuropathy at the elbow. Muscle Nerve 1995;18(3):336–40.
12. Rhee EK, England JD, Sumner AJ. A computer simulation of conduction block: effects produced by actual block versus interphase cancellation. Ann Neurol 1990;28(2):146–56.
13. Olney RK. Consensus criteria for the diagnosis of partial conduction block. Muscle Nerve 1999;22(Suppl 8):S225–9.
14. Kothari MJ, Heistand M, Rutkove SB. Three ulnar nerve conduction studies in patients with ulnar neuropathy at the elbow. Arch Phys Med Rehabil 1998; 79(1):87–9.
15. Caliandro P, Foschini M, Pazzaglia C, et al. IN-RATIO: a new test to increase diagnostic sensitivity in ulnar nerve entrapment at elbow. Clin Neurophysiol 2008; 119(7):1600–6.
16. Raynor EM, Shefner JM, Preston DC, et al. Sensory and mixed nerve conduction studies in the evaluation of ulnar neuropathy at the elbow. Muscle Nerve 1994; 17(7):785–92.
17. Kwon HK, Lee HJ, Hwang M, et al. Amplitude ratio of ulnar sensory nerve action potentials in segmental conduction study: reference values in healthy subjects and diagnostic usefulness in patients with ulnar neuropathy at the elbow. Am J Phys Med Rehabil 2008;87(8):642–6.
18. Caliandro P, Pazzaglia C, Granata G, et al. Re: Amplitude ratio of ulnar sensory nerve action potentials in segmental conduction study. Am J Phys Med Rehabil 2008;87(12):1053–4.
19. Herrmann DN, Preston DC, McIntosh KA, et al. Localization of ulnar neuropathy with conduction block across the elbow. Muscle Nerve 2001;24(5):698–700.
20. Venkatesh S, Kothari MJ, Preston DC. The limitations of the dorsal ulnar cutaneous sensory response in patients with ulnar neuropathy at the elbow. Muscle Nerve 1995;18(3):345–7.
21. Friedrich JM, Robinson LR. Prognostic indicators from electrodiagnostic studies for ulnar neuropathy at the elbow. Muscle Nerve 2011;43(4):596–600.
22. Campbell WW, Pridgeon RM, Riaz G, et al. Sparing of the flexor carpi ulnaris in ulnar neuropathy at the elbow. Muscle Nerve 1989;12(12):965–7.
23. Wu JS, Morris JD, Hogan GR. Ulnar neuropathy at the wrist: case report and review of literature. Arch Phys Med Rehabil 1985;66(11):785–8.

24. Olney RK, Hanson M. AAEE case report #15: ulnar neuropathy at or distal to the wrist. Muscle Nerve 1988;11(8):828–32.
25. Olney RK, Wilbourn AJ. Ulnar nerve conduction study of the first dorsal interosseous muscle. Arch Phys Med Rehabil 1985;66(1):16–8.
26. Kothari MJ, Preston DC, Logigian EL. Lumbrical-interossei motor studies localize ulnar neuropathy at the wrist. Muscle Nerve 1996;19(2):170–4.
27. McIntosh KA, Preston DC, Logigian EL. Short-segment incremental studies to localize ulnar nerve entrapment at the wrist. Neurology 1998;50(1):303–6.
28. Stewart JD. Median nerve. In: Focal peripheral neuropathies. West Vancouver (Canada): JBJ Publishing; 2010. p. 194–259.
29. Morris HH, Peters BH. Pronator syndrome: clinical and electrophysiological features in seven cases. J Neurol Neurosurg Psychiatry 1976;39(5):461–4.
30. Bilge T, Yalaman O, Bilge S, et al. Entrapment neuropathy of the median nerve at the level of the ligament of Struthers. Neurosurgery 1990;27(5):787–9.
31. Gross PT, Tolomeo EA. Proximal median neuropathies. Neurol Clin 1999;17(3):425–45.
32. Bilecenoglu B, Uz A, Karalezli N. Possible anatomic structures causing entrapment neuropathies of the median nerve: an anatomic study. Acta Orthop Belg 2005;71(2):169–76.
33. Gross PT, Jones HR Jr. Proximal median neuropathies: electromyographic and clinical correlation. Muscle Nerve 1992;15(3):390–5.
34. Bridgeman C, Naidu S, Kothari MJ. Clinical and electrophysiological presentation of pronator syndrome. Electromyogr Clin Neurophysiol 2007;47(2):89–92.
35. Kiloh LG, Nevin S. Isolated neuritis of the anterior interosseous nerve. Br Med J 1952;1(4763):850–1.
36. Nakano KK, Lundergran C, Okihiro MM. Anterior interosseous nerve syndromes. Diagnostic methods and alternative treatments. Arch Neurol 1977;34(8):477–80.
37. Wong L, Dellon AL. Brachial neuritis presenting as anterior interosseous nerve compression–implications for diagnosis and treatment: a case report. J Hand Surg Am 1997;22(3):536–9.
38. Rosenberg JN. Anterior interosseous/median nerve latency ratio. Arch Phys Med Rehabil 1990;71(3):228–30.
39. Vucic S, Yiannikas C. Anterior interosseous nerve conduction study: normative data. Muscle Nerve 2007;35(1):119–21.
40. van Alfen N, van Engelen BG. The clinical spectrum of neuralgic amyotrophy in 246 cases. Brain 2006;129(Pt 2):438–50.
41. Stewart JD. Radial nerve. In: Focal peripheral neuropathies. West Vancouver (Canada): JBJ Publishing; 2010. p. 314–47.
42. Carlson N, Logigian EL. Radial neuropathy. Neurol Clin 1999;17(3):499–523.
43. Rinker B, Effron CR, Beasley RW. Proximal radial compression neuropathy. Ann Plast Surg 2004;52(2):174–80.
44. Kaplan PE. Posterior interosseous neuropathies: natural history. Arch Phys Med Rehabil 1984;65(7):399–400.
45. Watson BV, Brown WF. Quantitation of axon loss and conduction block in acute radial nerve palsies. Muscle Nerve 1992;15(7):768–73.
46. Mondelli M, Morana P, Ballerini M, et al. Mononeuropathies of the radial nerve: clinical and neurographic findings in 91 consecutive cases. J Electromyogr Kinesiol 2005;15(4):377–83.
47. Malikowski T, Micklesen PJ, Robinson LR. Prognostic values of electrodiagnostic studies in traumatic radial neuropathy. Muscle Nerve 2007;36(3):364–7.

48. Stewart JD. Nerves arising from the brachial plexus. In: Focal peripheral neuropathies. West Vancouver (Canada): JBJ Publishing; 2010. p. 162–93.
49. Goslin KL, Krivickas LS. Proximal neuropathies of the upper extremity. Neurol Clin 1999;17(3):525–48.
50. Spindler HA, Felsenthal G. Sensory conduction in the musculocutaneous nerve. Arch Phys Med Rehabil 1978;59(1):20–3.
51. Kraft GH. Axillary, musculocutaneous and suprascapular nerve latency studies. Arch Phys Med Rehabil 1972;53(8):383–7.
52. Trojaborg W. Motor and sensory conduction in the musculocutaneous nerve. J Neurol Neurosurg Psychiatry 1976;39(9):890–9.
53. Buschbacher RM, Weir SK, Bentley JG, et al. Normal motor nerve conduction studies using surface electrode recording from the supraspinatus, infraspinatus, deltoid, and biceps. PM R 2009;1(2):101–6.
54. Merrell CA, Merrell KL. A variation of musculocutaneous neuropathy: implications for electromyographers. PM R 2010;2(8):780–2.
55. Aiello I, Serra G, Traina GC, et al. Entrapment of the suprascapular nerve at the spinoglenoid notch. Ann Neurol 1982;12(3):314–6.
56. Kopell HP, Thompson WA. Pain and the frozen shoulder. Surg Gynecol Obstet 1959;109(1):92–6.
57. Post M, Mayer J. Suprascapular nerve entrapment. Diagnosis and treatment. Clin Orthop Relat Res 1987;(223):126–36.
58. Liveson JA, Bronson MJ, Pollack MA. Suprascapular nerve lesions at the spinoglenoid notch: report of three cases and review of the literature. J Neurol Neurosurg Psychiatry 1991;54(3):241–3.
59. Lee BC, Yegappan M, Thiagarajan P. Suprascapular nerve neuropathy secondary to spinoglenoid notch ganglion cyst: case reports and review of literature. Ann Acad Med Singapore 2007;36(12):1032–5.
60. Boykin RE, Friedman DJ, Zimmer ZR, et al. Suprascapular neuropathy in a shoulder referral practice. J Shoulder Elbow Surg 2011;20(6):983–8.
61. Kaplan PE. Electrodiagnostic confirmation of long thoracic nerve palsy. J Neurol Neurosurg Psychiatry 1980;43(1):50–2.

Electrodiagnostic Evaluation of Lower Extremity Mononeuropathies

Vera Fridman, MD[a,b,*], William S. David, MD, PhD[a,b]

KEYWORDS

- Neuropathy • Nerve conduction studies • Electromyography
- Lower extremity

When approaching patients with suspected mononeuropathies of the lower extremity, the electromyographer is confronted with the challenge of differentiating lesions involving a single nerve from those involving the lumbosacral plexus, the lumbosacral nerve roots, or a more diffuse nerve process such as a polyneuropathy or polyradiculopathy. Distinguishing among these possible localizations requires a carefully crafted set of electrodiagnostic studies that are tailored to the individual patient's symptoms. When the abnormalities found localize the process to an individual nerve it is important to define the type of injury (axonal vs demyelinating) and to assess the severity of nerve damage, which may be useful for prognostication for the patient. This article emphasizes the role of electromyography (EMG) in determining the anatomic localization in patients with lower extremity symptoms and suspected lower limb mononeuropathies through a series of illustrative clinical vignettes.

GENERAL COMMENTS
Is EMG Necessary?

Whether electrodiagnostic studies are useful in the evaluation of patients with lower extremity signs and symptoms depends on the specific clinical scenario and the therapeutic considerations. For example, when a patient presents with signs and symptoms suggestive of a simple, uncomplicated lumbosacral radiculopathy, observation may represent the best initial response. If the patient does not improve, or if surgery

Dr Fridman has nothing to disclose.
Dr David has served as a consultant for Apnex Medical and Pfizer.
[a] Department of Neurology, Neuromuscular Diagnostic Center, Massachusetts General Hospital, Charles River Plaza, Suite 820, 165 Cambridge Street, Boston, MA 02114, USA
[b] Department of Neurology, Harvard Medical School, 25 Shattuck Street, Boston, MA 02115, USA
* Corresponding author. Neuromuscular Diagnostic Center, Massachusetts General Hospital, Charles River Plaza, Suite 820, 165 Cambridge Street, Boston, MA 02114.
E-mail address: vfridman@partners.org

Neurol Clin 30 (2012) 505–528
doi:10.1016/j.ncl.2011.12.004   **neurologic.theclinics.com**
0733-8619/12/$ – see front matter © 2012 Published by Elsevier Inc.

is being contemplated because of intractable pain or the presence of unacceptable weakness, a magnetic resonance (MR) imaging scan is often obtained. If the MR imaging findings are unrevealing or equivocal, or if there is a concern that the process may not involve the root, electrophysiologic studies are indicated. Although electro-diagnostic studies are helpful to identify a radiculopathy, the studies become more useful in localization with progressively more distal limb lesions and are generally war-ranted for any patient with a suspected lower extremity mononeuropathy.

What Can EMG Accomplish?

There are several important goals of an EMG in the evaluation of patients with a sus-pected lower extremity mononeuropathy. First, EMG can establish that a physiologi-cally relevant nerve injury exists. Lower extremity symptoms can emanate from numerous structures, including bone, tendon, and muscle. It is important to verify with EMG testing that the symptoms are neurogenic in origin.

Second, and perhaps most importantly, EMG can help anatomically to localize the site of injury to a specific nerve and at the same time assess for or exclude a process involving the root or plexus. Because nerve fascicles can selectively be injured at various locations, proximal lesions (root or plexus) can often masquerade as distal (nerve) lesions. The classic example is a patient with a sciatic neuropathy or sacral plexopathy who presents with foot drop, mimicking a peroneal neuropathy. In these scenarios, the fibers destined to form the peroneal nerve are preferentially affected at a proximal location, resulting in the clinical presentation that resembles a peroneal neuropathy. Defining the anatomic localization of an injury is important because the relevant potential causes of the underlying process vary by site of nerve involvement (**Table 1**).

Third, EMG can shed light on the timing of an injury (**Box 1**). The presence or absence of spontaneous activity, distribution of spontaneous activity, and alterations of motor unit potential morphology can assist in defining the chronicity of an injury as acute, subacute, or chronic.

Abnormal spontaneous activity in the form of fibrillation potentials emerges at vari-able times, depending on the distance between the site of injury and the muscle

Table 1
Possible causes of different nerve localizations involving the lower limb

Lumbosacral Radiculopathy or Polyradiculopathy	Lumbosacral Plexopathy	Lower Limb Mononeuropathy
Herniated intervertebral disk	Hip/pelvic trauma or surgery	External compression
Degenerative spondylosis	Retroperitoneal hematoma	Stretch
Tumors	Neoplasm	Trauma/fractures
Meningitis, nerve sheath tumors, other primary/ secondary	Diabetes (radiculoplexus neuropathy)	Penetrating or closed
Infectious	Idiopathic radiculoplexus neuropathy	Cysts/tumors
Herpes zoster, Lyme, cytomegalovirus, epidural abscess	Psoas abscess	Perioperative
Inflammatory (sarcoid)	Radiation	Vasculitis
Diabetes	Obstetric	Injections
Radiation		Compartment syndromes
Ischemic (dural arteriovenous malformations)		

Box 1
Needle EMG findings related to temporal course of a nerve injury

Acute

    Decreased recruitment of motor unit action potentials (MUAPs) only

Subacute

    Fibrillation potentials/positive sharp waves (PSWs)

    Increased percentage of polyphasic MUAPs

Subacute to chronic

    Fibrillation potentials/PSW

    Increased percentage of high-amplitude, long-duration MUAPs

Chronic

    ± Fibrillation potentials/PSWs

    High-amplitude, long-duration MUAPs

---

studied (**Box 2**). Muscles in closer proximity to the site of nerve injury show abnormalities earlier than those that are more distal.

Fourth, electrodiagnostic studies may provide information regarding the underlying pathophysiology of a nerve injury. Specifically, localized injuries can result in focal demyelination or axonal disruption. When performing motor nerve conduction studies, the former can manifest as differential amplitude reduction (conduction block) across a site of injury, the latter as a global amplitude reduction. Defining the pathophysiology of nerve injury can help define the severity of the injury and has important prognostic implications; predominantly demyelinating injuries may recover over weeks to months, whereas axonal injuries may take significantly longer (depending on the severity and site of injury). The outcome (full extent of recovery) is also less certain with axonal loss lesions.

General Approach to Patients with Suspected Lower Extremity Mononeuropathies

The usefulness of all laboratory studies and diagnostic procedures increases if these studies are obtained for specific reasons and to address a particular question. Similarly, EMGs should be hypothesis driven and designed to investigate a specific question or suspected diagnosis. The referring diagnosis, supplemented by a brief history and physical examination, generates an initial differential diagnosis. The electrodiagnostic examination can then be structured to confirm or exclude various diagnostic considerations. Although the present intent is to provide an algorithmic approach to the patient with lower extremity mononeuropathies, in reality it is important to remain flexible and

---

Box 2
Timing of the occurrence of spontaneous activity (in a lumbosacral radiculopathy)

Paraspinal muscles: 10–14 days

Proximal thigh muscles: 2–3 weeks

Leg muscles: 3–4 weeks

Distal leg and foot: 5–6 weeks

not constrained by any structured approach or recipe. As always, effective electrophysiologic studies are modified as the study ensues, based on a real-time analysis of the data as they are collected. Electrodiagnostic information must be interpreted within the context of the clinical picture. All final diagnoses must incorporate information drawn from the relevant history, physical examination findings, and imaging studies.

Motor Conduction Studies in Lower Extremity Disorders

In conventional motor conduction studies, recorded parameters include compound muscle action potential (CMAP) amplitudes, distal motor latencies, and conduction velocities. CMAP amplitudes may be reduced in nerve injuries relative to the severity of the injury and the degree of axonal disruption. Reduction in CMAP amplitudes can result from a lesion at any point along the lower motor neuron pathway (from the anterior horn cells to the individual nerve innervating the muscle being recorded from) (**Fig. 1**), and therefore cannot be used in isolation to definitively confirm a lower extremity mononeuropathy. However, in some preganglionic (root) injuries, CMAP amplitudes may be normal or only minimally reduced (unless multiple nerve roots are injured) because all muscles receive innervation from more than 1 nerve root; therefore, severe injury to 1 nerve root may only partially denervate a muscle that is being recorded from during a motor nerve conduction study.

Latencies and velocities are generally less helpful in the evaluation of focal lower extremity nerve injuries, unless the lesion is distal and the underlying pathophysiology involves focal demyelination (eg, tarsal tunnel syndrome [TTS]). In that setting, focal slowing or showing a discrete site of conduction block can allow for the precise localization of an injury (eg, peroneal neuropathy at the fibular head).

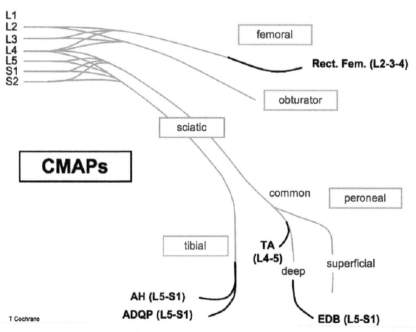

Fig. 1. Muscles used for recording CMAPs during lower extremity motor nerve conduction studies. The nerve (and roots) innervating the muscles are shown. ADQP, abductor digiti quinti pedis; AH, abductor hallucis; Rect. Fem, rectus femoris; TA, tibialis anterior. (*Courtesy of* V. Fridman MD, Boston, MA.)

Sensory Conduction Studies in Lower Extremity Disorders

In sensory conduction studies, recorded measurements include the amplitudes of the sensory nerve action potentials (SNAPs), distal sensory latencies, and sensory conduction velocities. SNAP amplitudes are useful in differentiating preganglionic (ie, root) from postganglionic (eg, plexus or nerve) injuries; SNAP amplitudes are typically normal in the former and abnormal in the latter. Therefore, in lower extremity mononeuropathies, SNAP amplitudes recorded from the lower extremity nerve involved are typically low or absent (**Fig. 2**). Important exceptions exist, which are illustrated in the subsequent case studies. As described later, sensory latencies and velocities are less useful unless the injury is distal and the underlying pathophysiology is demyelinating, in which case focal slowing may allow for the precise localization of an injury (eg, asymmetric focal slowing of a medial plantar sensory or mixed nerve response in the rare case of TTS).

Needle EMG in Lower Extremity Disorders

In evaluating the patient with suspected focal lower extremity mononeuropathies, needle EMG is vital to localization efforts. The pattern of abnormalities (which muscles are normal and which are abnormal) forms the basis of our approach (**Fig. 3**). However, there are several caveats related to interpreting needle EMG findings. Positive findings (ie, abnormalities in a muscle) are more helpful than negative findings (ie, a normal muscle). For example, finding fibrillation potentials in the extensor hallicus longus, in the appropriate clinical situation, might argue strongly for an L5 radiculopathy or peroneal neuropathy. However, the absence of abnormalities does not argue against these localizations, particularly if abnormal spontaneous activity is documented in at least 2 other relevant muscles. Needle EMG evaluation of the lumbar paraspinal muscles

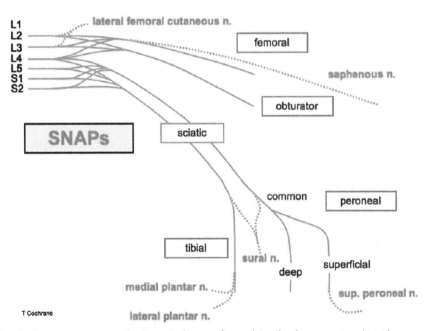

Fig. 2. Sensory nerve conduction studies performed in the lower extremity. The nerves through which the sensory fibers course are shown. (*Courtesy of* V. Fridman MD, Boston, MA).

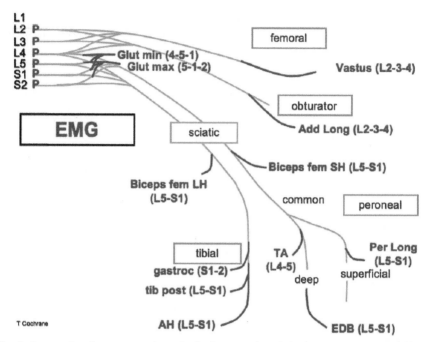

Fig. 3. Innervation (by nerve and root) of select muscles of the lower extremity. Add long, adductor longus; AH, abductor hallucis; Biceps fem LH, long head of the biceps femoris; Biceps fem SH, short head of the biceps femoris; gastroc, medial gastrocnemius; Glut max, gluteus maximus; Glut min, gluteus minimus; Per long, peroneus longus; TA, tibialis anterior; tib post, tibialis posterior. (*Courtesy of* V. Fridman MD, Boston, MA.)

represents another important example. In patients with a suspected lumbosacral radiculopathy, the detection of abnormal spontaneous activity in the paraspinal muscles provides strong evidence for a preganglionic injury; however, failure to detect spontaneous activity does not exclude a root injury, because paraspinal abnormalities may be identifiable in only 50% of patients with radiculopathy. The same fascicular phenomenon may occur with lesions involving individual nerves, such as when peroneal innervated muscles are preferentially affected (more than tibial innervated muscles) in sciatic neuropathies.

Some findings are more reliable than others. Abnormal spontaneous activity in the form of fibrillation potentials and PSWs is relatively easy to identify and allows the electrophysiologist to identify an abnormality with more confidence. Remodeled motor unit potentials in the form of high-amplitude, long-duration potentials are important markers of chronic nerve injury. However, such changes may be difficult to discern when the alterations are subtle, as can occur in long-standing lumbosacral spinal stenosis. MUAP morphology also varies as a function of age, and the electromyographer must take this into account when judging the normality of MUAP parameters. Very mild mononeuropathies that show only an increased percentage of polyphasic motor unit potentials or subtle recruitment abnormalities may be more difficult to confirm.

The identification of abnormalities on needle examination can assist greatly in our localization efforts. By proceeding in a methodical, distal to proximal fashion, it is often possible to identify how high an injury resides along the proximal-distal axis, thereby permitting the differentiation among a mononeuropathy, plexopathy, or radiculopathy.

In the following cases, we show the electrodiagnostic approach to several types of mononeuropathies of the lower extremity and discuss ways of distinguishing these nerve lesions from more proximal injury at the level of the lumbosacral plexus or lumbosacral nerve roots. We describe the electrophysiologic approach to common clinical presenting symptoms: the floppy foot, the buckling knee, and the painful foot.

LOWER EXTREMITY NERVE ANATOMY

The nerves of the lower extremity originate from the L1 to S3 nerve roots. After exiting the spinal cord, fibers originating from the L1 to L4 segments join to form the lumbar plexus in the retroperitoneum. The upper lumbar plexus gives rise to the ilioinguinal and genitofemoral nerves as well as the lateral cutaneous nerve of the thigh. The femoral and obturator nerves originate at the lower lumbar plexus. The sacral plexus is formed by S1 to S4 innervated fibers with an additional contribution from the L4/5 nerve roots (the lumbosacral trunk). The sacral plexus gives rise to the superior and inferior gluteal nerves, the pudendal nerve, the sciatic nerve, and the posterior cutaneous nerve of the thigh.

Obturator Nerve

The obturator nerve (supplied by the L2–4 roots) passes through the psoas muscle and travels posterior to the common iliac vessels to the obturator foramen, through which it enters the thigh. It supplies the gracilis, the 3 hip adductors (magnus, longus and brevis), and the obturator internus.

Femoral Nerve

The femoral nerve also originates from the L2 to 4 roots. After passing through the lower lumbar plexus it travels behind the psoas muscle (which it innervates) and passes underneath the inguinal ligament lateral to the femoral artery. It then divides into its motor and sensory branches, supplying the 4 heads of the quadriceps muscles (vastus medialis, vastus lateralis, vastus intermedius, rectus femoris) and the sartorius muscle and providing sensory innervation to the anterior thigh. The nerve ends in the saphenous nerve, which supplies sensation to the medial aspect of the calf.

Sciatic Nerve

The sciatic nerve is composed of S1 to S3 fibers as well as L4 to 5 fibers, which joined the sacral plexus by way of the lumbosacral trunk. After exiting the pelvis the nerve travels between the piriformis and obturator internus muscles. The sciatic nerve has also been observed to pass through the piriformis muscle itself. Through most of its course, the nerve contains 2 distinct nerve bundles: one containing fibers destined for the common peroneal nerve and one containing fibers destined for the tibial nerve. Above the knee, the tibial nerve portion of the sciatic nerve innervates the semitendinosus, semimembranosus, and the long head of the biceps femoris. It also offers partial innervation to the adductor magnus (which is in addition supplied by the obturator nerve). The only muscle innervated by the peroneal division of the sciatic nerve is the short head of the biceps femoris. The physical division of the sciatic nerve into the common peroneal and tibial nerves occurs just above the popliteal fossa.

Peroneal (Fibular) Nerve

The common peroneal (fibular) nerve splits into its 2 divisions (deep and superficial) at the level of the fibular neck. The superficial peroneal nerve supplies the peroneus longus and peroneus brevis muscles, which are responsible for foot eversion. It also supplies sensation to the lateral calf and dorsum of the foot. The deep division of the nerve innervates the tibialis anterior, extensor hallucis, peroneus tertius, extensor digitorum longus, and extensor digitorum brevis (EDB) muscles. The deep peroneal nerve also offers sensory supply to the first web space.

Tibial Nerve

The tibial nerve supplies all of the muscles of the posterior compartment of the leg, including the soleus, tibialis posterior, flexor digitorum longus, flexor hallucis longus medial gastrocnemius, and lateral gastrocnemius muscles. It also supplies all of the intrinsic muscles of the foot, with the exception of the EDB muscle. The tibial nerve terminates in the calcaneal, medial plantar, and lateral plantar branches, which arise at the level of the medial malleolus.

CLINICAL VIGNETTES: THE FLOPPY FOOT

Patients with foot drop or a floppy foot are commonly referred to the neurodiagnostics laboratory. A floppy foot can be caused by disorders of muscle, the neuromuscular junction, the deep peroneal nerve, the common peroneal nerve, the sciatic nerve, the lumbosacral plexus, the L4/L5 nerve roots, the anterior horn cells (as seen in motor neuron disease), or the upper motor neuron pathways. Electrodiagnostic studies can assist greatly in identifying a peripheral nervous system cause of foot drop and, when a neurogenic cause is confirmed, can help to localize the process. Once the injury is localized, it is possible to generate a reasonable differential diagnosis that helps to target further evaluation and therapy.

The initial electrodiagnostic approach to a patient with foot drop should include peroneal and tibial motor conduction studies (see **Fig. 1**), sural and superficial peroneal sensory conduction studies (see **Fig. 2**), and a needle examination of distal and proximal lower extremity muscles. The electrodiagnostic pattern of abnormalities with different localizations of causes of foot drop is summarized in **Table 2**.

Floppy Foot 1

A 29-year-old man presented to the EMG laboratory with foot drop. Seven days previously, he was helping a friend with a roofing job and had spent many hours in a squatting position. The nerve conduction study and needle EMG findings in this patient are shown in **Tables 3A** and **3B** and in **Fig. 4**.

Interpretation of floppy foot 1: common peroneal neuropathy

This case shows findings of a common peroneal neuropathy located at the fibular head (site B in **Fig. 5**). The only abnormality observed in the motor conduction studies is the presence of a conduction block at the fibular head in the peroneal motor study (see **Fig. 4**). The sensory conduction studies are normal, including the superficial peroneal study. The superficial peroneal sensory response may be normal because the predominant pathophysiology of the lesion is focal demyelination at the fibular head, and the sensory conduction studies (stimulating and recording sites) are performed distal to the site of injury. This pattern is also consistent with a hyperacute (within the first 3–5 days) axonal injury at the fibular head, before the CMAP and SNAP amplitudes have begun to drop; however, in this case, it is known that the injury occurred 7 days before the study. Another possibility is that the lesion is fascicular in nature, involving the motor but not the sensory fibers of the common peroneal nerve. Sparing of the superficial peroneal sensory fibers has recently been described[1] in a group of patients with electrophysiologically proven common peroneal neuropathies (many of whom had significant axonal loss).

Table 2
EMG localization of foot drop

	Deep Peroneal	Common Peroneal	Sciatic	Lumbosacral Plexus	L5 Root
Abnormal nerve conduction study					
Peroneal, motor	X	X	X	X	X
Tibial, motor			X	X	X
Superficial peroneal, sensory		X	X	X	Usually normal, but may be abnormal
Sural, sensory			X	X	
EMG abnormalities					
Tibialis anterior	X	X	X	X	X
Extensor hallucis	X	X	X	X	X
Peroneus longus		X	X	X	X
Tibialis posterior			X	X	X
Flexor digitorum			X	X	X
Short head biceps femoris			X	X	X
Gluteus medius				X	X
Lumbar Paraspinals					X

The identification of a conduction block at the fibular head (see **Fig. 4**) when recording from the EDB muscle was essential to localization in this study. In addition to a decrease in the motor amplitude between 2 sites of stimulation, focal demyelination can be confirmed by showing slowing of the peroneal motor conduction velocity across the fibular head. In cases in which conduction block or focal slowing cannot be shown with conventional peroneal motor conduction studies (recording from the EDB), or if the peroneal motor response is unobtainable at the EDB muscle, peroneal motor conduction studies recording from the tibialis anterior muscle could be performed in an effort to show focal slowing or conduction block.[2] Recording from the tibialis

Table 3A
Nerve conduction study findings in patient with floppy foot 1

Nerve (Recording Site)	Latency	Amplitude	Velocity
Peroneal Motor (EDB)			
Ankle	NL	NL	
Below fibular head	NL	NL	NL
Above fibular head	NL	↓↓↓	–
Tibial motor (AH)			
Ankle	NL	NL	
Knee	NL	NL	NL
Sural sensory	NL	NL	NL
Superficial peroneal sensory	NL	NL	NL

Abbreviations: AH, abductor hallucis; NL, normal; ↓↓↓, severely reduced.

Table 3B
Needle EMG findings in patient with floppy foot 1

Muscle	Spontaneous	MUAP Morphology	Recruitment
Medial gastrocnemius	NL	NL	NL
Tibialis posterior	NL	NL	NL
Tibialis anterior	NL	NL	↓↓↓ Reduced
Peroneus longus	NL	NL	↓↓↓ Reduced
Short head of biceps femoris	NL	NL	NL
Gluteus medius	NL	NL	NL

Abbreviations: NL, normal; ↓↓↓, severely reduced.

anterior can be especially helpful in determining prognosis, as tibialis anterior function often has more clinical relevance than that of the EDB.[3]

As shown in this case, the needle examination of a suspected peroneal neuropathy should include at least 1 deep peroneal and 1 superficial peroneal innervated muscle below the knee. In this case the tibialis anterior and peroneus longus muscles were

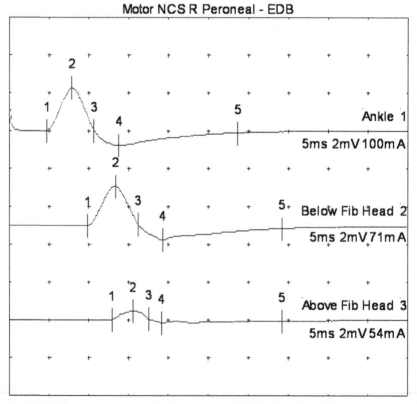

Fig. 4. Peroneal motor nerve conduction study, recording from the EDB showing a partial focal conduction block at the fibular head. This finding signifies segmental demyelination rather than axonal injury and indicates an excellent prognosis (expected recovery within 2–3 months). (*Data from* Refs.[2–4]) (*Courtesy of* V. Fridman MD, Boston, MA.)

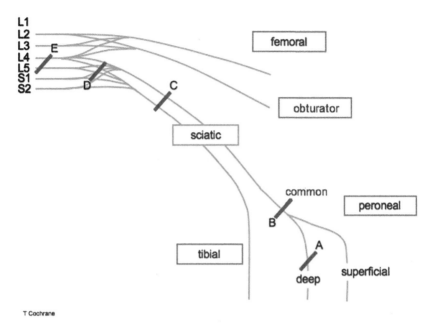

T Cochrane

Fig. 5. Sites of peripheral nerve lesions that may result in foot drop. (*Courtesy of* V. Fridman MD, Boston, MA.)

sampled. In addition, it is often useful to examine the short head of the biceps femoris muscle, which receives innervation from the peroneal division of the sciatic nerve above the knee (and hence proximal to the fibular head). Abnormalities seen in this muscle therefore localize the lesion to the level of the sciatic nerve or more proximally. Distal tibial innervated muscles (such as the medial gastrocnemius or tibialis posterior) are also typically sampled. Involvement of these muscles indicates that the injury extends beyond the distribution of the peroneal nerve and provides further support that the injury is at or proximal to the sciatic nerve. If a conduction block is not clearly shown on the nerve conduction studies, the examiner also has to consider the possibility of an L5 radiculopathy. This condition can be assessed by examining proximal L5 innervated muscles (such as the gluteus medius or tensor fascia lata). If the clinical history and electrical findings suggest the presence of a lumbar radiculopathy, the paraspinal muscles can also be examined in an effort to confirm a preganglionic localization.

The only abnormalities noted on needle EMG in this case were reduced recruitment (a rapid MUAP firing rate with few MUAPs firing) in 2 muscles, the tibialis anterior (deep peroneal nerve), and peroneus longus (superficial peroneal nerve). Involvement of both branches of the peroneal nerve indicates that the lesion lies proximal to the bifurcation of these 2 branches, and must involve the common peroneal nerve (or higher). When taken together with the finding of conduction block seen at the fibular head, a common peroneal neuropathy is confirmed (see site B in **Fig. 5**). The absence of spontaneous activity or alteration of MUAP morphology indicates 1 of 2 possibilities: either the injury is acute (insufficient time for spontaneous activity to appear and for MUAP remodeling to occur) or the lesion is purely demyelinating in nature. We were told that the injury occurred only 7 days before the current study and thus did not expect abnormal spontaneous activity to be present. Given the preservation of the peroneal distal motor amplitude as well as the presence of focal demyelination it is reasonable to postulate that no significant axonal injury was present and that the patient had a good prognosis (recovery within months of injury).[2–4]

Floppy Foot 2

A 44-year-old man presented to the EMG laboratory with foot drop which had begun 1 month previously. He discovered weakness on awakening on the floor after a drinking binge. The nerve conduction study and needle EMG findings in this patient are shown in **Tables 4A** and **4B**.

Interpretation of floppy foot 2: common peroneal neuropathy

This case also shows evidence of a common peroneal neuropathy, and is similar to the previous case but with a few differences (see site B in **Fig. 5**). As in the previous case, abnormalities are confined to the distribution of the common peroneal nerve. However, in this case the peroneal CMAP amplitude is reduced after stimulation at all sites, without an identified conduction block, suggesting a severe axonal injury. The superficial peroneal sensory response is also absent, providing support for a post-ganglionic injury. As mentioned earlier, we typically assume SNAPs to be normal in root injuries because the dorsal root ganglia (and the sensory neuron cell bodies contained within) reside in the intervertebral foramen, usually protected from herniated disks. However, the dorsal root ganglia can occasionally be positioned more proximally in the spinal canal, where they may be vulnerable to injury. A reduction in the superficial peroneal SNAP has specifically been described in the context of L5 radiculopathies, and therefore an abnormality in this nerve conduction study does not definitively confirm a postganglionic localization.[5]

The needle examination reveals abnormalities in the same 2 muscles as the previous case, with the added finding of abnormal spontaneous activity. This finding independently confirms the presence of axonal disruption and indicates that the injury is at least a few weeks old. However, the absence of alterations in MUAP morphology implies that the injury is less than several months old.

Two further points should be made. Although the presence of focal conduction block in floppy foot 1 allowed for a precise localization of the lesion along the peroneal nerve, in this case of an axonal lesion without focal conduction block, it was not possible to confidently localize the lesion to a precise site along the nerve. The lesion could have occurred anywhere at or proximal to the divergence of the deep and

Table 4A
Nerve conduction study findings in patient with floppy foot 2

Nerve	Latency	Amplitude	Velocity
Peroneal motor (EDB)			
Ankle	NL	↓↓↓	
Below fibular head	NL	↓↓↓	NL
Above fibular head	NL	↓↓↓	NL
Tibial motor (AH)			
Ankle	NL	NL	
Knee	NL	NL	NL
Sural sensory	NL	NL	NL
Superficial peroneal sensory	Absent	Absent	Absent

Abbreviations: NL, normal; ↓↓↓, severely reduced.

Table 4B Needle EMG findings in patient with floppy foot 2			
Muscle	Spontaneous	MUAP Morphology	Recruitment
Medial gastrocnemius	NL	NL	NL
Tibialis posterior	NL	NL	NL
Tibialis anterior	↑	NL	↓↓↓
Peroneus longus	↑	NL	↓↓↓
Short head of biceps femoris	NL	NL	NL
Gluteus medius	NL	NL	NL
Vastus medialis	NL	NL	NL

Abbreviations: NL, normal; ↑, presence of abnormal spontaneous activity; ↓↓↓, severely reduced.

superficial peroneal branches. For this reason, a more extensive needle examination to evaluate for evidence of a more proximal lesion was especially important. Muscles innervated by the sciatic nerve (eg, short head of the biceps) as well as proximal muscles that share the same root innervation with the 2 affected muscles (eg, gluteus medius) were sampled. Because needle EMG abnormalities were not observed in the short head of the biceps, a muscle supplied by the peroneal division of the sciatic nerve above the fibular head, one can argue that this pattern of EMG findings is consistent with an injury at the fibular head. However, one must be cautious in interpreting electrodiagnostic data in this situation, because proximal injuries can mimic more distal ones through selective injury to individual nerve fascicles. It is important to incorporate the clinical history and physical examination findings, which in this individual strongly suggested a common peroneal neuropathy at the fibular head.

Both cases 1 and 2 reflect common peroneal neuropathies at the fibular head (see location B in **Fig. 5**). However, because of the severe axonal disruption identified in case 2, the prognosis for recovery was less favorable.

Peroneal neuropathy is the most common mononeuropathy in the lower extremity. The most common mechanism of injury is compression at the fibular head. Other causes of peroneal neuropathy include trauma, application of tight casts, and improper positioning during surgical procedures. Repeated stretch injury can occur with frequent leg crossing and rapid weight loss can make the nerve vulnerable to minor trauma or compression. Less common causes include ischemic injury in the setting of mononeuritis multiplex and compressive masses such as nerve tumors or ganglion cysts.[2,4]

Floppy Foot 3

A 23-year-old man presented to the EMG laboratory with foot drop, which had begun when he sustained a gunshot injury to the posterior thigh 5 weeks previously. The nerve conduction study and needle EMG findings in this patient are shown in **Tables 5A** and **5B**.

Interpretation of floppy foot 3: sciatic neuropathy

In this case, the cause of the foot drop was an injury to the sciatic nerve (see site C in **Fig. 5**). Similar to cases 1 and 2, abnormalities were recorded in the peroneal CMAPs. However, the motor conduction studies now showed reduced amplitudes of the tibial CMAPs, implying a lesion proximal to the bifurcation of the peroneal and tibial nerves in the region of the knee (ie, sciatic nerve or higher). The reduced SNAPs implied a postganglionic injury involving nerves or plexus. In addition to the absent superficial

Table 5A			
Nerve conduction study findings in patient with floppy foot 3			
Nerve	**Latency**	**Amplitude**	**Velocity**
Peroneal motor (EDB)			
Ankle	Absent	Absent	
Below fibular head	Absent	Absent	Absent
Above fibular head	Absent	Absent	Absent
Tibial motor (AH)			
Ankle	NL	↓↓	
Knee	NL	↓↓	NL
Sural sensory	Absent	Absent	Absent
Superficial peroneal sensory	Absent	Absent	Absent

Abbreviations: NL, normal; ↓↓, moderately reduced.

peroneal SNAP, the sural SNAP was also unobtainable, which also indicated a lesion outside the distribution of the peroneal nerve and suggested a more proximal site of injury (sciatic nerve or sacral plexus).

In addition to showing abnormalities in the peroneal nerve innervated muscles, the needle examination now revealed findings in nonperoneal muscles (the medial gastrocnemius and tibialis posterior). These observations provided independent confirmatory data for the presence of a more proximal injury localized to the sciatic nerve or higher. The abnormalities noted in the short head of the biceps also supported this diagnosis. Based on these results, a sciatic neuropathy or more proximal lumbosacral plexopathy were possibilities. The normal needle examination of the gluteus medius might have supported a sciatic neuropathy as opposed to a plexopathy, but negative findings must be interpreted with caution. If a plexopathy was strongly suspected, other hip girdle muscles, such as the tensor fascia lata and gluteus maximus, might have been examined.

In this case, given the clinical history, a sciatic neuropathy was strongly suspected. The peroneal division of the sciatic nerve was disproportionately injured, accounting for the clinical presentation of a foot drop (mimicking a peroneal nerve injury). Such fascicular injuries are commonly seen after sciatic nerve trauma in adults and have recently also been described in children.[6–8] Based on the needle EMG findings, the injury would be classified as subacute. Because of the observation of severe axon loss, prognosis was likely unfavorable.

Table 5B			
Needle EMG findings in patient with floppy foot 2			
Muscle	**Spontaneous**	**MUAP Morphology**	**Recruitment**
Medial gastrocnemius	↑	NL	↓
Tibialis posterior	↑	NL	↓
Tibialis anterior	↑	None	None
Short head of biceps femoris	↑	None	None
Vastus medialis	NL	NL	NL
Gluteus medius	NL	NL	NL
Lumbar paraspinals	NL	–	–

Abbreviations: NL, normal; ↑, presence of abnormal spontaneous activity; ↓, mildly reduced.

Sciatic neuropathies are uncommon. Partial injuries to the nerve are more common than complete ones. The most common cause of sciatic neuropathy is retroperitoneal or pelvic bleeding, which occurs most commonly in patients who have undergone surgery or are being treated with anticoagulants. The proximity of the sciatic nerve to the posterior aspect of the hip joint makes it especially vulnerable after hip surgery. Less common causes include nerve ischemia (as seen in mononeuritis multiplex), nerve tumors, and vascular malformations.[4,6–8]

Floppy Foot 4

A 72-year-old woman presented to the EMG laboratory with foot drop, which had occurred 3 months previously after hip surgery for a pelvic fracture. The nerve conduction study and needle EMG findings in this patient are shown in **Tables 6A** and **6B**.

Interpretation of floppy foot 4: sacral plexopathy

This study is similar to case 3 and the same comments apply (see site D in **Fig. 5**). However, case 4 is different in 2 respects. First, in addition to all of the abnormal muscles recorded in case 3, the needle examination also showed abnormalities in the gluteus medius. The gluteus medius is supplied by the superior gluteal nerve, which originates proximal to the sciatic nerve. Therefore, this finding implicated a lesion at the level of the plexus or roots. The abnormal SNAPs and normal paraspinal muscle examination supported a postganglionic (ie, plexus) localization. Second, there had been remodeling of the MUAPs in the form of high-amplitude, long-duration units. This finding implied an injury that was at least several months old.

As in case 3, those fibers destined to form the peroneal nerve more distally were disproportionately affected. This situation is commonly seen in plexus injuries. In both case 3 and case 4, the patients presented with a foot drop simulating a peroneal neuropathy. This situation once again shows that proximal injury can mimic distal mononeuropathies by disproportionately affecting specific nerve fascicles.

Floppy Foot 5

A 46-year-old man suffered sudden back pain on lifting a couch. Three days later he developed a mild foot drop, which did not improve over the ensuing month. The nerve conduction study and needle EMG findings in this patient are shown in **Tables 7A** and **7B**.

| **Table 6A** ||||
| **Nerve conduction study findings in patient with floppy foot 4** ||||
Nerve	Latency	Amplitude	Velocity
Peroneal motor (EDB)			
Ankle	Absent	Absent	
Below fibular head	Absent	Absent	Absent
Above fibular head	Absent	Absent	Absent
Tibial motor (AH)			
Ankle	NL	↓	
Knee	NL	↓	NL
Sural sensory	Absent	Absent	Absent
Superficial peroneal sensory	Absent	Absent	Absent

Abbreviations: NL, normal; ↓, mildly reduced.

Table 6B
Needle EMG findings in patient with floppy foot 4

Muscle	Spontaneous	MUAP Morphology	Recruitment
Medial gastrocnemius	↑	↑	↓↓↓
Tibialis posterior	↑	↑	↓↓↓
Tibialis anterior	↑	None	None
Short head of biceps femoris	↑	None	None
Gluteus medius	↑	↑	↓↓
Vastus medialis	NL	NL	NL
Lumbar paraspinals	NL	–	–

Abbreviations: NL, normal; ↑, presence of abnormal spontaneous activity; ↓↓, moderately reduced; ↓↓↓, severely reduced.

Interpretation of floppy foot 5: L5 radiculopathy

In this case, the motor and sensory conduction studies were normal. The needle examination revealed findings in 2 distal muscles supplied by different nerves: the tibialis anterior muscle (peroneal nerve) and the tibialis posterior muscle (tibial nerve). As discussed earlier, this finding argues for a more proximal lesion localized to the sciatic nerve or higher. The normal SNAPs favored a preganglionic (ie, root) localization and the abnormal needle EMG examination of the paraspinal muscles supported this (see site E in **Fig. 5**). The sparing of the gluteus medius muscle might have been the result of fascicular sparing, and in some cases, particularly if abnormalities are not identified in the paraspinals, needle examination of another proximal L5 muscle such as the tensor fascia lata may be helpful to support a root lesion. The presence of abnormal spontaneous activity but normal MUAP morphology indicated an injury older than several weeks but younger than several months.

CLINICAL VIGNETTES: THE BUCKLING KNEE

Another common referral to the electrodiagnostic laboratory is the patient with quadriceps weakness and knee instability. Such patients often buckle when attempting to bear weight on the affected limb. Causes of quadriceps weakness include injuries localized to the femoral nerve, lumbar plexus, or upper lumbar to midlumbar roots.

Table 7A
Nerve conduction study findings in patient with floppy foot 5

Nerve	Latency	Amplitude	Velocity
Peroneal motor (EDB)			
Ankle	NL	NL	
Below fibular head	NL	NL	NL
Above fibular head	NL	NL	NL
Tibial motor (AH)			
Ankle	NL	NL	
Knee	NL	NL	NL
Sural sensory	NL	NL	NL
Superficial peroneal	NL	NL	NL

Abbreviation: NL, normal.

Table 7B
Needle EMG findings in patient with floppy foot 5

Muscle	Spontaneous	MUAP Morphology	Recruitment
Medial gastrocnemius	NL	NL	NL
Tibialis posterior	↑	NL	↓↓↓
Tibialis anterior	↑	NL	↓↓↓
Gluteus medius	NL	NL	NL
Vastus medialis	NL	NL	NL
Lumbar paraspinals	↑	–	–

Abbreviations: NL, normal; ↑, presence of abnormal spontaneous activity; ↓↓↓, severely reduced.

The goal of the electrophysiologic evaluation is to distinguish among these possibilities. In contrast to the evaluation of foot drop, fewer commonly performed nerve conduction studies are used to evaluate patients with a buckling knee. The nerve conduction studies that can be used to evaluate the femoral nerve include the femoral motor study recording from the rectus femoris and the saphenous sensory study. Both of these responses are technically more challenging to perform and often generate small-amplitude responses. It is therefore essential to study the contralateral side for comparison. A convincing unilateral abnormality of the saphenous SNAP suggests a lesion involving the femoral nerve or the lumbosacral plexus. In cases in which there is strong suspicion for an upper lumbar plexopathy the lateral femoral cutaneous nerve sensory response can also be obtained. Like the saphenous SNAP, the lateral femoral cutaneous sensory response often has a low amplitude, requiring careful side-to-side comparison studies for accurate interpretation.

To exclude the possibility of more widespread injury (lumbosacral polyradiculopathy or panplexopathy) the routine lower extremity motor conduction studies are typically performed (peroneal and tibial CMAPs and sural SNAP). With an isolated injury to the femoral nerve these studies are expected to be normal.

The needle examination of suspected femoral neuropathy begins with the quadriceps muscles and the iliopsoas muscle. The latter allows for localization either distal or proximal to the inguinal ligament. If abnormalities are detected, the hip adductors are sampled to evaluate for a more proximal localization (nerve root or upper plexus).

The pattern of findings on nerve conduction studies and needle EMG in different localizations of patients with a buckling knee is summarized in **Table 8**.

Buckling Knee 1

A 31-year-old woman had been experiencing frequent falls after the delivery of her first child. She presented to the EMG laboratory 6 weeks after symptom onset. The nerve conduction study and needle EMG findings in this patient are shown in **Tables 9A** and **9B**.

Interpretation of buckling knee 1: femoral neuropathy
In this case, the only abnormality recorded in the nerve conduction studies was an absent saphenous SNAP, which implies a postganglionic injury located distal to the root (eg, at the level of the plexus or femoral nerve). Femoral motor nerve conduction studies were not performed. The needle examination showed subacute abnormalities restricted to muscles supplied by the distal femoral nerve, below the inguinal ligament (site B in **Fig. 6**). Abnormalities in the iliopsoas muscle would have suggested a proximal femoral injury, because the branch to the iliopsoas muscle arises proximal to the

Table 8				
EMG localization of the buckling knee				
	Femoral Distal	Femoral Proximal	Plexus	L2–L4 Root
Abnormal nerve conduction study				
Femoral, motor	X	X	X	X
Saphenous sensory	X	X	X	
Lateral femoral cutaneous, sensory			X	
EMG abnormalities				
Vastus medialis	X	X	X	X
Vastus lateralis	X	X	X	X
Iliopsoas		X	X	X
Adductors			X	X
Lumbar Paraspinals				X

inguinal ligament. Had abnormalities been present in the hip adductors or tibialis anterior muscle, a more proximal localization (such as a lumbar plexopathy) would have been considered.

Although not shown in this case, femoral motor nerve conduction studies can also be performed by stimulating at the level of the groin and recording at the rectus femoris muscle (see **Fig. 1**). The nerve travels deep at this location and supramaximal stimulation can be difficult to achieve, often requiring stimulation with a monopolar needle. Side-to-side comparison studies are essential to proper interpretation of the study. The femoral compound muscle potential amplitude (CMAP) can provide an objective measure of the degree of axonal loss and can aid in prognostication. Patients with a femoral CMAP 50% of greater of the contralateral side show clinical improvement within 1 year.[9]

Femoral neuropathies are rare. Common causes include trauma and surgical procedures. In particular, the lithotomy position can increase the risk of nerve stretch or compression. Hematomas resulting from catheter placement into the femoral artery or retroperitoneal bleeding can also compress the nerve. Mononeuritis multiplex, mass lesions, and neoplastic nerve infiltration are other diagnostic considerations.

Table 9A			
Nerve conduction study findings in patient with buckling knee 1			
Nerve	Latency	Amplitude	Velocity
Peroneal motor (EDB)			
Ankle	NL	NL	
Below fibular head	NL	NL	NL
Above fibular head	NL	NL	NL
Tibial motor (AH)			
Ankle	NL	NL	
Knee	NL	NL	NL
Sural sensory	NL	NL	NL
Saphenous sensory	Absent	Absent	Absent
Saphenous sensory asymptomatic side	NL	NL	NL

Abbreviation: NL, normal.

Table 9B
Needle EMG findings in patient with buckling knee 1

Muscle	Spontaneous	MUAP Morphology	Recruitment
Medial gastrocnemius	NL	NL	NL
Tibialis anterior	NL	NL	NL
Vastus lateralis	↑	NL	↓↓↓
Vastus medialis	↑	NL	↓↓↓
Adductors	NL	NL	NL
Iliopsoas	NL	NL	NL
Lumbar paraspinals	NL	–	–

Abbreviations: NL, normal; ↑, presence of abnormal spontaneous activity; ↓↓↓, severely reduced.

Given the proximal origin of the nerve, nerve injury related to intra-abdominal disease should be considered.

Buckling Knee 2

A 56-year-old woman presented to the EMG laboratory with knee weakness. The symptoms had begun 2 weeks previously, soon after she began treatment with Coumadin for a deep venous thrombosis. The nerve conduction study and needle EMG findings in this patient are shown in **Tables 10A** and **10B**.

Interpretation of buckling knee 2: lumbar plexopathy

The nerve conduction studies reveal absent saphenous and lateral femoral cutaneous SNAPs, implying a postganglionic injury (nerve or plexus). Whereas the absent saphenous SNAP would have been consistent with a femoral nerve lesion (as in case 1), the

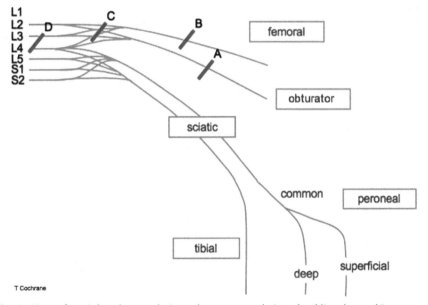

Fig. 6. Sites of peripheral nerve lesions that may result in a buckling knee. (*Courtesy of* V. Fridman MD, Boston, MA.)

Table 10A			
Nerve conduction study findings in patient with buckling knee 2			
Nerve	Latency	Amplitude	Velocity
Peroneal motor (EDB)			
Ankle	NL	NL	
Below fibular head	NL	NL	NL
Above fibular head	NL	NL	NL
Tibial motor (AH)			
Ankle	NL	NL	
Knee	NL	NL	NL
Sural sensory	NL	NL	NL
Saphenous sensory	Absent	Absent	Absent
Lateral femoral cutaneous sensory	Absent	Absent	Absent

Abbreviation: NL, normal.

absent lateral femoral cutaneous sensory response suggested a more proximal lesion because this nerve originates from the posterior divisions of the second and third lumbar roots, outside the distribution of the femoral nerve.

The needle examination, in addition to showing abnormalities in muscles supplied by the distal femoral nerve (as in case 1), showed abnormalities in the iliopsoas muscle. In addition, involvement of the adductor brevis (which is supplied by the obturator nerve) implied a more proximal injury. The abnormal muscles are supplied by different peripheral nerves, but they share a common myotome (L3/L4). Therefore, possible localizations include an L3/L4 radiculopathy versus a lumbar plexopathy. The absent SNAPs and normal paraspinal muscle needle EMG examination favored a plexopathy (see site C in **Fig. 6**). The history of Coumadin use in this case further raised concern for a compressive hematoma.

As illustrated in this case, lumbar plexopathies involve fibers destined to form both the obturator and femoral nerves more distally. Isolated lesions of the obturator nerve (see location A in **Fig. 6**) are rare and most often occur within the context of traumatic injury, pelvic surgery, or malignancy. Patients with obturator nerve injuries often present with medial thigh pain rather than frank sensory loss or weakness.[10,11] Needle examination in an isolated obturator neuropathy reveals abnormalities in the thigh

Table 10B			
Needle EMG findings in patient with buckling knee 2			
Muscle	Spontaneous	MUAP Morphology	Recruitment
Medial gastrocnemius	NL	NL	NL
Tibialis anterior	NL	NL	NL
Vastus lateralis	↑	None	None
Vastus medialis	↑	None	None
Adductors	↑	None	None
Iliopsoas	↑	NL	↓↓
Glut medius	NL	NL	NL
Lumbar paraspinals	NL	–	–

Abbreviations: NL, normal; ↑, presence of abnormal spontaneous activity; ↓↓, moderately reduced.

adductor muscles only, with a normal examination of the femoral innervated L3/4 muscles and lumbar paraspinal muscles. The adductor magnus muscle receives supply from both the obturator and the sciatic nerves, whereas the adductor longus and adductor brevis are innervated solely by the obturator nerve. For this reason the adductor longus and brevis are the preferred muscles for examination.

Buckling Knee 3

A 50-year-old electromyographer slipped on a rock while portaging a canoe. He experienced sudden-onset back tightness and a day later developed severe leg pain. In the subsequent days he began to have frequent falls and referred himself to the EMG laboratory for an evaluation. The nerve conduction study and needle EMG findings in this patient are shown in **Tables 11A** and **11B**.

Interpretation of buckling knee 3: L3/4 radiculopathy

Following the logic in previous discussions, involvement of the vastus lateralis and adductor brevis implicated a proximal lesion at the level of the lumbar plexus or L3/L4 root. The normal SNAPs and abnormal paraspinal needle EMG examination suggested a preganglionic (root) injury. The needle examination findings were consistent with a subacute radiculopathy.

CLINICAL VIGNETTE: THE PAINFUL FOOT

A 45-year-old woman presented with an insidious onset of foot pain. She had sustained an ankle fracture 5 years before the onset of her symptoms. The patient was referred to the EMG laboratory for evaluation of TTS (see site D in **Fig. 6**). The nerve conduction study findings in this patient are shown in **Table 12**.

Interpretation of Painful Foot: Distal Tibial Neuropathy (TTS)

TTS refers to entrapment of the posterior tibial nerve under the flexor retinaculum at the ankle. It is at this point that the tibial nerve divides into its 3 terminal branches: the calcaneal nerve, which supplies sensation to the heel; the medial plantar branch, which innervates the abductor hallucis, flexor digitorum brevis, and flexor hallucis brevis muscles and supplies sensation to the medial sole; and the lateral plantar nerve, which supplies sensation to the lateral sole and innervates the adductor hallucis, abductor digiti quinti pedis, flexor digiti quinti pedis, and the interossei muscles.

Table 11A
Nerve conduction study findings in patient with buckling knee 3

Nerve	Latency	Amplitude	Velocity
Peroneal motor (EDB)			
Ankle	NL	NL	
Below fibular head	NL	NL	NL
Above fibular head	NL	NL	NL
Tibial motor (AH)			
Ankle	NL	NL	
Knee	NL	NL	NL
Sural sensory	NL	NL	NL
Saphenous sensory	NL	NL	NL

Abbreviation: NL, normal.

Table 11B
Needle EMG findings in patient with buckling knee 3

Muscle	Spontaneous	MUAP Morphology	Recruitment
Medial gastrocnemius	NL	NL	NL
Tibialis anterior	NL	NL	NL
Vastus lateralis	↑	NL	NL
Adductors	↑	NL	NL
Iliopsoas	NL	NL	NL
Lumbar paraspinals	↑	–	–

Abbreviations: NL, normal; ↑, presence of abnormal spontaneous activity.

Compression at the tarsal tunnel can cause injury to any of the 3 terminal branches in isolation or combination.

TTS is rare. More common causes of focal foot pain include arthritic changes, ligamentous injury, plantar fasciitis, or a polyneuropathy (when the symptoms are bilateral). The electrophysiologic evaluation of possible TTS focuses on excluding injury at other sites within the peripheral nervous system such as the S1 nerve roots, the sacral plexus, or the sciatic nerve, because injury at all of these locations can present with similar symptoms. A proximal tibial neuropathy can also be considered, although the tarsal tunnel is the most common site of tibial mononeuropathy.[12]

In this case, all of the routine nerve conduction studies were normal. In addition to the routine tibial CMAP recording at the abductor hallucis muscles, a motor study recording at the abductor digiti minimi pedis was also performed and found to be normal. This study was performed to identify slowing of the distal motor latency, which

Table 12
Nerve conduction study findings in the patient with painful foot

Nerve	Latency	Amplitude	Velocity
Peroneal motor (EDB)			
Ankle	NL	NL	
Below fibular head	NL	NL	NL
Above fibular head	NL	NL	NL
Tibial motor (AH)			
Ankle	NL	NL	
Knee	NL	NL	NL
Tibial motor (ADMP)			
Ankle	NL	NL	
Knee	NL	NL	NL
Sural sensory	NL	NL	NL
Superficial peroneal sensory	NL	NL	NL
Medial plantar	↑	↓↓	
Lateral plantar	↑	↓↓	
Medial plantar asymptomatic side	NL	NL	
Lateral plantar asymptomatic side	NL	NL	

Abbreviations: ADMP, abductor digiti minimi pedis; AH, abductor hallucis; NL, normal; ↑, presence of abnormal spontaneous activity; ↓↓, moderately reduced.

provides support for a distal tibial neuropathy. The asymmetry in the amplitudes and latencies in the mixed medial and lateral plantar nerve conduction studies compared with the asymptomatic sides helped to confirm the suspected diagnosis of distal tibial neuropathy at the level of the tarsal tunnel. Mixed nerve studies of the lateral and medial plantar nerves (see **Fig. 2**) are believed to be more sensitive than tibial motor conduction studies in confirming TTS.[12] The plantar mixed nerve studies are used in a similar fashion to the mixed nerve studies used in the evaluation of median neuropathies at the wrist. Mixed plantar responses are obtained by stimulating the medial and lateral aspects of the sole of the foot while recording posterior to the medial malleolus (at the location of the tibial nerve).

In this case the examiner did not choose to perform a needle examination to confirm the suspected diagnosis of a distal tibial neuropathy because this had already been established by nerve conduction studies. In cases in which TTS is strongly suspected and nerve conduction studies are unrevealing a needle EMG of the abductor hallucis and abductor quinti pedis muscles can be performed.[12] However, EMG abnormalities of these muscles can also result from fascicular lesions at more proximal locations.

The most common cause of TTS is trauma resulting in ankle fractures or dislocations. The symptoms often develop years after the initial injury. Rheumatoid arthritis has also been reported as a risk factor.

SUMMARY

The cases described in this article show the role of electrodiagnostic testing in the evaluation of lower extremity mononeuropathies. When used in conjunction with the patient's clinical history and physical examination, nerve conduction studies and needle EMG can aid in determining whether a lower limb mononeuropathy is present (and exclude a root or plexus lesion), determine localization along the nerve involved, assess the underlying pathophysiology of nerve injury (axonal vs demyelinating), and determine the timing of the injury (acute, subacute, or chronic). The absence of abnormalities must be interpreted with caution when determining the site of injury, because fascicular lesions are common. Technical limitations as well as the relative timing of study to symptom onset must always be considered for accurate interpretation.

ACKNOWLEDGMENTS

We would like to thank Thomas Cochrane, MD (Assistant Professor, Harvard Medical School) for providing the illustrations presented in this chapter.

REFERENCES

1. Kang PB, Preston DC, Raynor EM. Involvement of superficial peroneal sensory nerve in common peroneal neuropathy. Muscle Nerve 2005;31:725–9.
2. Katirji B, Wilbourn AJ. Common peroneal mononeuropathy: a clinical and electrophysiologic study of 116 lesions. Neurology 1988;38:1723–8.
3. Masakado Y, Kawakami M, Suzuki K, et al. Clinical neurophysiology in the diagnosis of peroneal nerve palsy. Keio J Med 2008;57:84–9.
4. Katirji B. Electrodiagnostic approach to the patient with suspected mononeuropathy of the lower extremity. Neurol Clin 2002;20:479–501.
5. Levin KH. L5 radiculopathy with reduced superficial peroneal sensory responses: intraspinal and extraspinal causes. Muscle Nerve 1998;21:3–7.

6. Sunderland S. The relative susceptibility to injury of the medial and lateral popliteal divisions of the sciatic nerve. Br J Surg 1953;41:300–2.

7. Srinivasan J, Ryan MM, Escolar DM, et al. Pediatric sciatic neuropathies: a 30-year prospective study. Neurology 2011;76:976–80.

8. Yuen EC, So YT, Olney RK. The electrophysiological features of sciatic neuropathy in 100 patients. Muscle Nerve 1995;18:414–20.

9. Kuntzer T, van Melle G, Regli F. Clinical and prognostic features in unilateral femoral neuropathies. Muscle Nerve 1997;20:205–11.

10. Sorenson EJ, Chen JJ, Daube JR. Obturator neuropathy: causes and outcome. Muscle Nerve 2002;25:605–7.

11. Busis N. Femoral and obturator neuropathies. Neurol Clin 1999;17(3):633–53.

12. Atul T, Patel MD, Kenneth Gaines MD, et al. Usefulness of electrodiagnostic techniques in the evaluation of suspected tarsal tunnel syndrome: an evidence-based review. Muscle Nerve 2005;32:236–40.

Electrodiagnosis of Peripheral Neuropathy

Mark A. Ross, MD

KEYWORDS

- Peripheral neuropathy • Nerve conduction studies
- Electromyography • Axonal • Demyelinating
- Temporal dispersion • Conduction block • Polyneuropathy

The evaluation of the patient with suspected peripheral neuropathy involves consideration of multiple sources of information, including the clinical history, neurologic examination, electrodiagnostic (EDX) studies, and laboratory studies. In some cases genetic studies, radiographic studies, and tissue biopsy are necessary to diagnose the specific etiology of the peripheral neuropathy. Although the findings on the EDX study may occasionally suggest a specific etiology, more often the study helps to better characterize and categorize the features of the neuropathy rather than identify the cause. Thus, the EDX study serves as a critical initial diagnostic study for all patients suspected of having peripheral neuropathy because it provides multiple important clues about several aspects of the patient's neuropathy. The roles of EDX studies are discussed here and are summarized in **Box 1**.

CONFIRMATION OF PERIPHERAL NERVE DISEASE

One of the most useful roles of the EDX study is to confirm abnormalities demonstrated on the neurologic examination and to serve as support for the clinical suspicion of neuropathy. In addition, the EDX study may reveal abnormalities that cannot be detected on physical examination alone. For example, the EDX study may show slowed conduction velocities in a patient with subjective sensory loss but a normal neurologic examination, or show fibrillation potentials or motor unit potential abnormalities in muscles that are not weak on clinical examination. It is estimated that a muscle does not become weak until the supplying nerve loses 50% of its axons. However, fibrillation potentials can be detected when only a small number of motor axons are lost. The clinical sensory examination involves subjective reporting by the patient, and may be unreliable in some patients. Nerve conduction studies (NCS) provide objective quantified measurements of sensory nerve conduction and, when

EMG Laboratory, Department of Neurology, Mayo Clinic Arizona, 13400 East, Shea Boulevard, Scottsdale, AZ 85259, USA
E-mail address: ross.mark@mayo.edu

Neurol Clin 30 (2012) 529–549
doi:10.1016/j.ncl.2011.12.013
0733-8619/12/$ – see front matter © 2012 Elsevier Inc. All rights reserved.

neurologic.theclinics.com

Box 1
Roles of electrodiagnostic studies in evaluating peripheral neuropathy

Confirmation and localization

    Confirm peripheral nerve disease

    Localize nerve disease

Assessment of fiber-type involvement

    Motor

    Large sensory

    Small fiber: sensory and autonomic

Determining the distribution of nerve involvement

    Distal symmetric

    Polyradiculoneuropathy

    Multiple mononeuropathies (mononeuropathy multiplex)

    Upper extremity predominant

Identifying the underlying pathophysiologic process

    Axon loss

    Demyelination

    Mixed

    Channelopathy

Determining the severity of fiber involvement

    Mild

    Moderate

    Severe

Monitoring recovery or treatment effect

---

abnormal, help to confirm a disorder involving the peripheral nerves. The EDX study may also be normal and may serve to argue against the possibility of peripheral nerve disease as the basis of the patient's symptoms. However, interpretation of a normal EDX study must be made carefully in light of the patient's clinical presentation.

The approach to localization of abnormalities on EDX studies involves combined interpretation of the results of NCS and the needle electromyography (EMG) examination. The combination of findings on sensory NCS, motor NCS, and needle EMG can help to confirm a peripheral neuropathy and assess for other potential sites of localization.

Sensory Nerve Conduction Studies

Sensory nerve studies are particularly helpful for localization to the peripheral nerve, because an abnormal sensory nerve action potential (SNAP) indicates disease that is localized at or distal to the dorsal root ganglion. Reduced amplitude of SNAPs in multiple upper and lower extremity nerves is a reliable indicator of peripheral nerve disease. Sensory NCS are also abnormal with disease localized to the brachial or lumbosacral plexus regions, but are typically spared when nerve disease is localized to the nerve root level. For example, bilateral L5-S1 radiculopathies may cause distal weakness and sensory loss with reduced or absent ankle reflexes, mimicking a distal symmetric peripheral neuropathy. If a patient with distal lower extremity sensory symptoms has normal sensory NCS, the possibility of multiple lumbosacral radiculopathies or a polyradiculopathy should be considered.

Motor Nerve Conduction Studies

Reduced amplitude of the compound muscle action potential (CMAP) is also seen in peripheral nerve disease, but is much less specific for peripheral nerve disease than reduced-amplitude SNAPs. The CMAP may be reduced with other conditions including anterior horn cell disease, radiculopathy, plexopathy, neuromuscular transmission disorders, and myopathy. However, motor NCS may show several other abnormalities besides reduced-amplitude CMAPs, which help to localize the disease process to the peripheral nerve. Examples include prolonged distal latencies, slowed conduction velocities, temporal dispersion, conduction block, and F wave abnormalities, which indicate a disorder involving the peripheral nerves and are not typically seen in other locations. These features are discussed in detail in the section on demyelinating neuropathy.

Needle EMG

The needle EMG findings can also help with localization of peripheral nerve disease. Abnormalities that suggest a neurogenic process include fibrillation potentials and enlarged, complex motor unit potentials with reduced recruitment. The distribution of abnormalities on the needle examination helps to define the pattern of peripheral nerve disease. The typical neuropathy patterns are discussed in the section on distribution of peripheral nerve disease.

DETERMINATION OF TYPE OF NERVE FIBER INVOLVED

Peripheral nerves contain multiple specific fiber types including motor fibers, large sensory fibers carrying joint position and proprioceptive information, small sensory fibers carrying pain and temperature modalities, and autonomic fibers. Peripheral neuropathies may selectively involve one fiber type or, more commonly, simultaneously involve multiple types of nerve fibers. In cases where multiple types of nerve fibers are involved, there may be one fiber type that is most predominantly affected. The pattern of fiber-type involvement can help to suggest etiology of the neuropathy, because certain disorders are known for their fiber-type predilection.[1] **Table 1** lists selected causes of peripheral neuropathy by pattern of fiber-type involvement. This listing is intended to be illustrative but not inclusive, because of the vast number of causes of peripheral neuropathy. Some disorders that cause neuropathy may manifest with different, rather than uniform or consistent, clinical patterns of presentation of neuropathy. For example, diabetes can cause a mononeuropathy, multiple mononeuropathies, distal symmetric neuropathy, plexopathy, or a single or multiple root radiculopathy. Other examples of disorders that are well known to produce multiple different patterns of peripheral nerve disease include Guillain-Barré syndrome (GBS), chronic inflammatory demyelinating polyneuropathy (CIDP), Sjögren syndrome, human immunodeficiency virus, and renal disease.

Peripheral neuropathies with severe involvement of large sensory fibers or their ganglia produce a unique clinical picture of sensory ataxia.[2] Disorders that cause sensory ataxic neuropathies are summarized in **Box 2**. The neuropathy involving small sensory fibers may be associated with many disorders and often occurs as an

Table 1		
Etiology of neuropathy suggested by involvement of predominant fiber types		
Motor	**Sensory**	**Autonomic**
Guillain-Barré syndrome	Diabetes	Amyloidosis
CIDP	Uremia	Diabetes
Multifocal motor neuropathy	Alcohol	Guillain-Barré syndrome
Charcot-Marie-Tooth disease	HIV	Porphyria
Myeloma	Paraneoplastic	Hereditary sensory neuropathy
Diabetes	Sjögren syndrome	
Diphtheria	Connective tissue diseases	
	Toxins/medications	
	Vitamin B12 deficiency	

Abbreviations: CIDP, chronic inflammatory demyelinating polyradiculopathy; HIV, human immuno-deficiency virus.

idiopathic condition.[3] Disorders causing a small-fiber sensory neuropathy are summarized in **Box 3**.

The routine NCS and needle EMG examination that are performed as part of a standard electrodiagnostic study evaluate only the large motor and large sensory fibers. Small sensory and autonomic fibers are not assessed with the standard techniques and, therefore, patients with small-fiber neuropathies will typically demonstrate normal EMG studies. The evaluation of the small sensory nerve fibers and autonomic fibers requires additional tests, discussed later.

ASSESSMENT OF THE DISTRIBUTION OF NERVE INVOLVEMENT

The distribution of nerve involvement in the different peripheral neuropathies can be categorized into a few different patterns. Although these patterns can often be defined

Box 2
Disorders causing sensory neuropathy and ataxia
Acute onset
Idiopathic sensory neuropathy
GBS variant
Subacute onset
Paraneoplastic neuropathy
Platinum-based chemotherapy
Sjögren syndrome
Pyridoxine toxicity
Chronic
Chronic idiopathic ataxic neuropathy
Tropical ataxic neuropathy (human T-lymphotropic virus type 1)
Hereditary sensory neuropathies
Mitochondrial neuromyopathy

Box 3
Disorders associated with small-fiber neuropathy pattern

Diabetes mellitus

Impaired glucose tolerance

Alcohol abuse

Antineoplastic agents

Renal failure

Sjögren syndrome

Systemic lupus erythematosus

Sarcoidosis

Monoclonal gammopathy

Hepatitis C virus

Human immunodeficiency virus

Celiac disease

Amyloidosis (hereditary and acquired)

Cancer (paraneoplastic)

Hereditary sensory and autonomic neuropathy

Fabry disease

Tangier disease

---

on clinical grounds, findings on electrodiagnostic studies can confirm the suspected clinical distribution or sometimes identify subtle findings to indicate a pattern not suspected clinically. Defining the pattern of nerve involvement is helpful in categorizing the neuropathy and narrowing the list of possible causes.

Distal Symmetric Pattern

The most common pattern of neuropathy is a distal symmetric pattern whereby the initial symptoms begin symmetrically in the distal lower extremities and the severity of nerve deficits gradually diminishes in the proximal limbs. The electrodiagnostic abnormalities mirror the clinical distribution of symptoms and signs with NCS and needle EMG abnormalities greatest distally.

When the underlying pathophysiology in this pattern is axonal loss, the amplitudes of the lower extremity motor and sensory NCS become reduced. In early stages of neuropathy there may be minimal abnormalities in the nerves of the distal lower extremity, whereas the upper extremity nerve studies remain normal. With more advanced disease, the abnormalities become more severe in the lower extremities and abnormalities are also seen in upper extremity nerves. Although the severity of amplitude loss is often consistent with the severity of the disease, some patients with very low or absent distal responses may only have mild clinical symptoms or findings.

Needle examination demonstrates a distal gradient of abnormalities. Fibrillation potentials and chronic neurogenic motor unit potential changes are typically most severe in distal muscles, such as the intrinsic foot muscles, anterior tibialis, or medial gastrocnemius. In mild cases of peripheral neuropathy, the only abnormalities detected on needle examination may be in the foot muscles. In some cases, the foot muscles may show fibrillation potentials and the distal leg muscles may only show motor unit potential abnormalities. With more severe disease, similar abnormalities may be seen in muscles of the proximal lower extremity and distal upper extremity. Although many patients with a distal symmetric axonal peripheral neuropathy will demonstrate fibrillation potentials, in patients in whom the neuropathy is long-standing and in which reinnervation may be keeping up with denervation, fibrillation potentials may not be present or may only be sparse.

The distal symmetric neuropathy pattern is the most common presentation of neuropathy. Identifying this pattern by EDX testing is helpful for confirming a neuropathy, but because so many conditions produce this pattern, it is of limited help in suggesting the origin of the neuropathy.

Polyradiculoneuropathy

The polyradiculoneuropathy pattern refers to a process with combined involvement of distal and proximal nerves and the nerve roots. The distal involvement may be confluent or multifocal, and symmetric or asymmetric. The proximal involvement may include proximal nerves, nerve roots, or cranial nerves. This pattern of nerve illness may be seen in acquired inflammatory neuropathies such as GBS and CIDP. This pattern also occurs in patients with diabetic peripheral nerve disease, and may occur with other disorders that cause multifocal nerve involvement.

The EDX findings in the polyradiculoneuropathy pattern may initially appear similar to those of a distal symmetric neuropathy. On NCS, the distal CMAP and SNAP amplitudes may be reduced and, in cases of demyelinating polyradiculopathies, the conduction velocities may be slowed with increased temporal dispersion. Although the findings may be symmetric, asymmetry with selective involvement of individual nerves may also occur. The needle EMG demonstrates fibrillation potentials and long-duration motor unit potentials in not only distal limb muscles, as in the distal symmetric neuropathies, but also in proximal limb and paraspinal muscles.

Multiple Mononeuropathies

The pattern of multiple mononeuropathies, also known as mononeuropathy multiplex, represents an important pattern of peripheral nerve disease whereby the neuropathic manifestations occur in the territory of individual nerves, often with a stepwise progression, rather than simultaneously involving distal nerves symmetrically. The underlying disease mechanism typically involves nerve ischemia, nerve infiltration, or multifocal nerve inflammation. Disorders, which are known to commonly manifest with a multiple mononeuropathy pattern, are listed in **Box 4**.

The EDX approach to the evaluation of patients with suspected multiple mononeuropathies involves testing multiple nerves and muscles to demonstrate the multifocal and asymmetric pattern of neuropathy. The abnormal findings on NCS and needle EMG can be localized to an individual nerve territory while a neighboring nerve traveling in the same limb is spared. However, in severe or chronic cases, the stepwise involvement of multiple, bilateral lower extremity nerves over time may result in a clinical picture that is similar to a distal symmetric polyneuropathy. Side-to-side comparison of NCS and needle EMG in the lower extremity may identify subtle differences in the degree of abnormalities within nerves (eg, peroneal more severe than tibial), helping to raise the suspicion of multiple mononeuropathies. Most cases of multiple mononeuropathies produce findings of axonal loss on EDX testing. Exceptions include hereditary neuropathy with liability to pressure palsies (HNPP) or multifocal acquired demyelinating sensory and motor neuropathy (MADSAM).

Box 4
Neuropathies causing a pattern of multiple mononeuropathies

Axon loss

    Vasculitis

    Amyloidosis

    Lymphoma

    Diabetes

    Sarcoidosis

    Leprosy

Demyelination

    CIDP

    GBS

    Multifocal motor neuropathy

    Hereditary liability to pressure palsies

Upper Extremity Predominant Pattern

The vast majority of peripheral neuropathies begin in the lower extremities. When a neuropathy manifests initially or predominantly in the upper extremities, the clinician should immediately recognize that this represents an unusual pattern. When clinical findings are isolated to the upper extremities, EDX should assess for individual upper extremity mononeuropathies, such as carpal tunnel syndrome or an ulnar mononeuropathy, and also explore the lower extremity for abnormalities that are not clinically evident. Generalized disorders that may present with an upper extremity onset pattern of peripheral neuropathy are summarized in **Box 5**.

DEFINING THE PATHOPHYSIOLOGIC PROCESS OF A NEUROPATHY

Peripheral neuropathies may be the result of 2 main pathophysiologic processes: primary loss of axons or primary demyelination. Although either of these processes may be the only pathologic feature, many patients have evidence of a combination of both. The EDX findings can often indicate which type of pathologic process is present; however, there is not always a direct correlation between the suspected pathophysiology on EDX and the findings on nerve biopsy.

Box 5
Disorders causing a predominant neuropathy pattern in the upper extremity

Lead intoxication

Porphyria

Vasculitis

Chronic inflammatory demyelinating neuropathy

Multifocal motor neuropathy

Hereditary liability to pressure palsies

Axon Loss

Axon loss is the most common pathophysiologic process seen in peripheral neuropathies. Axon loss is a general term used to describe the net effect of degeneration of axons, which may be caused by many different underlying causes. The manifestations of axon loss on EDX studies are related to the loss of nerve fibers, and are summarized in **Table 2**. The main finding on NCS in axonal neuropathies is a reduction of the CMAP and SNAP amplitudes, which reflects the loss of motor or sensory axons, respectively. In axonal-loss peripheral neuropathies, there is relative preservation of conduction velocity. However, when axon loss results in a severe loss of many large myelinated, faster-conducting fibers, as revealed by a low-amplitude CMAP, the conduction velocity can also be slowed. Therefore, caution should be taken in interpreting a peripheral neuropathy as demyelinating in the context of low-amplitude CMAPs. The degree of slowing of conduction velocity that distinguishes demyelination from axon loss has been related to the CMAP amplitude. If the CMAP amplitude is greater than 80% of the lower limit of normal, the conduction velocity must be slower than 80% of the lower limit of normal to be considered within the demyelinating range. If the CMAP amplitude is less than 80% of the lower limit of normal, the velocity should be less than 70% of the lower limit of normal to be considered demyelinating.[4] However, when CMAP amplitudes become severely reduced, this rule may not be reliable.

Demyelination

Compared with axon loss, pure or primary demyelination is an uncommon mechanism of peripheral neuropathy. The myelin covering on large myelinated nerve fibers allows for rapid conduction of action potentials via the process of saltatory conduction. When myelin is reduced or absent, the conduction of action potentials is slowed and may even fail. Demyelination may produce several distinctive findings on NCS that are summarized in **Table 2**. Although reduced-amplitude CMAPs and SNAPs are commonly seen with axon-loss neuropathies, reduced amplitude or even absent CMAPs and SNAPs may occur when severe demyelination involves the most distal nerve segments. The demonstration of conduction block is only possible when the most distal nerve segments are relatively free of demyelination.

Conduction velocity slowing
The most common manifestation of demyelination is very slow conduction velocities and prolonged distal latencies, with preservation of the CMAP and SNAP amplitudes.

Table 2
Electrodiagnostic features of axon loss and demyelination

Finding	Axon Loss	Demyelination
Reduced SNAP amplitude	+++	+
Reduced CMAP amplitude	+++	+
Conduction block or increased temporal dispersion	−	+
Prolonged distal latency	± (slight)	+++
Slowed conduction velocities	± (mild)	+++
Prolonged F-wave latency	±	+++
Fibrillation potentials	++	+

As already mentioned, the degree of velocity slowing required for evidence of demyelination is at least 70% to 80% of the lower limit of normal, depending on the CMAP amplitude.

Conduction block

Other NCS features of demyelination include conduction block and temporal dispersion of the CMAP. Conduction block refers to failure of an action potential to propagate through a structurally intact axon. This block occurs as a result of loss of a section of myelin along the nerve, which prevents action potentials from jumping between nodes of Ranvier. Instead, the current in an action potential dissipates in the demyelinated nerve segment. Although the physiologic action potential does not pass beyond the demyelinated segment, if the distal axon is intact and has normal myelin covering, the distal axon may still conduct impulses normally if stimulated electrically. The general NCS finding that establishes conduction block in a motor nerve is a reduced amplitude (and area) of the CMAP with proximal stimulation and relatively large amplitude when the nerve is stimulated distally (**Fig. 1**).

The degree of amplitude difference between proximal and distal sites that is necessary to define conduction block has been debated, and many criteria exist.[5] An inherent difficulty in defining conduction block is the inability to know the degree to which phase cancellation due to temporal dispersion accounts for reduction of the CMAP amplitude obtained with proximal stimulation. For this reason, the duration (time from initial takeoff from baseline to the time of return to baseline of the final negative component) of the CMAP is incorporated into the definition of conduction block. One definition for definite conduction block requires that the increase in the duration of the CMAP obtained with proximal stimulation be less than 30%. The degree of

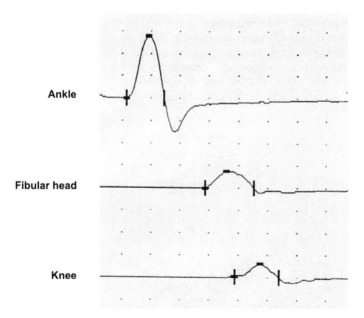

Fig. 1. Conduction block in the peroneal nerve localized below the fibular head stimulation site in an 11-year-old boy with hereditary liability to pressure palsies (with deletion of the PMP-22 gene). The location of conduction block is distal to the more common compression site above the fibular head.

amplitude reduction of the CMAP obtained with proximal stimulation for definite conduction block is greater than 50% for the median and ulnar nerves, and greater than 60% for the peroneal and tibial nerves.[6] To be confident of conduction block, there should be no technical barrier to supramaximal stimulation of the proximal nerve segment such as a very deeply located nerve. Likewise, there should be no physiologic variant such as a Martin Grüber anastomosis that might cause low amplitude with proximal stimulation of the ulnar nerve. When technical factors have clearly been eliminated, a mild, partial conduction block may be present when there is a 20% or greater amplitude reduction between distal and proximal stimulation in some nerves (eg, peroneal, ulnar, and median). In addition, a very mild, partial conduction block may be better identified with short-segment incremental stimulation over 2-cm nerve segments, during which a 10% reduction in CMAP amplitude and area may indicate a mild block.[7]

Increased temporal dispersion

Temporal dispersion is another NCS manifestation of multifocal demyelination, and refers to a prolongation in the CMAP negative peak duration with proximal nerve stimulation in comparison with distal stimulation (**Fig. 2**). Increased temporal dispersion results when action potentials traveling in different axons pass through demyelinated nerve segments and become desynchronized in their arrival at the recording electrodes, resulting in the CMAP having an excessively long duration and an irregularly contoured waveform. Criteria for identifying increased temporal dispersion include a greater than 30% increase in the CMAP negative peak duration obtained with proximal stimulation compared with distal stimulation.[8]

F-wave latency prolongation

Abnormalities of the F wave are common in demyelinating neuropathies. The F wave is a late motor response that occurs from backfiring of antidromically conducted action potentials from the site of motor nerve stimulation. Consequently, the action potentials giving rise to the F wave traverse the most proximal portions of the motor nerve. Therefore, the F wave is a good study method to assess proximal nerve conduction. The specific F-wave abnormalities that are suggestive of a demyelinating neuropathy include marked prolongation of latency, absence or decreased persistence of F waves

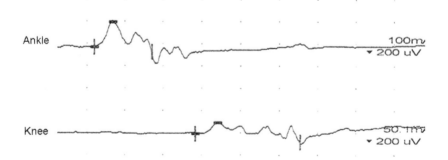

Fig. 2. Temporal dispersion in the peroneal nerve of a 67-year-old man with distal acquired demyelinating symmetric neuropathy. The lower extremity motor conduction velocities were in the range of 12 to 15 m/s. Despite clear EDX evidence of demyelination in motor nerves, he had only mild weakness of toe extensors.

in the context of a preserved distal CMAP amplitude (suggesting a proximal conduction block), and increased chronodispersion.

The degree of F-wave latency prolongation necessary to consider demyelination is in the range of 120% to 150% of the upper limit of normal, or 7 to 8 standard deviations from the normal mean.[4,6] Decreased persistence refers to a decreased number of F waves obtained in a series of 10 to 20 stimuli. The lower limit of normal is estimated to be 50% for the upper extremities, 80% for the tibial nerve, and only about 10% for the peroneal nerve.[6] However, some normal individuals have F-wave persistence values below these levels, therefore low F-wave persistence should be interpreted cautiously and be rarely used as the only criterion for demyelination. Chronodispersion refers to the latency difference between the shortest and longest F-wave values. Excessive chronodispersion might be present at a time when the minimum F-wave latency is still normal, and thus could be an early indicator of demyelination. The published values for the upper limit of normal have varied.[9] A simplified approach is to consider the upper limit of normal for chronodispersion to be 6.5 milliseconds for the upper extremities and 9.5 milliseconds for the lower extremities. It should be noted that abnormal F waves are not specific for demyelinating neuropathy, as F waves can be prolonged with other disorders that affect the proximal nerve or nerve root. Marked prolongation of F waves is not typical in distal symmetric polyneuropathies.

Needle EMG examination

The needle EMG examination may at times provide additional evidence to suggest a demyelinating neuropathy. Most distal muscles that are weak from an axon-loss neuropathy show some fibrillation potentials. The absence of fibrillation potentials in a weak muscle can be a clue that demyelination rather than axon loss is the chief reason for muscle weakness. However, very slowly progressive, chronic axonal neuropathies may have evidence of reinnervation, with large motor unit potentials but minimal or no fibrillations.

Although the presence of fibrillation potentials is a helpful clue that points toward axonal loss, it does not exclude the possibility of a demyelinating neuropathy, as many demyelinating neuropathies may be accompanied by secondary axon loss. In some demyelinating neuropathies characterized by conduction block, the needle EMG will demonstrate reduced recruitment of voluntary motor unit potentials. Another finding that suggests a demyelinating neuropathy is the inability to sustain motor unit potentials during voluntary muscle contraction. This phenomenon, known as rate-dependent conduction block or activity-dependent conduction block, is caused by a failure of demyelinated nerve fibers to sustain high-frequency impulses due to longer refractory periods.[10] The patient generates a brief burst of motor unit potentials that cannot be sustained (**Fig. 3**). However, after a brief rest of several seconds the patient can generate another similar bust of motor unit potentials.

Inherited versus acquired demyelination

Features of a primary demyelinating neuropathy can occur with inherited (eg, Charcot-Marie-Tooth [CMT] type 1a) or acquired (eg, CIDP) neuropathies. The findings on NCS can often help point toward an inherited or acquired process. In inherited demyelinating neuropathies, because the loss or dysfunction of myelin is usually uniform along the nerves the NCS demonstrate relatively uniform conduction velocity slowing or prolongation of distal latency, without increased temporal dispersion or conduction block.

Many EDX criteria for acquired demyelinative neuropathy have been proposed, with variable requirements for conduction block, temporal dispersion, slow conduction

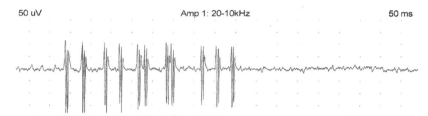

50 uV   Amp 1: 20-10kHz   50 ms

Fig. 3. Activity-dependent conduction block of motor unit potentials. A burst of voluntary motor unit potentials is recorded in the tibialis anterior of a 60-year-old man with multifocal acquired demyelinating sensory and motor neuropathy. He was unable to sustain activation of voluntary motor unit potentials, but after a brief rest he was able to generate another burst.

velocity, prolonged distal latency, and F-wave abnormalities.[4,6,8,11–14] In general, these criteria have required that multiple EDX features of demyelination are present in multiple nerves. Typically the common sites of entrapment neuropathies have been excluded from contributing to the evidence for demyelinative neuropathy. A commonly used set of EDX criteria for demyelinating neuropathy in GBS is shown in **Box 6**.[11] To meet criteria, a patient must have at least 3 of the 4 EDX findings listed in **Box 6**.

Mixed Axon Loss and Demyelination

A third designation of nerve injury represents an intermediate category in which mixed features of axon loss and demyelination are present, but the evidence favoring one category over the other is insufficient to be certain. A recent classification uses the term neuropathic to describe this category of neuropathy.[6] In fact, many peripheral

---

Box 6
EMG criteria for demyelinating neuropathy in GBS

Motor NCV	*Two or More Nerves:*
	CMAP ≥50%: NCV <90% LLN
	CMAP ≤50%: NCV <80% LLN
Motor DL	*Two or More Nerves:*
	CMAP > LLN: >115 ULN
	CMAP < LLN: >125% ULN
CB	*One or More Nerves:*
	P/D CMAP amplitude ratio: <0.7 or
	Unequivocal temporal dispersion
F latency	*One or More Nerves:*
	>125% ULN

Note: 3 of the 4 features must be present.
Abbreviations: CB, conduction block; DL, distal latency; LLN, lower limit of normal; NCV, nerve conduction velocity; P/D, proximal/distal; ULN, upper limit of normal.
Data from Albers JW, Kelly JJ. Acquired inflammatory demyelinating polyneuropathy: clinical and electrodiagnostic features. Muscle Nerve 1989;12:435–51.

neuropathies fall into this category. For example, in many neuropathies there is some reduction in the CMAP and SNAP amplitudes with a moderate degree of conduction velocity slowing that does not meet clear criteria for primary demyelination. In addition, needle EMG demonstrates features of axonal loss with long-duration motor unit potentials, with or without fibrillation potentials.

Channelopathy

Peripheral nerve disease can also be caused by impaired function of sodium or potassium ion channels.[15,16] Several marine toxins may cause rapid onset of neuropathy after seafood ingestion by interfering with sodium ion function. Tetrodotoxin and saxitoxin block sodium channels, and ciguatoxin causes prolonged activation of sodium channels. The EDX studies in these neuropathies usually show reduced amplitude of motor and sensory responses, slow conduction velocities, and prolonged F waves.[17–19] Hereditary disorders of sodium ion channel function have been associated with sensory neuropathies and primary erythromelalgia. Impaired peripheral nerve function may also be caused by antibodies to voltage-gated potassium channels as seen in Isaac syndrome or neuromyotonia. In this disorder, peripheral nerves are hyperexcitable. The main EDX feature of Isaac syndrome is high-frequency discharges known as neuromyotonic discharges, as well as myokymic discharges, seen on needle examination.

DEFINING THE SEVERITY OF FIBER INVOLVEMENT

There is no universally accepted EDX classification scheme for calculating severity of nerve disease. However, EDX studies can provide a good estimate of the severity of neuropathy. The number and distribution of nerves involved provides a general overview of severity. For example, a neuropathy involving only the sural nerve would be considered a mild neuropathy compared with one that involves multiple nerves in the legs and arms. Furthermore, there is often a discrepancy in the EDX severity and the severity of the patient's subjective symptoms. For example, a patient with CMT disease type 1a may only have minimal clinical weakness and no subjective sensory complaints, yet the NCS may show conduction velocities in the teens and absent sensory responses diffusely. By contrast, a patient with complaints of severe paresthesias or neuropathic pain may only demonstrate mild abnormalities on NCS.

In the case of an axon-loss neuropathy, the degree of reduction of motor and sensory responses can help to estimate severity of peripheral nerve disease. Completely absent motor and sensory responses indicates a severe neuropathy, whereas mildly slow conduction velocities or mildly prolonged distal latencies and mostly normal amplitude motor and sensory responses would be considered a mild neuropathy. The needle EMG examination can also help to gauge the severity of axon-loss neuropathy. Abundant fibrillation potentials indicate muscle fiber denervation and the relative lack of reinnervation, and represent a more severe abnormality than a muscle that shows enlarged motor unit potentials and no fibrillation potentials.

In demyelinating neuropathies, the number of nerves involved and the degree of conduction block can serve to estimate the severity of neuropathy. Prolonged distal latencies and slow conduction velocities are less helpful for estimating disease severity, as these features do not correlate well with neurologic deficits.

MONITORING RECOVERY OR TREATMENT EFFECT

When a patient recovers from peripheral neuropathy either through treatment of an underlying illness causing the neuropathy or with immune-modulating therapy for acquired demyelinating neuropathies, the EDX abnormalities usually improve. Using parameters such as a summated CMAP amplitude, by which the amplitude of the 4 routinely performed motor NCS (median, ulnar, peroneal, and tibial) are summated to provide a single value, may be one objective measure that can be followed to assess for improvement. However, in many neuropathies, even with treatment and stabilization of the symptoms, the EDX studies often show persistent abnormalities and do not usually completely return to normal.

PLANNING THE EDX STUDY

The initial EDX studies in patients with suspected neuropathy should always include motor and sensory NCS and needle EMG studies. The initial selection of nerves and muscles to study is guided by the clinical presentation of the individual patient. The NCS are selected in the region of the patient's predominant clinical symptoms. For most patients, symptoms and neurologic abnormalities on examination are greatest in the lower extremities, and a leg is usually selected as the site to begin the evaluation. If the leg studies are abnormal, NCS are performed in the arm to determine the extent of nerve involvement. If the patient has upper extremity predominant symptoms, NCS are started in the arm. If a patient's clinical presentation is symmetric, it is reasonable to perform NCS on one side only. If the presentation is asymmetric or a mononeuritis multiplex pattern, comparing studies of involved nerves with uninvolved nerves in the opposite limb serves to demonstrate the multifocal nature of the nerve disease.

Typically NCS are performed before the needle examination, and serve to give an overview of the fiber types involved and the severity of involvement. After the results of the initially selected NCS are reviewed, a decision is made as to whether additional NCS are needed. Next, the needle examination is performed. This examination should include muscles in the distal and proximal limbs, based on the pattern of clinical involvement. For patients with a distal symmetric pattern of neuropathy, muscles in the distal leg are typically studied first. If the distal leg muscles show normal results, a distal foot muscle (such as the abductor hallucis or first dorsal interosseus pedis) is studied to evaluate for abnormalities that may be confined to the most distal nerve distribution. If the distal leg muscles show abnormalities, the needle examination is carried up to the proximal leg muscles to determine the extent of proximal involvement. In some cases, the lumbosacral and thoracic paraspinal muscles are studied to determine if there is evidence of involvement of the nerves at the root level. Commonly performed NCS and muscles examined on needle EMG for assessment of peripheral neuropathy are listed in **Table 3**.

NORMAL EDX STUDIES AND NEUROPATHY

The patient with distal sensory symptoms and normal EDX studies deserves special consideration. One interpretation of this circumstance is that the patient does not have evidence of peripheral nerve disease. Such an interpretation may be true, but the possibility of peripheral neuropathy still exists despite normal studies. There are 2 main considerations for which peripheral neuropathy may be present despite normal EDX studies. One is that the patient may have peripheral neuropathy in an early stage, and the amplitude of SNAPs or CMAPs has declined but has not yet dropped below the lower limit of normal. The evolution of abnormalities on EDX studies may occur slowly over several years, and thus performing follow-up studies 6 to 12 months after the initial study may help to monitor for progression. The second possibility is that the patient may have a small-fiber peripheral neuropathy, which cannot be assessed by routine EDX studies. Evaluation of small-fiber neuropathy involves additional testing.

Table 3
Commonly performed EDX studies for assessment of peripheral neuropathy

Study	Comments
Nerve Conduction Studies (Recording Site)	
Peroneal motor (extensor digitorum brevis)	
Tibial motor (abductor hallucis)	
Sural	Performed in most patients
Medial plantar	Performed in patients aged <60 y, or in those with only mild sensory symptoms
Median sensory (index finger)	Performed if lower extremity NCS are abnormal
Ulnar motor (abductor digiti minimi)	Performed if lower extremity NCS are abnormal
Needle EMG	
Anterior tibialis	Performed in most patients
Medial gastrocnemius	Performed in most patients
Abductor hallucis or first dorsal interosseous pedis	Performed to look for distal involvement or demonstrate distal gradient
Tensor fascia lata or gluteus medius Gluteus maximus Lumbosacral paraspinals	If distal muscles abnormal to assess lumbosacral radiculopathies or polyradiculopathy
First dorsal interosseus (hand)	

SELECTED NEUROPATHIES
Small-Fiber Neuropathy

Small-fiber neuropathy typically presents with painful feet. The pain is often described as burning and is usually associated with dysesthesias.[20,21] In addition, disorders affecting small fibers may also be associated with dysfunction of the peripheral autonomic nerves, and patients may experience orthostatic hypotension, bowel or bladder dysfunction, impotence, or anhidrosis.

Although sensory symptoms are prominent in small-fiber neuropathies, the routine EDX studies are typically normal because they assess only large, myelinated fibers. Other studies that can be used to help with the diagnosis include quantitative sensory testing[21] and other tests of autonomic function.[22,23] Another study that may be helpful for diagnosis of small-fiber neuropathy is a skin biopsy, which evaluates epidermal nerve fiber density. Reduced epidermal nerve fiber density is considered a characteristic finding that supports the diagnosis of small-fiber neuropathy.[24–26]

Diabetes

Diabetes is a common cause of peripheral neuropathy. Patients with impaired glucose tolerance (IGT) may also develop peripheral neuropathy, which is particularly well established in the case of small-fiber neuropathy.[27,28] Patients with diabetes may develop many different types of neuropathy, the most common of which is a distal symmetric, predominantly sensory neuropathy. The EDX studies show evidence of an axon-loss neuropathy with mildly slowed conduction velocities, and reduced amplitude of motor and sensory responses with a distal gradient. Other forms of neuropathy that may occur in diabetes include a small-fiber neuropathy, a predominantly autonomic neuropathy, an isolated cranial neuropathy, an isolated painful truncal neuropathy, or a polyradiculoneuropathy.

Assessment of autonomic neuropathy typically involves specialized tests of autonomic function performed in a laboratory designed for autonomic testing.[22] For clinicians without ready access to an autonomic laboratory, several cardiovascular autonomic tests can be performed at bedside without special equipment.[29] The sympathetic skin response (SSR), also known as the peripheral autonomic surface potential, can provide assessment of distal sudomotor function.[30] Although the SSR provides less information than other sudomotor tests such as the quantified sudomotor axon reflex test and the thermoregulatory sweat test, the SSR can be performed with routine EDX equipment.

The cranial neuropathies that occur in diabetes involve the oculomotor, abducens, trochlear, and facial nerves. The occulomotor neuropathy in diabetes usually spares the pupil. This has been attributed to the superficial location of the papillary parasympathetic fibers in the third nerve. Most diabetic cranial neuropathies are diagnosed clinically without EDX studies. A facial mononeuropathy can be assessed with facial NCS and needle EMG of facial muscles.

Diabetic polyradiculoneuropathy may take several forms.[31] The more common form is characterized by acute or subacute onset of asymmetric proximal lower extremity weakness, accompanied by pain involving the thigh or back. Sensation is usually preserved in the region of pain. The weakness is often moderate to severe, and muscle atrophy develops. Significant weight loss may occur. The disorder is most often called diabetic amyotrophy. Other names for the condition include diabetic polyradiculopathy and diabetic polyradiculoplexopathy. The EDX studies may reveal that the patient has an underlying distal symmetric axon-loss sensorimotor polyneuropathy. Whether or not there is evidence of a distal neuropathy, the needle examination shows denervation and neurogenic motor unit potentials distributed in any of the proximal lower extremity and pelvic muscles and, often, the lumbosacral paraspinal muscles. The onset of recovery is delayed and may occur in the range of 1 to 2 years from onset. The less common form of diabetic polyradiculopathy is a painless symmetric proximal muscle weakness, which may represent a form of CIDP occurring in patients with diabetes.

Charcot-Marie-Tooth Disease

CMT disease is the most common hereditary neuropathy, with prevalence estimated to be 1 in 2500.[32] The typical phenotype involves slowly progressive distal lower extremity weakness and atrophy, high arches (pes cavus), and a family history of other affected members. Sensory deficits are mild, and the patient usually does not have positive sensory symptoms such as tingling or paresthesias. There are many subtypes of CMT disease, with extensive classification now based on genetic studies.[32,33]

Historically, EDX studies have played a key role in classification of CMT patients, with CMT disease type 1 showing a demyelinative pattern and CMT disease type 2 showing an axon-loss pattern. The most common type of CMT disease is CMT type 1A, which has a demyelinative pattern with uniformly slow nerve conduction velocity (NCV), less than 38 m/s in the upper extremities. Other forms of type 1 CMT disease, including CMT type 1B and CMT type 1X, also have very slow NCV. Type 2 CMT patients have an axon-loss picture on EDX studies.

As mentioned earlier, an important use of EDX studies is to help differentiate the acquired demyelinative neuropathies, such as GBS and chronic inflammatory demyelinating neuropathy, from hereditary demyelinating neuropathies. The underlying basis for making this distinction is that hereditary neuropathies tend to have uniform changes affecting all nerves, whereas acquired neuropathies have varying degrees of demyelination with a multifocal distribution of nerve involvement.[34] Hence, a patient with an acquired demyelinating neuropathy may have some nerves that show severe abnormalities and other nerves that appear to be unaffected. Likewise, conduction block and temporal dispersion of the CMAP are commonly seen in acquired demyelinative neuropathies and are not typical of hereditary neuropathies.[34]

An important exception to these rules is HNPP. This hereditary neuropathy is known to have multifocal demyelinative changes, including conduction block and temporal dispersion of the CMAP. Patients with HNPP may have several different forms of peripheral nerve disease. The classic history, leading to the descriptive name of this disorder, is that of multiple recurrent nerve palsies. Episodes often occur on awakening or may be related to physical activity. Often the nerve palsies can be localized to physiologic compression sites where the nerve may be especially predisposed to injury. **Fig. 3** shows conduction block in the peroneal nerve in a patient with HNPP, which is localized distal to the common site of compression above the fibular head. Other patterns of nerve disease seen in HNPP include a distal symmetric motor neuropathy, brachial plexopathy, chronic mononeuropathies, and an asymptomatic carrier state.[35]

Guillain-Barré Syndrome

GBS is an immune-mediated inflammatory neuropathy, which usually presents as an acute motor neuropathy with minor sensory involvement and varying degrees of autonomic involvement.[36,37] The progression typically ends by 4 weeks, although some cases of subacute GBS may progress up to 8 weeks. A characteristic laboratory finding is an elevated spinal fluid protein with few white blood cells. The EDX studies usually show evidence of demyelination.[36,37] In very early stages, the EDX studies may be normal or may show limited abnormalities. Some patients have an axonal variant of GBS characterized by rapidly progressive weakness, inexcitable nerves, and poor prognosis. These cases differ greatly from the typical demyelinating form of GBS and were thus controversial when first reported in 1986.[38] Years later, it was recognized that similar cases of acute flaccid paralysis occurred in epidemics in the summer months in northern China, and these cases were designated acute motor axonal neuropathy (AMAN) and acute motor sensory axonal neuropathy (AMSAN).[39,40] These axonal variants constitute only about 5% of GBS patients in North America and Europe, but account for up to 50% of cases from Japan, northern China, and Central and South America.[41] The prognosis tends to be poor, but some cases of AMAN may have rapid recovery. The EDX studies in AMAN typically show reduced-amplitude CMAPs with normal distal motor latencies and normal conduction velocities. Patients with AMSAN have reduced amplitude or absent SNAPs in addition to the reduced amplitude motor responses.

Chronic Inflammatory Demyelinative Neuropathy

CIDP is an acquired, predominantly motor, neuropathy that is similar to GBS in many ways. Most patients have evidence of a demyelinative neuropathy on EDX studies, and elevated spinal fluid protein.[8,13] CIDP differs from GBS in several respects including the time course of the illness, lack of autonomic involvement, rare cranial nerve or respiratory muscle weakness, and the response to different treatments.[35] The onset of CIDP is typically gradual, and progression continues beyond 8 weeks. Occasionally patients with CIDP have an initial presentation identical to GBS, and the chronic nature of the illness is only apparent when discontinuation of immune-modulating treatment leads to relapse. Many different EDX criteria for CIDP have been developed,[4,8,13,14] most of which require evidence of demyelination in multiple nerves. The American Academy of Neurology (AAN) research criteria defined specific criteria for demyelination in CIDP.[4] The AAN criteria list 4 EDX features of demyelination including partial conduction block, slow motor conduction velocity, prolonged distal motor latency, and prolonged or absent F waves. To meet the criteria, the patient must have 3 of the 4 EDX features. For slow velocity, prolonged distal latency, and prolonged F waves, the EDX abnormality must be present in 2 different nerves. Conduction block is required in only 1 nerve.

The AAN research criteria for CIDP were rigorous and designed for research specificity rather than clinical sensitivity. A recent set of EDX criteria is reported to have high sensitivity and specificity for CIDP.[14] These criteria require the following: (1) recordable CMAPs must exist in 75% or more of motor nerves; and (2) more than 50% of motor nerves must show abnormal distal latency, abnormal conduction velocity, or abnormal F-wave latency. If the AAN criteria were applied to patients diagnosed with CIDP by these criteria, only 11% would have met the AAN criteria. This finding confirms the lack of utility of the AAN criteria in clinical practice.

Many variants of CIDP have been described,[42] including MADSAM, distal acquired demyelinating symmetric neuropathy, CIDP associated with another illness such as diabetes, a sensory variant of CIDP, and an axonal form of CIDP.

Multifocal Motor Neuropathy

Multifocal motor neuropathy (MMN) is a rare chronic, motor neuropathy characterized by demyelination of motor nerves with relative or complete sparing of sensory nerves.[10] The disorder presents with gradual onset and slowly progressive asymmetric weakness. The upper extremities are involved more often than the lower extremities. The weakness is often in the distribution of 1 or more individual nerves with neighboring nerves not being involved. The EDX studies often show evidence of conduction block in motor nerves with sparing of sensory nerve conduction across the same nerve segment. The sites of conduction block in MMN are often in atypical locations rather than at physiologic compression sites. Some patients may have the typical clinical syndrome without evidence of conduction block.[43] The diagnosis of MMN may also be helped by positive titers of anti-GM1 antibody, although the antibody is only present in only 40% to 50% percent of cases.

Critical-Illness Neuropathy

Critical-illness neuropathy is a sensorimotor axonal neuropathy that develops in patients who have suffered a critical illness. Such patients usually have a prolonged stay in the intensive care unit with multiorgan failure.[44] The illness often comes to attention when it is discovered that the patient cannot be weaned from a ventilator, or when the patient regains consciousness after a prolonged coma or encephalopathy and is found to have significant weakness. The EDX studies show an axon-loss process with reduced amplitude of CMAPs and SNAPs, and mildly slow conduction velocities.[45] Conduction velocities may become quite slow if the amplitude of motor responses is markedly reduced. The needle examination shows distal predominant changes consisting of fibrillation potentials and enlarged, complex motor unit potentials.

Vasculitic Neuropathy

Vasculitis involving peripheral nerves may occur as part of a systemic vasculitis or isolated vasculitis involving the peripheral nervous system. Peripheral neuropathy is common in systemic vasculitis and may sometimes be the initial manifestation. The pattern of mononeuritis multiplex is particularly common in vasculitis, and should prompt consideration of this possibility. With vasculitic peripheral neuropathy, there is a high incidence of involvement of the peroneal and ulnar nerves. The nature of nerve injury in vasculitis is ischemia with nerves undergoing infarction at points of ischemia. If such a patient undergoes EDX studies in the first few days after onset, the NCS may give the false impression of a demyelinating neuropathy, due to the apparent finding of conduction block. Although nerve infarction causes an axon-loss injury, if the EDX studies are performed within a few days of onset the distal degeneration of the axons has not yet occurred. In this setting, the amplitude of the motor response with distal stimulation will be normal and the amplitude with stimulation proximal to the infarct will be very low or absent. This conduction-block pattern is attributable to axonal injury and insufficient time for distal axonal degeneration, and should not be mistaken for a demyelinative nerve injury. An additional point about vasculitic neuropathy is that a distal symmetric or asymmetric pattern may also occur. A review of biopsy-proven vasculitic neuropathy cases revealed that only about half had clinical features of a mononeuritis multiplex pattern and that 36% had a distal symmetric pattern.[46] Thus, the absence of a mononeuropathy multiplex pattern does not exclude the possibility of vasculitic neuropathy.

SUMMARY

Electrodiagnostic studies are an important component of the evaluation of patients with suspected peripheral nerve disorders. The pattern of findings and the features that are seen on the motor and sensory NCS and needle EMG can help to identify the type of neuropathy, define the underlying pathophysiology (axonal or demyelinating), and ultimately help to narrow the list of possible causes. Criteria for axonal and demyelinating neuropathies should always be carefully considered when interpreting the EDX findings in patients with neuropathy in order to accurately define the pathophysiology.

REFERENCES

1. Donofrio PD, Albers JW. AAEM minimonograph #34; polyneuropathy; classification by nerve conduction studies and electromyography. Muscle Nerve 1990; 13(10):889–903.
2. Sheikh SI, Amato AA. The dorsal root ganglion under attack: the acquired sensory ganglionopathies. Pract Neurol 2010;10:326–34.
3. Lauria G. Small fibre neuropathies. Curr Opin Neurol 2005;18:591–7.
4. Ad Hoc Subcommittee of the American Academy of Neurology AIDS Task Force. Research Criteria for diagnosis of chronic inflammatory demyelinating polyneuropathy (CIDP). Neurology 1991;41:617–8.
5. Pfeiffer G, Wicklein EM, Wittig K. Sensitivity and specificity of different conduction block criteria. Clin Neurophysiol 2000;118(8):1388–94.
6. Tankisi H, Pugdahl K, Fuglsang-Frederiksen A, et al. Pathophysiology inferred from electrodiagnostic nerve tests and classification of polyneuropathies. Suggested guidelines. Clin Neurophysiol 2005;116:1571–80.
7. Olney RK. Consensus criteria for the diagnosis of partial conduction block. Muscle Nerve 1999;8:225–9.
8. Van den Bergh PY, Pieret F. Electrodiagnostic criteria for acute and chronic inflammatory demyelinating polyradiculoneuropathy. Muscle Nerve 2004;29(4): 565–74.
9. Fisher MA. F-waves-physiology and clinical uses. Scientific World Journal 2007;7: 144–60.

10. Kaji R. Physiology of conduction block in multifocal motor neuropathy and other demyelinating neuropathies. Muscle Nerve 2003;27:285–96.
11. Albers JW, Kelly JJ. Acquired inflammatory demyelinating polyneuropathy: clinical and electrodiagnostic features. Muscle Nerve 1989;12:435–51.
12. Albers JW, Donofrio PD, McGonagle TK. Sequential electrodiagnostic abnormalities in acute inflammatory demyelinating polyneuropathy. Muscle Nerve 1985;8: 528–39.
13. Barohn RJ, Kissel JT, Warmolts JR, et al. Chronic inflammatory demyelinating polyradiculoneuropathy. Clinical characteristics, course, and recommendations for diagnostic criteria. Arch Neurol 1989;46:878–84.
14. Koski CL, Baugmarten M, Magder LS, et al. Derivation and validation of diagnostic criteria for chronic inflammatory demyelinating polyneuropathy. J Neurol Sci 2009;277:1–8.
15. Kullmann DM. Neurological channelopathies. Annu Rev Neurosci 2010;33: 151–72.
16. Graves TD, Hanna MG. Neurological channelopathies. Postgrad Med J 2005;81: 20–32.
17. Oda K, Araki K, Totoki T, et al. Nerve conduction study of human tetrodotoxin. Neurology 1989;39:743–5.
18. Long RR, Sargent JC, Hammer K. Paralytic shellfish poisoning: a case report and serial electrophysiologic observations. Neurology 1990;40:1310–2.
19. Cameron J, Flowers AE, Capra MF. Electrophysiological studies on ciguatera poisoning in man (Part II). J Neurol Sci 1991;101:93–7.
20. Mendell JR, Sahenk Z. Painful sensory neuropathy. N Engl J Med 2003;348: 1243–55.
21. Magda P, Latov N, Renard MV, et al. Quantitative sensory testing; high sensitivity in small fiber neuropathy with normal NCS/EMG. J Peripher Nerv Syst 2002;7: 225–8.
22. Stewart JD, Low PA, Fealey RD. Distal small fiber neuropathy: results of tests of sweating and autonomic cardiovascular reflexes. Muscle Nerve 1992;15:661–5.
23. Malik RA, Veves A, Tesfaye S, et al. Small fibre neuropathy: role in the diagnosis of diabetic sensorimotor polyneuropathy. Diabetes Metab Res Rev 2011;27: 678–84.
24. McArthur JC, Stocks EA, Hauer P, et al. Epidermal nerve fiber density: normative reference range and diagnostic efficiency. Arch Neurol 1998;55:1513–20.
25. Lauria G, Morbin M, Lombardi R, et al. Axonal swellings predict the degeneration of epidermal nerve fibers in painful neuropathies. Neurology 2003;61:631–6.
26. Hlubocky A, Wellik K, Ross MA, et al. Skin biopsy for diagnosis of small fiber neuropathy: a critically appraised topic. Neurologist 2010;16(1):61–3.
27. Hoffman-Synder C, Smith BE, Ross MA, et al. The value of oral glucose tolerance test in the evaluation of chronic idiopathic axonal polyneuropathy. Arch Neurol 2006;63(8):1075–9.
28. Rajabally YA. Neuropathy and impaired glucose tolerance: an updated review of the evidence. Acta Neurol Scand 2011;124:1–8.
29. Ewing DJ, Campbell IW, Clarke BP. Assessment of cardiovascular effects in diabetic autonomic neuropathy and prognostic implications. Ann Intern Med 1980; 92:308–11.
30. Vetrugno R, Liguori R, Cortelli P, et al. Sympathetic skin response: basic mechanisms and clinical applications. Clin Auton Res 2003;13:256–70.
31. Amato AA, Barohn RJ. Diabetic lumbosacral polyradiculoneuropathies. Curr Treat Options Neurol 2001;3:139–46.

32. Reilly MM, Murphy SM, Laurá M. Charcot-Marie-Tooth disease. J Peripher Nerv Syst 2011;16:1–14.
33. Patzko A, Shy ME. Update on Charcot-Marie-Tooth disease. Curr Neurol Neurosci Rep 2011;11:78–88.
34. Lewis RA, Sumner AJ. The electrodiagnostic distinction between chronic familial and acquired demyelinative neuropathies. Neurology 1982;32:592–6.
35. Stogbauer F, Young P, Kuhlenbaumer G, et al. Hereditary recurrent focal neuropathies: clinical and molecular features. Neurology 2000;54(3):546–51.
36. Trojaborg W. Acute and chronic neuropathies: new aspects of Guillain-Barré syndrome and chronic inflammatory demyelinating polyneuropathy, an overview and an update. Electroencephalogr Clin Neurophysiol 1998;107:303–16.
37. Van der Meché FG, Van Doorn PA, Meulstee J, et al. Diagnostic and classification criteria for the Guillain-Barré syndrome. Eur Neurol 2011;45:133–9.
38. Feasby TE, Gilbert JJ, Brown WF, et al. An acute axonal form of Guillain-Barré polyneuropathy. Brain 1986;109:1115–26.
39. Mckahn GM, Cornblath DR, Ho TN, et al. Clinical and electrophysiological aspects of acute paralytic disease of children and young adults in Northern China. Lancet 1991;338:333–42.
40. McKahn GM, Cornblath DR, Griffin JW, et al. Acute motor axonal neuropathy: a frequent cause of flaccid paralysis in China. Ann Neurol 1993;33:333–42.
41. Hughes RA, Cornblath DR. Guillain-Barré syndrome. Lancet 2005;366:1653–66.
42. Saperstein DS, Katz JS, Amato AA, et al. Clinical spectrum of chronic acquired demyelinating polyneuropathies. Muscle Nerve 2001;24(3):311–24.
43. Pakiam AS, Parry GJ. Multifocal motor neuropathy without overt conduction block. Neurology 1998;21:243–5.
44. Latranco N, Bolton CF. Critical illness polyneuropathy and myopathy: a major cause of muscle weakness and paralysis. Lancet 2011;10:931–41.
45. Zifko UA, Zipko HT, Bolton CF. Clinical and electrophysiological findings in critical illness polyneuropathy. J Neurol Sci 1998;159:186–93.
46. Olney R. AANEM minimonograph #38: neuropathies in connective tissue disease. Muscle Nerve 1992;15:531–42.

Electrodiagnostic Assessment of the Brachial Plexus

Mark A. Ferrante, MD[a,b,*]

KEYWORDS

- Brachial plexus • EMG • Sensory nerve conduction studies
- Motor nerve conduction studies • Root • Trunk • Division
- Cord

The brachial plexus, which supplies most of the upper extremity and shoulder and is one of the largest and most complex structures of the peripheral nervous system (PNS), has an inherent susceptibility toward trauma and other diseases. Its traumatic vulnerability directly reflects its superficial location and its position between 2 highly mobile structures—the neck and the arm—whereas its susceptibility toward other diseases is indirect, reflecting the disease susceptibility of structures adjacent to it (eg, lymph nodes, lung tissue, major blood vessels).[1,2] These susceptibilities combine to make disorders of the brachial plexus a frequent occurrence and, consequently, patients with brachial plexopathies frequently are encountered by electrodiagnostic (EDX) medicine providers. For these reasons, it is imperative that EDX medicine providers be able to identify, localize, and characterize brachial plexus lesions, determine the particular brachial plexus elements involved, characterize the lesions pathologically, determine their severity and prognosis for recovery, and properly plan follow-up studies based on the EDX findings.

Because of its size and complexity, there is no single nerve conduction study (NCS) or muscle assessable by needle electrode examination (NEE) that is capable of evaluating the brachial plexus in its entirety. Even the routine NCS and standard NEE screens do not adequately evaluate all of its elements. Consequently, nonroutine NCS and a more extensive NEE typically are required in its assessment. In addition, the contralateral, asymptomatic limb often must be studied so that relative abnormalities are not missed (discussed later). For these reasons, the EDX assessment of patients with brachial plexopathies typically is more time-consuming than that of other structures. Fortunately, however, because disorders involving the brachial plexus typically are focal in nature (ie, they do not involve it in its entirety), once the region of involvement is identified (by screening sensory NCS), the remainder of the assessment

a EMG Laboratory, Guadalupe Regional Medical Center, 1339 East Court Street, Suite 230, Seguin, TX 78155, USA
b Department of Neurology, University of Tennessee Health Science Center, Memphis, 855 Monroe Avenue, TN 38163, USA
* 3041 Saddlehorn Drive, Seguin, TX 78155.
E-mail address: mafmd1@gmail.com

Neurol Clin 30 (2012) 551–580
doi:10.1016/j.ncl.2011.12.005
0733-8619/12/$ – see front matter © 2012 Elsevier Inc. All rights reserved.

is tailored to that region, significantly lessening the time burden on the EDX provider. Thus, the anatomic complexity of this structure, and the focal nature of its lesions, combine to permit EDX providers to localize brachial plexus lesions with extreme accuracy (ie, to individual root, trunk, cord, division, or terminal nerve elements). When properly studied, in addition to localization, the EDX provider characterizes the lesion (ie, defines its pathology, pathophysiology, and severity). This information helps direct clinical management and, thus, often is critical to the referring physician.

The EDX assessment of the brachial plexus is the focus of this article. The article begins with a review of brachial plexus anatomy, pathology, and pathophysiology, as well as the EDX manifestations of the various pathophysiologies; it then concludes with our approach, a regional one, to the EDX assessment of these lesions.

ANATOMY OF THE BRACHIAL PLEXUS

The brachial plexus contains more than 100,000 individual nerve fibers.[1] As these fibers advance peripherally (inferolaterally) from the neck toward the axilla, they intermingle and exchange nerve fibers, giving rise to the individual components of the brachial plexus: 5 roots (C5 through T1), 3 trunks (upper, middle, and lower), 6 divisions (3 anterior and 3 posterior), 3 cords (lateral, posterior, and medial), and several terminal nerve branches (the latter are contiguous with the proximal aspects of some of the major nerve trunks of the upper extremity) (**Fig. 1**).

Roots

Anatomically, the dorsal and ventral rootlets exiting from each spinal cord segment fuse to form the dorsal and ventral roots, respectively. The dorsal and ventral roots traverse the intraspinal canal and enter the corresponding intervertebral foramen, where they fuse to form a *mixed spinal nerve*. Almost immediately after exiting the foramen, the mixed spinal nerve gives off a posteriorly directed branch, the *posterior primary ramus*, and then continues peripherally as the *anterior primary ramus* (APR). Anatomists consider the APR as the "roots" of the brachial plexus, whereas most physicians and surgeons dealing extensively with brachial plexus injuries define brachial plexus roots to include the APR, the posterior primary rami, the mixed spinal nerves, the dorsal and ventral roots, and the dorsal and ventral rootlets. Consequently, when the latter definition is used, avulsion injuries are brachial plexus lesions. Throughout this article, the more expansive definition of the term "root" is used. Thus, "C5 root" refers to the C5 dorsal and ventral rootlets and roots, the C5 mixed spinal nerve, and the C5 anterior and posterior primary rami, and "C5 APR" refers to the APR portion of the C5 root.

Although the brachial plexus typically is derived from the C5 through T1 roots, not infrequently the C4 and T2 roots also contribute nerve fibers to it. Whenever the C4 contribution is large and the T1 contribution is small, the brachial plexus is said to be *prefixed*; the term *postfixed* is applied when the C5 contribution is small and the T2 contribution is large.[3] Nerves arising from the APR include the nerves to the scalene and longus colli muscles (C5 through C8 APR); the long thoracic nerve, which innervates the serratus anterior (C5 through C7 APR); a portion of the phrenic nerve, which innervates the diaphragm (C5 APR); and a portion of the dorsal scapular nerve, which innervates the levator scapulae and rhomboideus major and minor muscles (C5 APR).[4] Because of their proximal location, these nerves cannot be studied using percutaneous stimulation applied at the supraclavicular fossa because stimulation at this site generates action potentials at the midtrunk level, which is distal to the APR.[5]

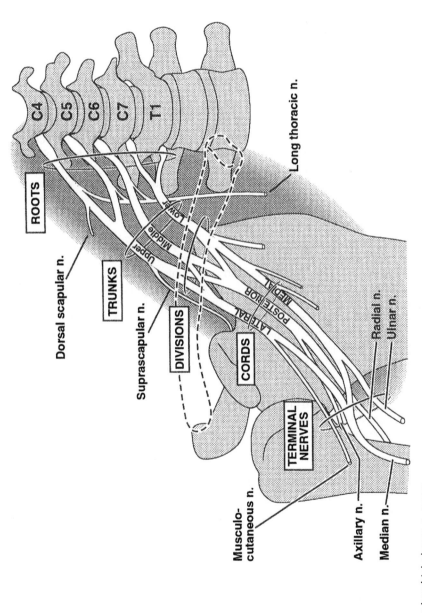

Fig. 1. The brachial plexus. n, nerve.

Trunks

These brachial plexus elements are named for their relationship to each other: the upper, middle, and lower trunks. The upper trunk is formed by the fusion of the C5 and C6 APR, the middle trunk is a continuation of the C7 APR, and the lower trunk results from the joining of the C8 and T1 APR. These elements are seldom anomalous, the middle trunk begins a direct extension of the C7 APR in 100%, and the upper and lower trunks are of classical formation in more than 90% and more than 95%, respectively.[6] The trunk elements give off 2 branches, both from the proximal aspect of the upper trunk: the nerve to the subclavius muscle and the suprascapular nerve.[4] The distal one-third of the trunk elements can be studied by percutaneous stimulation applied to the supraclavicular fossa. The proximal aspects of the trunks are not assessable by this technique.[5]

Divisions

In the anatomic position, the divisions lie behind the clavicle (ie, they are retroclavicular). Two divisions (1 anterior and 1 posterior) are derived from each trunk element after the latter divide into anteriorly and posteriorly directed processes. In general, the divisions do not give off any nerve branches.[4] Although assessable via percutaneous stimulation, the divisions seldom require EDX assessment because lesions restricted to this level are infrequent.

Cords

The cords are located in the axilla and are named for their relationship with the axillary artery. The lateral cord is formed by the fusion of the anterior divisions of the upper and middle trunks and contains fibers derived from the C5 through C7 roots; the posterior cord is formed by the joining of all 3 posterior divisions and contains fibers derived from the C5 through C8 roots; and the medial cord, which is simply a continuation of the anterior division of the lower trunk, contains fibers derived from the C8 and T1 roots. The lateral and medial pectoral nerves arise from the lateral and medial cords, respectively, just after the cords are formed. The lateral cord then gives off the musculocutaneous nerve and then terminates as the lateral head of the median nerve. The posterior cord gives off the subscapular, thoracodorsal, and axillary nerves and continues as the radial nerve. The medial cord gives off the medial brachial cutaneous, medial antebrachial cutaneous, and ulnar nerves; it then terminates as the medial head of the median nerve.[4] The cord elements can be studied by percutaneous stimulation.

Terminal Branches

Depending on the investigator, the number of terminal branches derived from the cords varies from 3 (median, radial, and ulnar) to 5 (the latter 3 nerves plus the musculocutaneous and axillary nerves). Because they all derive from the cords, we consider there to be 5 terminal branches. The median nerve is formed by the joining of the lateral and medial heads of the median nerve (from the lateral and medial cords, respectively), the radial nerve from the posterior cord, the ulnar nerve from the medial cord, the musculocutaneous nerve from the lateral cord, and the axillary nerve from the posterior cord.[4] The terminal branches of the brachial plexus can be studied by percutaneous stimulation.

Further Anatomic Commentary

Several other useful anatomic points warrant mention. First, although percutaneous stimulation cannot be used to assess brachial plexus elements proximal to the distal trunk level, proximal brachial plexus lesions involving the C5 through C7 motor nerve fibers can be localized via the NEE. For example, because the rhomboids and serratus anterior muscles are innervated by motor nerve fibers derived from the C5 through C7 APR, their involvement on NEE signifies that the responsible lesion must lie at or proximal to the APR level. Second, although the C8 and T1 APR elements do not give off any nerve branches, the C8 and T1 mixed spinal nerves contain preganglionic sympathetic fibers that, when interrupted, produce a Horner syndrome. Consequently, in the setting of a Horner syndrome, the lesion must lie at or proximal to the C8 and T1 mixed spinal nerves. Third, because the pectoral nerves are derived from the cord elements very proximally,[4] pectoral muscle involvement is more commonly associated with supraclavicular brachial plexus lesions than with infraclavicular lesions. Fourth, in general, the motor nerve fibers contained in root and trunk elements innervate both flexor and extensor muscles, whereas the motor fibers contained within a cord or terminal branch element innervate either flexor or extensor muscles, but not both. This difference reflects motor fiber rearrangements at the division level and explains why root and trunk lesions are more similar in appearance to each other than they are to infraclavicular lesions and, likewise, why cord and terminal nerve lesions are more similar in appearance to each other than they are to supraclavicular lesions.

THE CLASSIFICATION OF BRACHIAL PLEXUS LESIONS

The brachial plexus can be divided into various regions. Anatomically, because the divisions lie deep to the clavicle, the brachial plexus can be divided into a supraclavicular plexus (roots and trunks), a retroclavicular plexus (divisions), and an infraclavicular plexus (cords and terminal nerves). In a similar manner, brachial plexopathies are divided into supraclavicular and infraclavicular plexopathies lesions at the division level (retroclavicular plexopathies). As previously stated, lesions affecting supraclavicular elements resemble each other, as do infraclavicular lesions. This anatomic subdivision has significant clinical relevance because supraclavicular and infraclavicular plexopathies differ in their incidence, severity, and prognosis. Supraclavicular lesions are more common and, because of the nature of the lesions associated with them, tend to be more severe, which gives them an overall worse prognosis.[1,7,8] The supraclavicular plexus is further divided into 3 regions: the *upper plexus* (the upper trunk and the C5 and C6 roots), the *middle plexus* (the middle trunk and the C7 root), and the *lower plexus* (the lower trunk and the C8 and T1 roots). This distinction also has clinical relevance regarding incidence, severity, and prognosis. Upper plexus lesions have the highest incidence among supraclavicular plexopathies and typically occur in isolation. Most of these lesions are traumatic in etiology, especially closed traction.[9] Isolated lesions of the middle plexus are infrequent.[10,11] Nearly all middle plexus lesions are caused by traction,[10] although nontraumatic etiologies have also been reported.[11] The lower plexus is affected less often than the other 2 supraclavicular plexus regions. Upper plexus lesions tend to be less severe than lower plexus lesions because (1) their pathophysiology is more commonly demyelinating conduction block (ie, remyelination tends to be much more complete than axon regeneration), (2) their location is more proximate to the muscles they innervate (ie, they are more able to undergo reinnervation by axon regrowth), and (3) they are more frequently extraforaminal (ie, they are more amenable to surgical repair). Unlike upper plexus lesions, lower plexus lesions are (1) less frequently attributable to demyelinating conduction block (more commonly axon loss), (2) typically are farther from the muscles they innervate (less likely to undergo axon regrowth), and (3) are less frequently extraforaminal (less amenable or not amenable to surgical repair).[1] Thus, overall, lower plexus lesions tend to be more severe and, consequently, their prognosis is worse. For these reasons, despite initial equal severity, upper plexus lesions have more complete resolution than lower plexus lesions.[12] Consequently, a supraclavicular plexus lesion that initially involved all 3 of these regions (pan-supraclavicular plexopathy) equally may appear as a remote lower plexus lesion when studied years after the inciting event, owing to poor lower plexus recovery. The individual disorders associated with supraclavicular and infraclavicular plexopathies also differ. Supraclavicular plexopathies are primarily related to closed-traction injuries (eg, obstetric paralysis, motor vehicle accidents, burner syndrome), malpositioning on the operating table (eg, classic postoperative paralysis), rucksack palsy, neoplastic processes (especially lung or breast cancer), true neurogenic thoracic outlet syndrome, disputed thoracic outlet syndrome, and plexopathies following median sternotomy (eg, open heart surgery). Infraclavicular plexopathies are more frequently related to trauma (eg, gunshot and stab wounds, humeral head fractures, midshaft clavicular fractures, shoulder dislocations), radiation, medial brachial fascial compartment syndrome, crutch use, and iatrogenic causes (eg, shoulder operations, shoulder arthroscopy, axillary arteriograms, axillary regional anesthetic blocks). Isolated retroclavicular plexopathies are infrequent, even in the setting of clavicular fractures; the latter more commonly produce supraclavicular traction injuries. These entities have recently been reviewed.[13]

ELECTRODIAGNOSTIC MANIFESTATIONS OF THE VARIOUS PATHOPHYSIOLOGIC SUBTYPES

The nerve fibers studied by NCS and NEE are the larger, more heavily myelinated fibers. Although these fibers can be injured in many ways, their pathologic and pathophysiologic responses are limited. Regardless of cause, axon disruption causes the portion of the nerve fiber distal to the disruption site to undergo degeneration (termed Wallerian degeneration or axon loss).[14] Following axon disruption, but before Wallerian degeneration, the distal stump remains capable of conducting action potentials (up to 6 days for motor nerve fibers and 10 days for sensory nerve fibers). This phenomenon has profound consequences on the timing of the EDX study and on its interpretation (discussed in the next section). Nerve fiber lesions of lesser severity may disrupt only the myelin (demyelination). The pathophysiology associated with demyelination depends on whether the demyelinated fiber loses its ability to conduct action potentials (demyelinating conduction block) or conducts them at a slower rate (demyelinating conduction slowing). Each of these pathophysiologies has unique electrodiagnostic (and clinical) manifestations.

Axon Loss Lesions

Most brachial plexus lesions are axon loss in nature without accompanying focal demyelination (eg, avulsions, neoplastic processes). Less frequently, concomitant demyelination is present (early traumatic lesions). As previously stated, axon loss produces conduction failure. Because the amplitude reflects the total number of conducting fibers, conduction failure reduces the sensory nerve action potential (SNAP) and compound muscle action potential (CMAP) amplitude values. In contrast, because the latency and conduction velocity values reflect the conduction rate along only the fastest-conducting fibers, these values reflect only a small percentage of the stimulated nerve fibers. As a result, the calculated latency and conduction velocity values may be normal despite a severe axon loss lesion, demonstrating a significantly reduced motor response (low-amplitude CMAP). Once Wallerian degeneration occurs and the distal stump becomes incapable of conducting action potentials, the recorded amplitude is the same regardless of where the nerve is stimulated (ie, proximal to, at, or distal to the lesion) because the degenerated nerve fibers cannot generate or propagate action potentials in response to stimulation. Consequently, whether the lesion affects the cell body of origin of the axon (the motor neuron located in the spinal cord for the motor fiber or the sensory neuron located in the dorsal root ganglion (DRG) for the sensory fiber) or the axon itself, the effect that it has on the recorded SNAP or CMAP is the same. In our EDX laboratories, whenever the amplitude of the recorded response is less than the age-based, laboratory control value for that NCS, the response is considered *absolutely* abnormal. Whenever the recorded response amplitude is less than half of the size of the homologous response recorded from the contralateral side, it is termed *relatively* abnormal. On NEE, axon disruption results in motor unit action potential (MUAP) dropout (proportional to the number of disrupted motor axons) and fibrillation potentials (proportional to the number of denervated muscle fibers). Although motor unit loss is present from the time that the nerve fiber becomes disrupted, it may not be appreciable, even when the lesion is moderate in severity. Because most extremity muscles have an innervation ratio (ie, the average number of muscle fibers innervated per motor nerve fiber) of several hundred or more, several hundred or more fibrillation potentials are produced per disrupted motor nerve fiber. In general, fibrillation potentials appear about 3 weeks after motor nerve fiber disruption and, because of the innervation ratio, they can be quite prominent even when the lesion is only minimal in degree. Because axon loss lesions of the brachial plexus are on a continuum from minimal to extremely severe, their electrodiagnostic manifestations vary. With minimal lesions affecting both the sensory and motor fibers, fibrillation potentials may be observed in the setting of normal SNAPs and CMAPs. With more severe lesions, the appropriate SNAP amplitudes decrease. Greater severity next produces CMAP amplitude decline and concomitant MUAP dropout, although, as previously stated, the latter may not be appreciable until the lesion is at least moderate in degree of severity. At this point, the SNAP responses typically are low or absent. With even more severe lesions, the appropriate CMAP amplitudes decrease further and MUAP loss becomes more obvious. Of the 3 components of the EDX examination (ie, sensory NCS, motor NCS, NEE), the CMAP amplitudes are the most useful component for quantifying the amount of axon loss suffered by a nerve.[12] The sensory NCS tends overestimate the degree of severity; SNAP amplitudes frequently are very low or absent when fewer than half of the axons contained within the PNS element under study are affected. On NEE, fibrillation potentials typically overestimate the lesion, being prominent even with minimal degrees of axon loss (a reflection of the high innervation ratio of most limb muscles). In addition, on NEE, MUAP dropout is challenging to quantify and, for this reason, is not useful for severity estimation. Thus, before reinnervation via collateral sprouting, the CMAP amplitudes are the most reliable indicators of the amount of axon loss present, and the relationship is roughly linear. For example, if the value of the motor response amplitude from the symptomatic side is 5 mV whereas the value for the homologous response recorded from the asymptomatic side is 10 mV, then roughly 50% of the motor axons contained within the affected element are affected (discussed in more detail later in this article). Following reinnervation via collateral sprouting, although the CMAP value improves as more and more muscle fibers are reinnervated, the number of degenerated motor nerve fibers is unchanged; thus, at this point, the CMAP value underestimates the true percentage of motor nerve fibers affected.

The time elapsed between the inciting event and the performance of the EDX study is extremely important. Failure to consider this temporal relationship may result in significant misinterpretations of the EDX manifestations and erroneous, and often misleading, conclusions. In general, the CMAP amplitudes begin to decrease at about day 2 or 3 and reach their nadir by day 7, whereas the SNAP amplitudes begin to decrease about day 6 and reach their nadir about day 10 or 11. As already mentioned, fibrillation potentials usually do not appear until the beginning of the fourth week (ie, after day 21) after the inciting event. Although MUAP loss occurs immediately, it may not be appreciable unless the lesion is at least moderate in degree. Thus, when a patient with a severe upper trunk lesion is studied on day 6, the pattern of normal SNAPs and abnormal CMAPs may cause the lesion to be mistakenly localized to the intraspinal canal (eg, avulsion injury, radiculopathy). Following successful rein-nervation—either via progressive advancement of affected motor fibers from their injury site to the denervated muscle fibers (proximodistal regeneration) or via collateral sprouting from unaffected motor fibers—prolonged duration, heightened amplitude, or increased polyphasicity of the appropriate MUAPs may become apparent on NEE.

Prognostication is another important EDX function. For axon loss lesions, this usually is dictated by the potential for reinnervation, which can be determined by considering the grade of the injury, the distance between the injury site and the dener-vated muscle fibers, and the completeness of the lesion. The grade of the injury reflects the damage sustained by the supporting structures of the affected nerve (ie, the endoneurium, perineurium, and epineurium). When all of the supporting structures are affected, axon advancement cannot occur and, consequently, any reinnervation must occur by collateral sprouting or by surgical treatment of the injured nerve segment. When all of the supporting structures are spared, there is no impediment to proximodistal regeneration other than the distance between the lesion site and the denervated muscle fibers (discussed later in this article). In this setting, both collat-eral sprouting and proximodistal regeneration can occur. The length of nerve between the lesion site and the denervated muscle fibers determines the distance that the motor fibers must advance to reinnervate the denervated muscle fibers. In general, advancement occurs at a rate of about 1 inch per month and denervated muscle fibers survive for approximately 18 to 24 months in the denervated state. After this period has elapsed, the muscle fibers undergo fibrofatty degeneration and, from that point onward, can no longer be reinnervated. Consequently, whenever the denervated muscle fibers lie more than 24 inches from the injury site, reinnervation generally cannot occur by proximodistal regeneration. Rather, reinnervation must occur by collateral sprouting. The completeness of the lesion determines the potential for collateral sprouting. With complete lesions (ie, when all of the motor nerve fibers are disrupted), there are no unaffected nerve fibers from which collateral sprouting can occur. Thus, collateral sprouting requires that the lesion be incomplete. Hence, the more incomplete the lesion is, the better is its potential for reinnervation by this mech-anism. In summary, the best prognosis for motor recovery exists when (1) the support-ing structures are spared, (2) the distance between the lesion and the denervated muscle fibers is short, and (3) the lesion is incomplete. Because the end organs of the sensory nerve fibers do not undergo degeneration, there is no time limit for sensory nerve fiber regeneration. Consequently, if it requires more than 2 years for the sensory fibers to reach their end organs, reinnervation of the latter can still be successful. Clin-ically, the presence of SNAP amplitude decrement correlates with loss of large fiber sensory modalities (vibratory and proprioceptive perceptions). This also is true for CMAP amplitude decrement and clinical weakness. Not only does the degree of CMAP amplitude decrement have a linear relationship with the degree of motor nerve fiber disruption, but in the acute setting it also is correlated with the number of func-tioning muscle fibers. Consequently, when the CMAP recorded from an affected muscle is 50% less than that recorded from the contralateral side, then that muscle usually has lost about half of its strength, and when the CMAP is absent, the muscle usually is nearly or completely paralyzed. During motor NCS, the negative area under the curve parameter is even more accurate than is the amplitude for making these determinations.

When a significant axon loss lesion lies within the intraspinal canal (ie, proximal to the DRG), it may affect the motor and sensory fibers located there. Because the motor fibers project distally and are assessed by the motor NCS and NEE components of the EDX examination, their involvement is recognizable; however, because the sensory NCS assesses only the sensory neurons and their postganglionic sensory fibers, they are not identifiable by sensory NCS. Therefore, intraspinal canal lesions may affect the motor NCS and NEE components of the EDX examination, but not the sensory NCS; an exception exists when the DRG lies within the intraspinal canal.[15] This pattern also is observed with disorders restricted to muscle fiber (eg, distal myopathies), neuromuscular junction (eg, Lambert-Eaton myasthenic syndrome), or terminal motor branch (eg, early Guillain-Barre syndrome), as well as with axon loss lesions studied at a time (ie, 5–7 days after injury) when the motor response amplitudes are recognizably reduced by Wallerian degeneration but those of the sensory NCS are not yet affected. Although isolated CMAP abnormalities strongly suggest that the lesion lies at a site other than where the sensory and motor nerve fibers are contiguous, this statement does not apply to isolated SNAP abnormalities because sensory responses are more sensitive to axon loss lesions than are motor responses. For this reason, isolated SNAP abnormalities cannot be used to exclude motor axon involvement or to localize lesions to those PNS levels at which the motor and sensory nerve fibers are noncontiguous. Mild motor axon loss does not register on motor NCS and, after the fibrillation potentials associated with the denervated muscle fibers disappear (ie, after reinnervation), it is typically too subtle to be recognized by MUAP inspection during NEE. Once enough time has elapsed to allow for reinnervation by collateral sprouting, even previously severe motor nerve fiber loss may no longer be evident on motor NCS because enough muscle fibers have been reinnervated to normalize the recorded CMAP. Fortunately, however, such severe motor nerve fiber loss with subsequent reinnervation is permanently reflected on the NEE as increased duration MUAPs and a neurogenic MUAP recruitment pattern (ie, MUAPs firing in decreased numbers at rates more rapid than normally observable). Because the sensory NCSs are so sensitive toward axon loss processes, it is important to fully use them whenever an axon loss brachial plexopathy is suspected. As will be discussed later, the pattern of sensory NCS abnormalities can typically localize the lesion to an individual brachial plexus element. Because of the innervation ratio, before reinnervation, even small axon loss lesions result in large numbers of fibrillation potentials on NEE. At this stage, the distribution of fibrillation potentials also contributes to lesion localization. After reinnervation has occurred, however, MUAP changes (eg, duration, recruitment pattern) are more sensitive to motor fiber loss than are CMAP changes. In general, roughly 50% of the motor fibers must be lost before a neurogenic MUAP recruitment pattern becomes discernible.

Demyelinating Lesions

Demyelinating lesions may be focal (eg, carpal tunnel syndrome), multifocal (eg, multifocal motor neuropathy, radiation injury), or generalized (eg, hereditary motor sensory neuropathy) in distribution. Because the latter is not pertinent to a discussion of brachial plexus lesions, it is not discussed further. Unlike axon loss lesions, which induce pathologic changes distant to the disrupted axon and affect the NCS regardless of stimulation site, demyelinating lesions do not induce distant changes and, therefore, their recognition is stimulation site-dependent; they are identifiable only when the lesion lies between the stimulating and recording electrodes.

There are 2 types of pathophysiology associated with demyelination: demyelinating conduction slowing and demyelinating conduction block. With demyelinating conduction slowing, all of the impulses traverse the lesion site, albeit at an abnormally slower rate. Because all of the impulses ultimately reach their respective end organs, weakness and sensory loss are unexpected. For that reason, patients with this type of pathophysiology are asymptomatic with regard to negative phenomena (ie, numbness, weakness) and, consequently, seldom are referred to EDX laboratories. For this reason, this type of pathophysiology will not be discussed further. Unlike demyelinating conduction slowing, demyelinating conduction block, as the term implies, blocks the propagation of action potentials at the lesion site, thereby preventing them from reaching their end organs. As a result, this type of pathophysiology, when it affects a sufficient number of nerve fibers, is symptomatic, and the symptoms are similar to those produced by axon loss lesions, although the sensory deficits are limited to large fiber modalities and significant muscle atrophy is unexpected. Unlike axon loss, demyelinating conduction block is seldom observed in isolation. Instead, at least some accompanying axon loss usually is present. The rationale behind this finding is straightforward—any lesion severe enough to produce demyelinating conduction block along most of the affected nerve fibers generally is severe enough to produce axon loss in at least some of them.[16] When weakness has been present for 7 days (the time required for Wallerian degeneration–related motor NCS changes to appear with distal stump stimulation), significant demyelinating conduction block lesions are identified when the CMAP amplitude obtained with distal stimulation is significantly larger than the one obtained with proximal stimulation. Whenever both the recording and stimulating electrodes lie either proximal or distal to the demyelinating conduction block lesion, this amplitude discrepancy is not noted. When a demyelinating conduction block lesion lies distal to the stimulating and recording electrodes, the distal and proximal CMAP amplitudes will be equally reduced, thereby mimicking an axon loss process. Occasionally, it can be localized by stimulating more distally along the studied nerve; its presence is suspected whenever a significant amplitude decrement is not associated with the appropriate NEE findings.

When a significant demyelinating conduction block lies proximal to the stimulating and recording electrodes, the distal and proximal CMAP amplitudes appear normal. Clinically, however, the CMAP amplitudes are too preserved for the degree of weakness reported or observable and, for that reason, a more proximally located demyelinating conduction block should be suspected. It can be confirmed by discordance between the normal/near-normal CMAP amplitude recorded from the clinically weak muscle and the neurogenic MUAP recruitment pattern of it noted on NEE. In this setting, an attempt to localize the lesion by stimulating at more proximal sites (eg, axilla, supraclavicular fossa) is performed. Whenever the lesion lies proximal to the upper midtrunk level (ie, the most proximal stimulation site available for surface stimulation of the brachial plexus), a CMAP amplitude decrement will not be observed with surface stimulation. Nonetheless, its presence can be inferred based on the CMAP/NEE discordance just described. With demyelinating conduction block lesions, the degree of MUAP dropout should match the degree of CMAP amplitude decrement seen on stimulation proximal to the lesion site. Clinically, one should be aware that although most demyelinating conduction block lesions reflect acute trauma and are associated with a good prognosis, there are at least 2 *chronic* brachial plexus conditions in which demyelinating conduction block is the predominant pathophysiology and the prognosis is not good: the early and middle stages of radiation-induced plexopathy (these lesions later convert to axon loss and never resolve) and multifocal motor neuropathy and its variants (these lesions tend to be slowly progressive in nature and do not respond well to treatment).

ELECTRODIAGNOSTIC ASSESSMENT OF THE BRACHIAL PLEXUS

Each brachial plexus element, in addition to having its own *muscle domain* (ie, the muscles innervated by the motor nerve fibers comprising that element), has its own *SNAP domain* (ie, the sensory nerve fibers traversing it that subserve sensory NCS) and *CMAP domain* (ie, the motor nerve fibers traversing it that subserve motor NCS). Consequently, when injured, each element is associated with a unique pattern of EDX abnormalities (ie, SNAP, CMAP, and NEE abnormalities), the recognition of which permits lesion localization. As expected for a structure of its size, a complete brachial plexus assessment requires the performance of a large number of sensory and motor NCSs and an extensive NEE. All components of the EDX examination (ie, sensory and motor NCSs and NEE) must be performed, as each one complements the information obtained by the other 2. Omitting any one of these studies renders the examination incomplete, inadequate, and potentially misleading. The sensory NCSs are performed first because their sensitivity toward axon loss lesions makes them useful for identifying brachial plexus lesions. In addition, because the pathways through the brachial plexus that the sensory nerve fibers subserving each sensory NCS take are known, performing the sensory NCS first also localizes the lesion.[11] These pathways are illustrated in **Figs. 2–6**. The elements assessed by the sensory nerve fibers subserving the ulnar NCS recording from the fifth digit (Uln-D5) and the medial antebrachial cutaneous (MABC) NCSs are not shown because they are anatomically defined; they traverse the medial cord and lower trunk and then enter the C8 DRG and the T1 DRG, respectively. Following identification and localization of the lesion, the motor NCSs are performed. One of the most beneficial attributes of motor NCSs is their ability to quantify axon loss. In the setting of an axon loss lesion, before reinnervation has begun to occur, the amplitude and negative area under the curve values, when compared with the contralateral values, are the most useful parameters by which to estimate the percentage of motor axon loss, assuming that the contralateral responses are normal. Before reinnervation, the NEE is the most

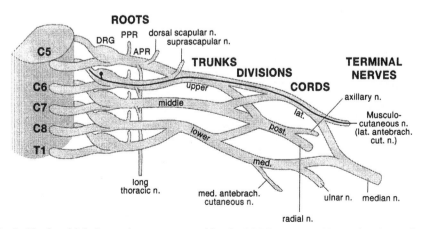

Fig. 2. The brachial plexus elements assessed by the LABC sensory NCS. antebrach, antebrachial; cut, cutaneous; lat, lateral; med, medial; n, nerve; post, posterior.

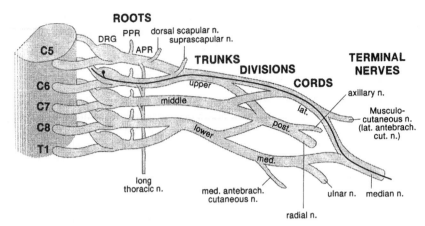

Fig. 3. The brachial plexus elements assessed by the Med-D1 sensory NCS. antebrach, ante-brachial; cut, cutaneous; lat, lateral; med, medial; n, nerve; post, posterior.

sensitive component for identifying motor axon loss. Unfortunately, the NEE has a tendency to mislocalize lesions more distally than their actual location. This occurs in 2 settings: (1) when partial proximal lesions mimic distal lesions and (2) when recovery is more complete proximally than distally. For example, when a lower trunk lesion spares the C8/radial nerve–innervated muscles (eg, extensor indicis proprius, extensor pollicis brevis), it mimics a medial cord lesion. Likewise, when a medial cord lesion spares the C8/median nerve–innervated muscles, it mimics an ulnar nerve lesion. In addition, when the denervated muscle fibers in the affected muscles are rein-nervated, they frequently are no longer recognized as being abnormal. When recovery begins proximally, only the more distally located muscles appear abnormal and the lesion appears to lie distal to its actual position.

ASSESSMENT OF INDIVIDUAL BRACHIAL PLEXUS ELEMENTS

Knowing which sensory and motor nerve fibers are contained within an individual brachial plexus element allows one to calculate its SNAP and CMAP domains. The

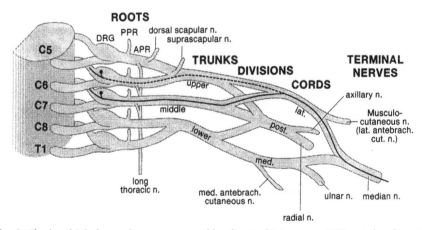

Fig. 4. The brachial plexus elements assessed by the Med-D2 sensory NCS. antebrach, ante-brachial; cut, cutaneous; lat, lateral; med, medial; n, nerve; post, posterior.

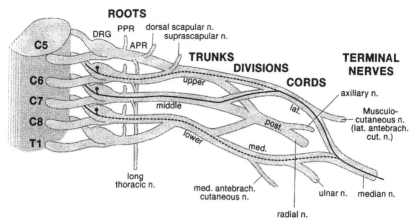

Fig. 5. The brachial plexus elements assessed by the Med-D3 sensory NCS. antebrach, ante-brachial; cut, cutaneous; lat, lateral; med, medial; n, nerve; post, posterior.

muscle domain of an individual brachial plexus element is calculated from the standard myotomal charts.[2,17-21] For example, the biceps muscle belongs to both the C5 and C6 myotomes. Thus, it receives its innervation from motor axons derived from the C5 and C6 anterior horn cells (AHCs). Based on known anatomy, these motor axons must traverse the C5 and C6 roots, the C5 and C6 mixed spinal nerves, the C5 and C6 APR, the upper trunk, the lateral cord, and the musculocutaneous nerve to reach the biceps muscle. Thus, each of these PNS elements includes the biceps muscle in its muscle domain, and their CMAP domains each include the musculocutaneous CMAP, recording biceps. The derivation of the SNAP domain for each brachial plexus element is more complicated.[11]

At this point, the SNAP, CMAP, and muscle domains of the individual brachial plexus elements are discussed. The median and ulnar palmar NCSs and the dorsal ulnar cutaneous response are omitted from the discussion because, with regard to brachial plexus lesions, they do not provide additional information not already realized

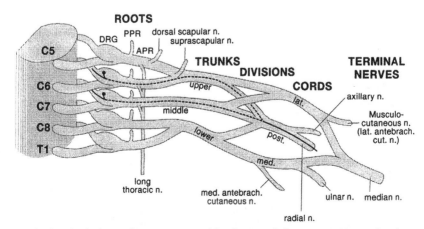

Fig. 6. The brachial plexus elements assessed by the S-Radial sensory NCS. antebrach, ante-brachial; cut, cutaneous; lat, lateral; med, medial; n, nerve; post, posterior.

by the standard sensory NCS. The SNAP domains of the trunk and cord elements are provided in **Box 1**.[11] The CMAP domains of the trunk and cord elements are provided in **Box 2**; they are derived from the muscle domains. The muscle domain of any brachial plexus element can be derived through anatomic reasoning. Thus, the muscle domain of any brachial plexus element is equivalent to the sum of the muscle domains of the elements forming it, minus the muscle domains of the elements departing from the latter elements before its formation. For example, the muscle domain of the upper trunk is equivalent to the sum of the muscle domains of the C5 and C6 roots (ie, the proximal elements forming the upper trunk) minus the sum of the muscle domains of the long thoracic (serratus anterior) and dorsal scapular (levator scapulae, rhomboideus major and minor) nerves (ie, the nerve branches exiting the C5 and C6 roots). Put

---

Box 1
The SNAP domains of the trunk and cord elements

Upper trunk
    LABC (100%)
    Med-D1 (100%)
    Radial (60%)
    Med-D2 (20%)
    Med-D3 (10%)

Middle trunk
    Med-D2 (80%)
    Med-D3 (70%)
    Radial (40%)

Lower trunk
    Uln-D5 (100%)
    MABC (100%)
    Med-D3 (20%)

Lateral cord
    LABC (100%)
    Med-D1 (100%)
    Med-D2 (100%)
    Med-D3 (80%)

Posterior cord
    Radial (100%)

Medial cord
    Uln-D5 (100%)
    MABC (100%)
    Med-D3 (20%)

Abbreviations: LABC, lateral antebrachial cutaneous NCS; MABC, medial antebrachial cutaneous NCS; Med-D1, median NCS recording from first digit; Med-D2, median NCS recording from second digit; Med-D3, median NCS recording from third digit; S-Radial, superficial radial NCS; Uln-D5, ulnar NCS recording from fifth digit.

Box 2
The CMAP domains of the trunk and cord elements

Upper Trunk
    Musc-biceps
    Ax-deltoid
    Radial-EDC
Middle Trunk
    Radial-EDC
Lower Trunk
    Median-APB
    Ulnar-ADM
    Ulnar-FDI
    Radial-EIP
    Radial-EDC
Lateral cord
    Musc-biceps
Posterior cord
    Ax-deltoid
    Radial-EDC
    Radial-EIP
Medial cord
    Median-APB
    Ulnar-ADM
    Ulnar-FDI

Abbreviations: Ax-deltoid, axillary NCS, recording deltoid; Median-APB, median NCS, recording abductor pollicis brevis; Musc-biceps, musculocutaneous NCS, recording biceps; Radial-EDC, radial NCS, recording extensor digitorum communis; Radial-EIP, radial NCS, recording extensor indicis proprius; Ulnar-ADM, ulnar NCS, recording abductor digiti minimi; Ulnar-FDI, ulnar NCS, recording first dorsal interosseous.

---

another way, if the root innervation of a particular muscle is known (myotome charts), then the pathway it traverses through the brachial plexus can be derived. For example, the biceps muscle is innervated by motor nerve fibers derived from the C5 and C6 spinal cord levels (ie, the biceps belongs to the C5 and C6 myotomes) via the musculocutaneous nerve. Thus, these motor nerve fibers traverse the C5 and C6 roots, the upper trunk, the lateral cord, and the musculocutaneous nerve to reach the biceps. Those muscles that we feel are most useful from the standpoint of the EDX examination can be derived using either approach and are included in **Box 3**.

C5 APR

There are no sensory nerve fibers traversing the C5 APR that can be assessed with a sensory NCS. Thus, there is no SNAP domain for this element. Its CMAP domain includes the musculocutaneous NCS, recording biceps (Musc-biceps), and the

| Box 3 |
| Useful muscles for NEE of the trunk and cord elements |

Upper Trunk

    Teres minor

    Levator scapulae

    Rhomboideii

    Deltoid

    Triceps

    Biceps

    Brachioradialis

    Pronator teres

    Extensor carpi radialis

    Flexor carpi radialis

    Pectoralis major

Middle Trunk

    Pronator teres

    Flexor carpi radialis

    Extensor carpi radialis

    Extensor digitorum communis

Lower Trunk

    Flexor carpi ulnaris

    Flexor digitorum profundus-4/5

    Extensor digitorum communis

    Extensor carpi ulnaris

    Extensor pollicis brevis

    Extensor indicis proprius

    Abductor digiti minimi

    First dorsal interosseous

    Abductor pollicis brevis

Lateral cord

    Biceps

    Brachialis

    Pronator teres

    Flexor carpi radialis

Posterior cord

    Latissimus dorsi

    Teres minor

    Deltoid

    Triceps

    Anconeus

Brachioradialis

Extensor carpi radialis

Extensor digitorum communis

Extensor carpi ulnaris

Extensor pollicis brevis

Extensor indicis proprius

Medial cord

Flexor carpi ulnaris

Flexor digitorum profundus-4/5

Flexor pollicis longus

Abductor digiti minimi

First dorsal interosseous

Abductor pollicis brevis

axillary NCS, recording deltoid (Ax-deltoid). Its muscle domain includes those muscles contained within the C5 myotome.

C6 APR

The sensory nerve fibers traversing the C6 APR subserve the lateral antebrachial cutaneous NCS (LABC; 100%), the median NCS recording from the first digit (Med-D1; 100%), the superficial radial NCS (S-Radial; 60%), the median NCS recording from the second digit (Med-D2; 20%), and the median NCS recording from the third digit (Med-D3; 10%).[11] Thus, these sensory NCSs are included in the C6 APR SNAP domain and, consequently, can be used in its assessment. As indicated by the accompanying percentage values, some of these studies are more reliable (ie, LABC, Med-D1, and S-Radial NCS) than others (Med-D2 and Med-D3 NCSs). Because the biceps and deltoid muscles belong to the C6 myotome, the CMAP domain of the C6 APR includes the Musc-biceps and the Ax-deltoid motor NCS. Its muscle domain includes those muscles belonging to the C6 myotome.

C7 APR

The sensory nerve fibers traversing the C7 APR subserve the Med-D2 (80%), the Med-D3 (70%), and the S-Radial (40%) sensory NCSs and, consequently, these sensory NCSs are included in its SNAP domain and are useful in its assessment.[11] The CMAP domain of the C7 APR includes the radial NCS, recording extensor digitorum communis (Radial-EDC) and its muscle domain includes those muscles belonging to the C7 myotome.

C8 APR

The sensory nerve fibers traversing the C8 APR subserve the ulnar NCS recording the fifth digit (Uln-D5; 100%) and the Med-D3 NCS (20%) and, hence, these sensory NCSs are contained in its SNAP domain.[11] The sensory nerve fibers comprising the MABC nerve predominantly traverse the T1 APR and, therefore, the MABC NCS is not included in the SNAP domain of the C8 APR.[11,22] The CMAP domain of the C8 APR includes the ulnar NCS recording abductor digiti minimi (Uln-ADM), the ulnar NCS recording first dorsal interosseous (Uln-FDI), the radial NCS recording extensor indicis proprius (Radial-EIP), and, to a lesser extent, the median NCS recording abductor pollicis brevis (Med-APB). Its muscle domain consists of those muscles belonging to the C8 myotome.

T1 APR

The sensory nerve fibers traversing the T1 APR subserve the MABC sensory NCS and, for that reason, this sensory NCS is included in its SNAP domain.[11,22] Its CMAP domain is the same as that of the C8 APR. Because the abductor pollicis brevis muscle receives innervation mostly from T1 AHCs,[11,12] the Median-APB study is a more reliable assessor of this element than are the ulnar motor NCSs. Its muscle domain consists of those muscles belonging to the T1 myotome, of which the abductor pollicis brevis and the flexor pollicis longus muscles tend to be the most reliable.

Upper Trunk

After the dorsal scapular and long thoracic nerve branches exit from the APR level of the brachial plexus, the C5 and C6 APRs join to form the upper trunk. Thus, the SNAP domain of the upper trunk is equal to the sum of the SNAP domains of the C5 and C6 APRs minus the SNAP domains of the 2 exiting nerves. Because there are no reliable sensory NCSs for the exiting nerves or for the C5 APR, the SNAP domain of the upper trunk is the same as that of the C6 APR. Because the CMAP domain of the C5 and C6 APRs are identical, the CMAP domain of the upper trunk is the same. The muscle domain of the upper trunk is equivalent to the muscle domains of the C5 and C6 APRs minus the muscle domains of the dorsal scapular and long thoracic nerves. The most useful muscles for the NEE of this element are provided in **Box 3**.

Middle Trunk

The middle trunk is a continuation of the C7 APR after it gives off a motor nerve branch to the long thoracic nerve. Thus, its SNAP and CMAP domains are the same as that of the C7 APR. Its muscle domain is equivalent to the C7 muscle domain minus the serratus anterior. The most useful muscles for the NEE of this element are provided in **Box 3**.

Lower Trunk

The lower trunk is formed by the fusion of the C8 and T1 APRs. Consequently, its SNAP, CMAP, and muscle domains are equivalent to the sum of those of the C8 and T1 APRs. The most useful muscles for the NEE of this element are provided in **Box 3**.

Lateral Cord

Anatomically, the lateral cord is formed from the anterior divisions of the upper and middle trunks after the suprascapular nerve branch is given off from the upper trunk. Consequently, its SNAP domain is equivalent to the SNAP domain of the upper trunk minus the SNAP domains of the exiting fibers (ie, the suprascapular nerve branch and the posterior division of the upper trunk) plus the SNAP domain of incoming nerve fibers (ie, the anterior division of the middle trunk). Thus, it includes the LABC, Med-D1, Med-D2, and Med-D3, but not the S-Radial sensory NCS. The CMAP domain of the lateral cord is equivalent to the CMAP domain of the upper trunk minus the CMAP domain of its posterior division plus the CMAP domain of the anterior division of the middle trunk. Thus, its CMAP domain includes the Musc-biceps motor NCS, but not the Ax-deltoid motor NCS. The muscle domain of the lateral cord is equivalent to the sum of the muscle domains of the upper trunk and the anterior division of the middle trunk minus the muscle domains of the suprascapular nerve and the posterior division of the upper trunk (ie, those C5 or C6 motor nerve fibers contributing to the subscapular, thoracodorsal, axillary, and radial nerves). The most useful muscles for the NEE of this element are provided in **Box 3**.

Posterior Cord

Anatomically, the posterior cord consists of the sum of the posterior divisions of all 3 trunks (ie, the subscapular, thoracodorsal, axillary, and radial nerves). Consequently, its SNAP, CMAP, and muscle domains are equivalent to those of these nerves. The most useful muscles for the NEE of this element are provided in **Box 3**.

Medial Cord

Anatomically, the medial cord represents the continuation of the anterior division of the lower trunk. Thus, its SNAP, CMAP, and muscle domains are equivalent to those of the lower trunk minus the SNAP, CMAP, and muscle domains of its posterior division. The most useful muscles for the NEE of this element are provided in **Box 3**.

Axillary Nerve

There are no reliable sensory NCSs that assess this nerve and, thus, there is no SNAP domain for this nerve. Its CMAP domain is the Ax-deltoid. Its muscle domain consists of the axillary nerve–innervated muscles.

Musculocutaneous Nerve

The sensory nerve fibers comprising the musculocutaneous nerve are assessed by the LABC sensory NCS, which is the only sensory NCS in its SNAP domain. Its CMAP domain consists of the Musc-biceps motor NCS and its muscle domain includes the musculocutaneous nerve–innervated muscles.

Radial Nerve

The S-Radial sensory NCS constitutes its SNAP domain, the Radial-EDC and Radial-EIP motor NCSs comprise its CMAP domain, and its muscle domain consists of those muscles innervated by the radial and posterior interosseous nerves.

Median Nerve

The Med-D1, Med-D2, and Med-D3 sensory NCSs make up its SNAP domain, the Med-APB motor NCS constitutes its CMAP domain, and its muscle domain consists of those muscles innervated by the median nerve.

Ulnar Nerve

The Uln-D5 sensory NCS constitutes its SNAP domain, the Ulnar-ADM and Ulnar-FDI motor NCS constitute its CMAP domain, and the muscles innervated by the ulnar nerve make up its muscle domain.

Medial Antebrachial Cutaneous Nerve

The MABC sensory NCS constitutes the SNAP domain of the medial antebrachial cutaneous nerve. There is no CMAP or muscle domain because this nerve contains only sensory nerve fibers.

Commentary

Based on the SNAP domains of the brachial plexus elements discussed previously, the pathways through the brachial plexus that the sensory nerve fibers under study traverse during the performance of the various sensory NCSs are known (see **Figs. 2–6**). As shown in these figures, each sensory NCS assesses more than one brachial plexus element and, consequently, each of these elements is being assessed when that particular study is performed. When more than one pathway is possible, the frequency for that pathway is provided (**Table 1**).[11] This knowledge is mandatory for localizing brachial plexus lesions. The individual pathways taken by the sensory nerve fibers under study for each of the 7 sensory NCSs used in brachial plexus assessment are discussed next.

- The LABC response assesses the LABC nerve, the musculocutaneous nerve, the lateral cord, the upper trunk, and the C6 APR 100% of the time (see **Fig. 2**).
- The Med-D1 response assesses the median nerve, the lateral cord, the upper trunk, and the C6 APR 100% of the time (see **Fig. 3**).
- The Med-D2 response assesses the median nerve and lateral cord 100% of the time, the upper trunk and C6 APR 20% of the time, and the middle trunk and C7 APR 80% of the time (see **Fig. 4**).
- The Med-D3 response assesses the median nerve 100% of the time, the lateral cord 80% of the time, the medial cord 20% of the time, the upper trunk and C6 APR 10% of the time, the middle trunk and C7 APR 70% of the time, and the lower trunk and C8 APR 20% of the time (see **Fig. 5**).
- The S-Radial response assesses the superficial radial nerve, the radial nerve, and the posterior cord 100% of the time; the upper trunk and C6 APR 60% of the time, and the middle trunk and C7 APR 40% of the time (see **Fig. 6**).
- The Uln-D5 response assesses the ulnar nerve, the medial cord, the lower trunk, and the C8 APR 100% of the time.
- The MABC response assesses the MABC nerve, the medial cord, the lower trunk, and the T1 APR 100% of the time.

Table 1
The frequency that axon loss lesions of individual brachial plexus elements are associated with particular sensory nerve conduction study abnormalities

Sensory NCS	Upper Trunk	Middle Trunk	Lower Trunk	Lateral Cord	Posterior Cord	Medial Cord
LABC, %	100	0	0	100	0	0
Med-D1, %	100	0	0	100	0	0
Med-D2, %	20	80	0	100	0	0
Med-D3, %	10	70	20	80	0	20
S-Radial, %	60	40	0	0	100	0
Uln-D5, %	0	0	100	0	0	100
MABC, %	0	0	100	0	0	100

Abbreviations: LABC, lateral antebrachial cutaneous NCS; Med-D1, median NCS recording from first digit; Med-D2, median NCS recording from second digit; Med-D3, median NCS recording from third digit; MABC, medial antebrachial cutaneous NCS; S-Radial, superficial radial NCS; Uln-D5, ulnar NCS recording from fifth digit.

AN APPROACH TO THE ELECTRODIAGNOSTIC ASSESSMENT OF THE BRACHIAL PLEXUS

Rather frequently, patients determined to have brachial plexopathies in the EDX laboratory were referred with some other diagnostic consideration, and the brachial plexus lesion became apparent during the EDX assessment. If only the diagnostic considerations put forth by the referring physician were sought, many of these brachial plexus lesions would have been missed. For example, when a patient with a lower trunk lesion is referred for EDX evaluation of a suspected ulnar neuropathy, if only ulnar sensory and motor NCSs are performed and only ulnar nerve–innervated muscles are sampled on NEE, then an incorrect confirmation will result. To avoid this pitfall, a more organized approach is required. Although the ideal approach would assess every brachial plexus element, this is impractical. Our approach is more regional in nature. It includes a "general survey" (**Box 4**), with subsequent studies based on the general survey findings. Although the general survey assesses all of the cord elements, it assesses the upper trunk only 20% of the time, and it does not assess the C5 or T1 roots; moreover, the assessed elements are not assessed equally. Rather, the general survey assesses the medial cord and lower trunk elements most extensively; the lateral cord, posterior cord, and middle trunk elements to a lesser extent; and the upper trunk element the least. Consequently, whenever an individual is referred for assessment of the brachial plexus or whenever the EDX findings suggest the presence of a brachial plexus lesion—especially an upper trunk lesion—additional NCSs are required. We first localize the lesion with the sensory NCS. Then, the pertinent motor NCSs are performed to grade the severity of the lesion. The NEE is performed last to verify the NCS conclusions and to further characterize the lesion.

Box 4
General survey of the upper extremity

Sensory NCS

    Med-D2

    S-Radial

    Uln-D5

Motor NCS

    Ulnar-ADM

    Median-APB

Needle Electrode Examination

    First dorsal interosseous

    Flexor pollicis longus

    Extensor indicis proprius

    Pronator teres

    Triceps (lateral head)

    Biceps

    Deltoid

    Cervical paraspinal muscles

Trunks

Regarding the trunk elements, the general survey best assesses the lower trunk and least assesses the upper trunk. Consequently, whenever upper trunk lesions are suspected, the general survey must be expanded. We typically add contralateral Med-D2 and S-Radial sensory NCSs (the ipsilateral NCSs are included in our general survey) and bilateral LABC and Med-D1 sensory NCSs (bilateral Med-D3 sensory NCS may also be required). If indicated, on the motor NCS portion of the EDX study, bilateral Musc-biceps and Ax-deltoid responses are added. These studies are also added whenever the patient is noted to have forearm flexion or upper extremity abduction weakness, or whenever reduced MUAP recruitment is seen on NEE of the biceps or deltoid muscles. On NEE, in addition to the general survey muscles, several muscles from the muscle domain of the upper trunk are added. Because the suprascapular nerve exits the upper trunk very proximally, whenever NEE abnormalities are detected in one of the spinati muscles, a lesion proximal to the upper trunk is more likely. In this setting, NEE of muscles innervated by nerves exiting the brachial plexus at the APR level is indicated, such as the serratus anterior (long thoracic nerve), the levator scapulae (dorsal scapular nerve), or the rhomboids (dorsal scapular nerve). Because brachial plexus lesions affect the upper trunk more frequently than any other brachial plexus element, additional studies typically are required.

When attempting to localize a lesion to the upper plexus, it is important to exclude a lateral cord localization. The sensory NCSs are the most helpful in this regard. With upper trunk lesions, the Med-D1 and LABC responses are abnormal (essentially 100% of the time), the Med-D2 response is less frequently abnormal (approximately 20% of the time), and the Med-D3 response is infrequently abnormal (approximately 10% of the time). Thus, with an upper trunk lesion, all 4 of these responses are expected to be abnormal only 2% ($1.0 \times 1.0 \times 0.2 \times 0.1 = 0.02$) of the time (ie, only 1 in 50 upper trunk lesions is expected to affect all 4 of these responses). With lateral cord lesions, however, all 4 responses tend to be abnormal ($1.0 \times 1.0 \times 1.0 \times 0.8 = 80\%$). Another helpful discriminator is the S-Radial sensory NCS, because it is affected approximately 60% of the time with upper trunk lesions but never with lateral cord lesions. Thus, when it is involved, the lesion cannot be localized to the lateral cord. The motor NCS also helps to discriminate between these 2 lesion sites. Whereas upper trunk lesions may affect both the Musc-biceps and the Ax-deltoid responses, lateral cord lesions never affect the Ax-Delt response. Consequently, if the Ax-deltoid response is affected, then the lesion cannot be restricted to the lateral cord. Differentiation by NEE uses the C5,6-radial and axillary nerve–innervated muscles (eg, brachioradialis; deltoid, teres minor), which can be affected with upper trunk lesions, but not by lateral cord lesions.

Evaluation of the middle trunk also requires expansion of the EDX study. To the general survey, we typically add the Med-D2 and radial sensory NCSs contralaterally and the Med-D3 sensory NCS bilaterally. Because of domain overlap between the middle trunk and the upper and lower trunks, all of the NCS and muscle studies comprising the middle trunk domains also assess one of the adjacent trunks (ie, there are no NCS or muscle studies unique to the middle trunk). With isolated middle trunk lesions, the LABC, Med-D1, Uln-D5, and MABC sensory responses are spared, whereas the Med-D2 and Med-D3 tend to be affected. The S-Radial response is not useful for differentiating a middle trunk lesion (affected about 40% of the time) from an upper trunk lesion (affected about 60% of the time). On motor NCS, bilateral Radial-EDC responses are added. On NEE, many muscles must be studied before one can conclude that a lesion involves only the middle trunk (fortunately, a rare event).

Again, there are no muscles contained solely in the muscle domain of the middle trunk (ie, *private* muscles) that are not also contained in the muscle domain of one of the adjacent trunks (ie, *shared* muscles). Nonetheless, isolated middle trunk lesions can be identified. Whenever only the shared muscles (ie, upper and lower trunk muscles that also belong to the middle trunk muscle domain) are affected and the private muscles of the upper and lower trunk are spared, the lesion most likely is restricted to the middle trunk. In our review of the EDX abnormalities associated with more than 417 brachial plexus lesions, we came across this pattern only once (an intraoperatively verified case caused by an idiopathic fibrotic process).[11]

Because the routine survey assesses the lower trunk element to a greater degree than the other 2 trunk elements, few additional studies are required in its EDX assessment. We typically add a contralateral Uln-D5 and bilateral MABC sensory NCS. Additional motor NCSs are not needed, although bilateral Radial-EIP responses may be helpful. We usually expand the NEE with radial (eg, extensor pollicis brevis), ulnar (eg, abductor digiti minimi), and median (eg, abductor pollicis brevis) nerve–innervated muscles. Differentiating a lower trunk lesion from a medial cord lesion can be challenging because most of the available studies assess both elements. There is no sensory NCS that distinguishes between these 2 sites. On motor NCS, an abnormal Radial-EIP response identifies a lower trunk lesion, but a normal response does not identify a medial cord lesion because of the possibility of a partial lower trunk lesion. For differentiating lower trunk lesions from medial cord lesions, the most helpful component of the EDX study is NEE of C8/radial nerve–innervated muscles (ie, extensor indicis proprius; extensor pollicis brevis). When affected, the lesion is accurately localized proximal to the medial cord (eg, lower trunk). As with the motor NCS, sparing of the C8-radial nerve–innervated muscles does not identify a medial cord lesion because a partial lower trunk lesion could also spare these muscles. This differentiation has profound clinical pertinence. For example, among individuals with ulnar sensory and motor nerve symptoms following median sternotomy, the question arises as to whether the symptoms reflect an ulnar neuropathy at the elbow or a C8 APR lesion. If only a focused ulnar nerve evaluation is performed, all of the C8 APR lesions will be falsely localized to the ulnar nerve.

Cords

Regarding the cord elements, as previously stated, the general survey is biased toward assessment of the medial cord. Consequently, whenever lateral cord lesions are suspected, the general survey is expanded. We usually add contralateral Med-D2 and S-Radial NCSs and bilateral LABC, Med-D1, and Med-D3 sensory NCSs. With lateral cord lesions, the LABC, Med-D1, Med-D2, and Med-D3 responses are usually abnormal, whereas with upper trunk lesions, only the LABC and Med-D1 responses are typically affected (discussed previously). A Bilateral Musc-biceps motor NCS may be helpful, especially if forearm flexion weakness has been recognized or if NEE abnormalities were noted in the biceps muscle. Unlike upper trunk lesions, which tend to affect both the Musc-biceps and the Ax-deltoid responses, lateral cord lesions can affect only the Musc-biceps response. Thus, the Ax-deltoid response is added and is expected to be normal with lateral cord lesions. On NEE, muscles from the upper trunk, lateral cord, and posterior cord are added to demonstrate that only muscles belonging to the muscle domain of the lateral cord are affected (ie, C5,6-radial and axillary nerve–innervated muscles are spared).

With suspected posterior cord lesions, we generally add a contralateral S-Radial sensory NCS, bilateral Ax-deltoid motor NCS, and one of the radial motor NCSs (ie, Radial-EDC or Radial-EIP) bilaterally. On NEE, additional radial and axillary nerve–innervated muscles are incorporated. Differentiation of a posterior cord lesion from a middle trunk lesion is important. On sensory NCS, the Med-D2 and Med-D3 sensory NCSs are helpful; they are always spared by posterior cord lesions, but commonly affected when the underlying lesion affects the middle trunk. On motor NCS, the Ax-deltoid and Radial-EIP responses are affected by posterior cord lesions but spared by middle trunk lesions. On NEE, the C7/median nerve–innervated muscles (ie, pronator teres, flexor carpi radialis) are spared with posterior cord lesions, but may be affected by middle trunk lesions.

With suspected medial cord lesions, we typically add a contralateral Uln-D5 and bilateral MABC sensory NCS. Bilateral Radial-EIP motor NCSs are helpful to differentiate a lower trunk process from a lesion affecting the medial cord. We usually expand the NEE with C8/radial (eg, extensor pollicis brevis), C8/ulnar (eg, flexor carpi ulnaris), and C8/median (eg, abductor pollicis brevis) nerve–innervated muscles. The NEE of the C8/radial nerve–innervated muscles (ie, extensor indicis proprius, extensor pollicis brevis) is mandatory for differentiating a medial cord lesion from a lower trunk lesion and is the best way to differentiate a postoperative ulnar neuropathy from a median sternotomy–related C8 APR lesion. The triceps muscle, contrary to popular belief, is not very helpful in this regard because it receives little C8-derived innervation; this explains why it is infrequently affected with both true neurogenic thoracic outlet syndrome (this syndrome affects the T1 > C8 APR) and with median sternotomy–induced brachial plexopathies (this disorder primarily affects the C8 APR).[23]

SUMMARY

Of the 4 major PNS plexuses, disorders of the brachial plexus are encountered far more frequently than those of the others. The EDX examination is probably the best procedure available by which to evaluate brachial plexus lesions. It provides localizing, pathologic, pathophysiologic, severity, and prognostic information. By localizing the lesion and identifying the underlying pathophysiology, it often predicts the underlying etiologic process, examples of which include (1) major T1 APR involvement with true neurogenic thoracic outlet syndrome; (2) C8 APR involvement with postmedian sternotomy brachial plexopathy; (3) supraclavicular demyelinating conduction block with classic postoperative paralysis (often confined to the upper plexus); (4) widespread infraclavicular demyelinating conduction blocks with radiation plexopathy; (5) severe progressive axon loss with neoplastic processes; (6) motor NCS abnormalities exceeding sensory NCS abnormalities for the same PNS segment with intraspinal canal lesions (eg, avulsions); (7) demyelinating conduction block with sparing of the pertinent sensory NCS with multifocal motor neuropathy; and (8) lack of EDX abnormalities with hysteria, conversion reactions, and malingering, as well as with disputed thoracic outlet syndrome. In addition, incorrect clinical considerations may be excluded (eg, when abnormal sensory responses are identified, an isolated radiculopathy is excluded).

CASE VIGNETTES

The following 3 cases serve to illustrate our approach to the diagnosis of brachial plexus lesions. This approach is useful whether the patient is referred with a suspected brachial plexus disorder or not. Because the pathophysiology underlying brachial plexopathies is not demyelinating conduction slowing, the associated latency and conduction velocity values were normal. Thus, only the amplitude values are provided in the tables. Values shown in parentheses represent the values recorded from the contralateral side.

Case 1

Clinical

A 58-year-old woman with a history of breast cancer is referred for right upper extremity pain and weakness. She was treated surgically 11 years earlier. She did not receive radiation therapy.

Screening sensory NCS

SNAP	Abnormal	Normal
Med-D2		26.3
S-Radial	4.0; (28.2)	
Uln-D5		12.7

The screening sensory NCSs show an abnormal S-Radial response, indicating that the responsible lesion involves the superficial radial nerve, radial nerve, posterior cord, upper plexus, or middle plexus. The normal Med-D2 and Uln-D5 responses do not shorten this list of possibilities. In the setting of an abnormal S-Radial or Med-D2 response, because the sensory fibers subserving these 2 studies emanate from the C6 or C7 DRG, the LABC and Med-D1 responses are added.

Added sensory NCSs

SNAP	Abnormal	Normal
LABC	No response	
Med-D1	No response	

The abnormalities indicate the upper plexus localization and exclude the superficial radial nerve, radial nerve, posterior cord, and middle plexus as potential lesion sites. Thus, at this point, the sensory NCSs have localized the lesion to the upper plexus. For this reason, the motor NCS survey will be expanded to include the Musc-biceps and Ax-deltoid NCSs (for severity assessment).

Screening and added motor NCSs

CMAP	Abnormal	Normal
Ulnar-ADM		8.0
Median-APB		7.1
Ax-deltoid	3.4; (7.4)	
Musc-biceps	2.5; (6.1)	

The motor NCS findings concur with the upper plexus localization and, based on the recorded values, suggest a lesion of moderate-severe degree. Several muscles in the upper plexus muscle domain were added, including those receiving innervation via the APR (to attempt to deduce the extent of the lesion).

NEE

The NEE showed features of acute (eg, fibrillation potentials) and chronic (eg, long-duration motor unit action potentials) motor axon loss in the following muscles identified as abnormal.

Abnormal: deltoid, brachioradialis, biceps, and pronator teres.

Normal: serratus anterior, infraspinatus, flexor pollicis longus (FPL), triceps, extensor indicis proprius (EIP), first dorsal interosseous (FDI), and paraspinals.

Sparing of the serratus anterior argues against an APR-level lesion, as does sparing of the spinati (because the suprascapular nerve exits the upper trunk just after its formation). Thus, the NEE examination suggests that the lesion involves the upper trunk region of the upper plexus. Normal rhomboids would also support a lesion distal to the APR level of the upper plexus. Following this EDX study, magnetic resonance imaging of the brachial plexus identified a mass involving the upper trunk that was ultimately shown to be recurrent breast cancer. Thus, this case represents a neoplastic brachial plexopathy.

Case 2

Clinical

A 26-year-old woman was referred for EDX assessment of thenar eminence atrophy that was noted by her sister. Further questioning revealed at least a 10-year history of intermittent aching along the medial aspect of her upper extremity and a recently history of intermittent tingling along the medial aspect of her forearm and hand when lying on her back.

Screening sensory NCS

SNAP	Abnormal	Normal
Med-D2		51.3
S-Radial		61.1
Uln-D5	16.0; (37.7)	

The amplitude value of the Uln-D5 response is normal but, in comparison with the other responses, is suspicious. For this patient's age, the lower limit of normal for the Med-D2 response is 20, for the S-Radial response is 17, and for the Uln-D5 response is 12. Thus, the Med-D2 response value is approximately 2.5 times the lower limit of normal, the S-Radial response is roughly 3.5 times the lower limit of normal, and the Uln-D5 response is only about 1.25 times the lower limit of normal. For this reason, the Uln-D5 response was compared with the response recorded on the contralateral asymptomatic side and identified as being relatively abnormal (ie, the side-to-side difference exceeded 50%). The value of the contralateral response value is about 3 times the lower limit of normal, similar to the ipsilateral values.

An abnormal Uln-D5 response is consistent with a lesion involving the ulnar nerve, the medial cord, or the lower plexus. In the setting of an abnormal Uln-D5, the MABC response is added.

Added sensory NCS

SNAP	Abnormal	Normal
	MABC	No response; (15.7)

If the MABC response had been normal, the dorsal ulnar cutaneous response could have been added for further localization but, because it was abnormal, this study was not required. The presence of an abnormal MABC indicates that the lesion lies in the medial cord or the lower plexus of the brachial plexus. Another feature of these responses is that the Uln-D5 response (C8-derived fibers) is only relatively abnormal, whereas the MABC response (T1-derived fibers) is absent. This pattern suggests that the lesion may involve the APR level of the brachial plexus because the T1 fibers (assessed by the MABC response) are involved to a greater extent than the C8 fibers (assessed by the Uln-D5 response). To differentiate a medial cord lesion from a lower plexus lesion, studies that assess the C8/radial motor nerve fibers are added because they traverse the lower plexus and the posterior cord, but not the medial cord. Thus, their involvement localizes the lesion to the lower plexus. For this reason, the routine motor NCSs are expanded to include the Radial-EIP study.

Screening and added motor NCS

CMAP	Abnormal	Normal
Ulnar-ADM		8.0; 10.3
Median-APB	1.5; (8.0)	
Radial-EIP		2.9; (4.1)
Ulnar-FDI		10.3; (14.7)

Of the 2 routine studies, the Median-APB response is quite abnormal and the Ulnar-ADM is normal. The Ulnar-FDI study was added to better assess the medial cord and lower plexus elements and was also normal. Although the ulnar and radial motor response values are smaller than those recorded from the contralateral side, they do not meet the criteria for a relative abnormality. Because the thenar eminence muscles receive a heavy T1 > C8 input, whereas the other studied muscles have a heavier C8 input, the T1 fibers again appear more affected than the C8 fibers, likewise suggesting an APR-level lesion. Thus, as this point, the lesion has not been further localized by the motor NCS. On NEE, muscles receiving C8/radial nerve innervation are added (eg, extensor indicis proprius; extensor pollicis brevis).

NEE
Abnormal: APB, FPL, FDI, flexor digitorum profundus (FDP)-4,5, EIP, extensor pollicis brevis (EPB).
   Normal: Deltoid, brachioradialis, biceps, triceps, pronator teres, paraspinals.
   Among the abnormal muscles, the APB was much more abnormal than the other muscles. Involvement of the C8/radial nerve–innervated muscles indicates that the lesion is indeed supraclavicular, that it involves the lower plexus, and that the T1 sensory and motor nerve fibers are affected out of proportion to the C8 fibers, again supporting an APR-level lesion. This pattern is commonly observed among patients with true neurogenic thoracic outlet syndrome, which is what this patient had. True neurogenic thoracic outlet syndrome is a condition in which a taut band extends from the first rib to either a C7 rib or an elongated C7 transverse process. The band deflects the lower plexus from below, angulating the T1 nerve fibers to a greater extent than the C8 nerve fibers, thereby rendering this constellation of EDX findings. The latter reflects the fact that most of the sensory and motor nerve fibers comprising the ulnar nerve derive from the C8 DRG and C8 AHCs, respectively, whereas those comprising the MABC and recurrent thenar motor branch derive predominantly from the T1 DRG and AHCs, respectively.[11,13]

Case 3

Clinical
A 71-year-old man underwent open heart surgery via a median sternotomy and, postoperatively, complained of hand weakness and numbness along the medial aspect of the hand. He was referred for EDX assessment of a suspected ulnar neuropathy.

Screening sensory NCS

SNAP	Abnormal	Normal
Med-D2		14.0
S-Radial		13.8
Uln-D5	NR	

The absent Uln-D5 response is consistent with an ulnar neuropathy or a brachial plexus lesion involving the medial cord or lower plexus. To better localize the lesion, the MABC sensory NCS is added.

Added sensory NCS

SNAP	Abnormal	Normal
MABC		11; (12)
Dorsal ulnar cutaneous	NR	

The MABC response was normal, arguing against a medial cord, lower trunk, or T1 APR lesion and supporting an ulnar nerve or C8 APR lesion. A partial lesion of the medial cord or lower trunk cannot be excluded. The dorsal ulnar cutaneous sensory NCS was added and was abnormal. Thus, if the lesion involves the ulnar nerve, it lies proximal to the wrist.

Screening and added motor NCS

CMAP	Abnormal	Normal
Ulnar-ADM	3.5; (10.0)	
Median-APB		7.1; (6.3)
Radial-EIP	0.8; (2.3)	
Ulnar-FDI	2.1; (8.9)	

The routine motor NCSs do not further define the localization of the lesion. The added Radial-EIP is abnormal, indicating that the lesion is supraclavicular and, thus, involves the C8 APR. The Ulnar-FDI was added to further assess the severity of the process. The 3 motor responses indicate that approximately 65% to 75% of the motor nerve fibers of the C8 APR are affected.

NEE

Abnormal: FDP-3,4, FDI, EIP, EPB, FPL.

Normal: Biceps, triceps, pronator teres, APB, paraspinals.

The abnormal muscles include those receiving C8/radial, C8/median, and C8/ulnar nerve innervation. If the referral diagnosis of postoperative ulnar neuropathy was assumed to be correct by the EDX provider and the NCSs were limited to ulnar sensory and motor NCSs and NEE of only ulnar nerve–innervated muscles of the hand and proximal forearm, then the lesion would have been mistakenly localized to the ulnar nerve and an unnecessary ulnar nerve transposition might have been performed. Whenever ulnar distribution features follow a median sternotomy, consideration should be given to postmedian sternotomy brachial plexopathy. It is postulated that the median sternotomy causes first rib rotation into the C8 APR or causes first rib fracture with impingement of the C8 APR by the fractured segment. In either case, the median sternotomy results in a traction injury of the lower plexus that involves the C8 APR disproportionately. Unless significant axon loss involves the dominant hand or causalgic pain develops, these lesions usually are treated conservatively.[13]

SUMMARY OF CASES

These 3 cases illustrate the localizing utility of the sensory NCS. Following the screening sensory NCS, if either the Med-D2 or S-Radial sensory responses are abnormal (both of which assess sensory nerve fibers derived from the C6 or C7 DRG), the LABC and Med-D1 sensory NCSs are added (the latter assess the lateral cord and the C6 fibers of the upper plexus). If the Uln-D5 sensory response is abnormal, then the MABC sensory NCS is added. If the MABC response is abnormal, then a dorsal ulnar cutaneous (DUC) study is not required because the lesion lies proximal to the ulnar nerve. If the MABC is normal, then the DUC study is added. If the DUC study were to be performed before the MABC study, regardless of whether it is normal or abnormal, the MABC study is still required. Following the sensory NCSs, the motor NCSs are used, both the routine screening studies and those dictated by the localization of the lesion identified during the sensory NCSs. The motor NCSs confirm the localization of the lesion and grade its severity before collateral sprouting (following reinnervation via collateral sprouting, the CMAP is normalized and the severity of the lesion is underestimated). The NEE confirms the localization and severity of the lesion while simultaneously characterizing it further.

REFERENCES

1. Wilbourn AJ. Brachial plexus disorders. In: Dyck PJ, Thomas PK, editors. Peripheral neuropathy, vol. 2. 4th edition. Philadelphia: Elsevier Saunders; 2005. p. 1339–73.
2. Stewart JD. Focal peripheral neuropathies. 2nd edition. New York: Raven Press; 1993.
3. Swash M. Diagnosis of brachial root and plexus lesions. J Neurol 1896;233: 131–5.
4. Clemente CD, editor. Gray's anatomy. 30th edition (American). Philadelphia: Lea & Febiger; 1985.
5. Ferrante MA, Wilbourn AJ. Basic principles and practice of electromyography. In: Younger DS, editor. Motor disorders. Philadelphia: Lippincott, Williams, Wilkins; 1999. p. 19–44.
6. Leffert RD. Brachial plexus injuries. London: Churchill Livingstone; 1985.
7. Birch R, Bonney G, Wynn Parry CB. Surgical disorders of peripheral nerves. London: Churchill Livingstone; 1998.
8. Kline DG, Hudson AR. Nerve injuries. Philadelphia: WB Saunders; 1995.
9. Coene LN. Mechanisms of brachial plexus lesions. Clin Neurol Neurosurg 1993; 95:S24–9.
10. Brunelli GA, Brunelli GR. A fourth type of brachial plexus injury: middle lesion (C7). Ital J Orthop Traumatol 1992;18:389–93.
11. Ferrante MA, Wilbourn AJ. The utility of various sensory conduction responses in assessing brachial plexopathies. Muscle Nerve 1995;18:879–89.
12. Wilbourn AJ. Electrodiagnosis of plexopathies. Neurol Clin 1985;3:511–29.
13. Ferrante MA. Brachial plexopathies: classification, causes, and consequences. Muscle Nerve 2004;30:547–68.

14. Waller A. Experiments on the section of the glossopharyngeal and hypoglossal nerves of the frog, and observations of the alterations produced thereby in the structure of their primitive fibres. Philos Trans R Soc Lond B Biol Sci 1850;140: 423–9.

15. Levin KH. L5 radiculopathy with reduced superficial peroneal sensory responses: intraspinal and extraspinal causes. Muscle Nerve 1998;21:3–7.

16. Wilbourn AJ, Ferrante MA. Clinical electromyography, Section 2 (Neurodiagnostic studies). Record. In: Joynt RJ, Griggs RC, editors. Baker's clinical neurology on CD-ROM. Philadelphia: Lippincott, Williams, Wilkins; 2000. p. 7592–8248. Chapter 5.

17. Liveson JA, Ma DM. Laboratory reference for clinical neurophysiology. Philadelphia: Davis; 1991. p. 415–23.

18. Liveson JA. Peripheral neurology: case studies in electrodiagnosis. Philadelphia: Davis; 1992. p. 36–42.

19. Kendall FP, McCreary EK, Provance PG. Muscles: testing and function. 4th edition. Baltimore (MD): Williams & Wilkins; 1993. p. 406–7.

20. Wilbourn AJ, Aminoff MJ. Radiculopathies. In: Brown WF, Bolton CF, editors. Clinical electromyography. 2nd edition. Boston: Butterworth-Heinemann; 1993. p. 175–205.

21. Perotto AO. Anatomical guide for the electromyographer: the limbs and trunk. 3rd edition. Springfield (IL): Charles C Thomas Publisher LTD; 1994. p. 305–7.

22. Levin KH, Wilbourn AJ, Maggiano HJ. Cervical rib and median sternotomy-related brachial plexopathies: a reassessment. Neurology 1990;50:1407–13.

23. Wilbourn AJ, Ferrante MA. Plexopathies. In: Pourmand R, editor. Neuromuscular diseases: expert clinicians' views. Boston: Butterworth Heineman; 2001. p. 493–527.

Approach to the Patient with Suspected Radiculopathy

Kerry H. Levin, MD

KEYWORDS

- Radiculopathy • Electrodiagnosis • Neuromuscular disorders
- Intraspinal canal lesion • EMG

Radiculopathy is one of the most common causes for referral to the electromyography (EMG) laboratory. Despite this, the value of electrodiagnosis in the assessment of possible radiculopathy is extremely variable. Depending on issues of patient selection, segmental level of involvement, and the electrodiagnostic modalities used, reports have suggested high and low correlation between electrodiagnostic testing and either neuroimaging or surgical localization.[1–3] Many patients referred to the laboratory have nonspecific symptoms that represent nonneurologic disorders because of musculoskeletal disease. Among patients with true radiculopathy, most have only radicular pain and sensory symptoms, which do not have electrophysiologic correlates measurable with standard nerve conduction studies (NCS) and needle electrode examination (NEE).

Electrodiagnostic testing is most valuable in the patient with motor or other focal neurologic deficits, such as muscle stretch reflex asymmetry. In this setting, electrodiagnostic testing can aid in the segmental localization of the lesion, and can provide information regarding the physiology (axon loss or conduction block), age, activity, and severity of the process. Electrodiagnostic testing can aid in the exclusion of other disorders masquerading as radiculopathy, and may be of value in the assessment of patients with postsurgical deficits, multisegmental neurologic deficits, or multilevel intraspinal structural changes.

The rational approach to the patient with suspected radiculopathy should incorporate data from various sources: the clinical history, general and neurologic examination, and imaging studies. In the patient with classic localizable symptoms of radiculopathy, focal neurologic deficits, and appropriately positioned structural abnormalities on neuroimaging studies, clinical decisions can be made without the confirmatory findings provided by the EMG examination. Unfortunately, it is usually

Department of Neurology, Desk S-90, Cleveland Clinic, 9500 Euclid Avenue, Cleveland, OH 44195, USA
E-mail address: levink@ccf.org

Neurol Clin 30 (2012) 581–604
doi:10.1016/j.ncl.2011.12.011
0733-8619/12/$ – see front matter © 2012 Elsevier Inc. All rights reserved.

not the case that the medical picture is completely clear, especially when pain hampers the reliability of muscle strength testing at the bedside. The following discussion explores the principles of electrodiagnosis in radiculopathy, and discusses various testing procedures and their relative value.

ANATOMY AND PATHOPHYSIOLOGY

In all, there are 31 pairs of spinal nerve roots: 8 cervical, 12 thoracic, 5 lumbar, 5 sacral, and 1 coccygeal. Each spinal nerve root is comprised of a dorsal (somatic sensory) root and a ventral (somatic motor) root, that join in the intraspinal region, just proximal to the neural (intervertebral) foramen (**Fig. 1**). In the extraspinal region, just distal to the neural foramen, the nerve root divides in two: a small posterior primary ramus that supplies innervation to the paraspinal muscles and skin of the neck and trunk, and a large anterior primary ramus that supplies innervation to the limbs and trunk, including intercostal and abdominal wall muscles.

Neural foramina are formed between each pair of vertebral bodies, and are bounded superiorly and inferiorly by pedicles, anteriorly by intervertebral disks and vertebral bodies, and posteriorly by facet joints (see **Fig. 1**). Through the neural foramina pass the spinal nerve roots, recurrent meningeal nerves, and radicular blood vessels. Cervical roots 1 through 7 enter the neural foramen above the vertebral body of the same number, such that the C3 root exits the spinal canal via the C2-3 neural foramen. Because there are only seven cervical vertebrae, the C8 root exits through the C7-T1 neural foramen. As a result, all thoracic, lumbar, and sacral roots exit below the vertebral body of the same number.

The blood supply to spinal nerve roots is provided by a capillary network derived from the radicular arteries. In the rat, in the transitional region between the peripheral and central nervous system (the root entry zone), blood vessels are positioned on the surface of rootlets and in interradicular spaces, but not in rootlets themselves. The

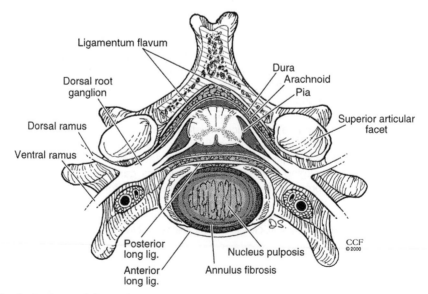

Fig. 1. Anatomy of the root.

density of capillaries is very high in the ventral nerve root entry zone.[4] Distal to the root-lets in rats, at the proximal and distal root levels, ventral root capillary density is higher than at the dorsal roots.[5]

Cell bodies of the motor nerve fibers reside in the anterior horns of the spinal cord, whereas those of the sensory nerve fibers reside in the dorsal root ganglia (DRG). DRG are in general located in a protected position within the neural foramina, and are not strictly speaking intraspinal. However, at the lumbar and sacral levels, there is a tendency for DRG to reside proximal to the neural foramina, in intraspinal locations. About 3% of L3 and L4 DRG are intraspinal, about 11% to 38% of L5 DRG are intra-spinal, and about 71% of S1 DRG are intraspinal, according to recent cadaver, radio-graphic, and magnetic resonance imaging (MRI) studies.[6,7] In the cervical region, the C5 and C6 DRG also have a tendency to reside in relative intraspinal locations.[8] When DRG are in intraspinal positions they are more exposed, and therefore vulnerable to injury. With disk or boney compression of DRG, or with disruption of sensory axons distal to DRG, sensory axons degenerate and sensory nerve action potential (SNAP) amplitude loss is seen on NCS.

Nerve root fibers are vulnerable to the same types of injury as other peripheral nerves: entrapment, compression, infiltration, ischemia, and transection. The likeli-hood of nerve root compression by disk rupture at lumbosacral levels may be increased by the presence of extrathecal dural and foraminal ligaments that anchor nerve roots and reduce their plasticity.[9] Mild injury may result in focal demyelination leading to conduction block or conduction velocity slowing along nerve root fibers. Axon loss at the root level results in wallerian degeneration along the whole course of affected nerve fibers. Conduction block and axon loss produce symptoms and neurologic deficits if a sufficient number of nerve fibers are affected. Conduction velocity slowing alone is insufficient to produce weakness or significant sensory loss, although sensory modalities requiring timed volleys of impulse transmission along their pathways, such as vibration and proprioception, can be altered.

NERVE CONDUCTION STUDIES

A number of factors reduce the sensitivity of NCS in the diagnosis of radiculopathy. First, most radiculopathies are caused by compression from disk protrusion or spon-dylosis, and result in damage to only a fraction of nerve root fibers, producing limited motor and sensory deficits. Second, in the acute setting, radiculopathy manifests itself most commonly by symptoms of pain and alteration of sensory perception. Sensory radiculopathy can only rarely be reliably localized segmentally by electro-diagnostic techniques. This is the case because symptoms of pain and paresthesia are primarily mediated through C-type sensory fibers that are too small to be studied by routine electrodiagnostic techniques, and because the peripheral processes of sensory root fibers remain intact with intraspinal lesions, so SNAPs remain normal. Third, the intraspinal location of most lesions makes it impossible to perform direct NCS on the nerve root proximal to the damaged segment, preventing the diagnosis of conduction block or focal conduction velocity slowing along the damaged segment of the root.

NCS are an important part of the routine electrodiagnostic work-up for radiculop-athy as a means to exclude other disorders that may coexist with radiculopathy or may clinically masquerade as radiculopathy. Such disorders include focal mono-neuropathies and polyneuropathy. The tibial H reflex is one NCS that is very useful to support the diagnosis of S1 radiculopathy.

Routine Studies

Sensory NCS performed along peripheral nerve trunks are characteristically normal in radiculopathy. The SNAP amplitude, distal latency, and nerve conduction velocity should not be affected in radiculopathy. The SNAP amplitude may be abnormal if DRG are affected in the pathologic process. In pathologic processes that infiltrate or extend from the intraspinal space into the neural foramen, such as malignancy, infection, or meningioma, DRG are damaged and wallerian degeneration along sensory axons occurs, resulting in SNAP amplitude loss. When DRG reside in an intraspinal location they become vulnerable to compression by disk protrusion and spondylosis. For this reason L5 radiculopathy can uncommonly be associated with loss of the superficial peroneal SNAP.[10] However, S1 radiculopathy is almost never associated with sural SNAP amplitude loss. Although S1 DRG are even more commonly intraspinal than L5 DRG, their intraspinal location is caudal to the L5-S1 disk space where most compressive S1 radiculopathies occur. When nerve root damage occurs distal to the neural foramen, SNAP amplitude is affected.[10,11]

Motor NCS are relatively insensitive in the diagnosis of motor radiculopathy for several reasons. First, most radiculopathies interrupt only a fraction of the total number of motor root fibers, whereas loss of close to 50% of motor axons in a nerve trunk is required to reliably establish a significant reduction in the compound muscle action potential (CMAP) amplitude compared with the same response on the uninvolved side.[12] Second, to identify an abnormality of CMAP amplitude in a motor radiculopathy, the muscle belly from which the CMAP is generated must be in the myotome of the injured root. For example, a severe C8 radiculopathy is expected to produce some change in the ulnar CMAP amplitude, recording from either the abductor digiti minimi or the first dorsal interosseus. In the C5 myotome, the musculocutaneous and axillary nerve trunks can be stimulated to assess CMAPs from the biceps and deltoid muscles, respectively. However, muscles in the C6 and C7 myotomes are not spatially isolated from muscles of other myotomes, and therefore CMAPs derived from them are unreliable. **Tables 1** and **2** outline the screening NCS that are performed for nonspecific arm and leg symptoms.

Table 1		
Nerve conduction studies performed for arm pain		
Nerve	**Recording Site**	**Root Distribution**
Sensory nerve conduction study		
Median	Digit 1	C6
	Digit 2	C6-7
	Digit 3	C7
Ulnar	Digit 4-5	C8 (T1)
Radial	Dorsal hand	C6 (7)
Lateral antebrachial cutaneous	Forearm	C6
Medial antebrachial cutaneous	Forearm	T1
Motor nerve conduction study		
Median	Thenar eminence	(C8) T1
Ulnar	Hypothenar eminence	C8 (T1)
Radial	Extensor digitorum communis	C8
Musculocutaneous	Biceps	C5-6
Axillary	Deltoid	C5-6

Table 2		
Nerve conduction studies performed for leg pain		
Nerve	**Recording Site**	**Root Distribution**
Sensory nerve conduction study		
Sural	Lateral ankle	S1
Superficial peroneal	Dorsum foot	L5
Saphenous	Medial foreleg	L3-4
Tibial H reflex	Foreleg	S1
Motor nerve conduction study		
Posterior tibial	Abductor hallucis	S1
Peroneal	Extensor digitorum brevis	L5 (S1)
Femoral	Rectus femoris	L3-4

Late Responses

Late responses (F wave and H reflex) are electrical stimulus-evoked motor potentials that can be used to measure the travel time of propagated nerve action potentials from a distal point of electrical stimulation along a peripheral nerve trunk, proximally to the spinal cord, and then back down the limb to a muscle belly innervated by the same peripheral nerve trunk. Theoretically, they make possible the assessment of conduction through the damaged segment of a nerve root, but there are several limitations. First, because the traditional measurement is latency, the sensitivity is low because even severe slowing over a short segment usually does not prolong the total latency enough to be significant. Second, as long as a few nerve fibers conduct normally through a damaged segment, a normal "shortest" latency is recorded, even in the presence of severe nerve root damage. Finally, late responses, such as F waves, are of limited value in the diagnosis of radiculopathy because they are not recorded along sensory nerve fibers, and are useless in the assessment of sensory symptoms.

F Wave

The F wave was first described by McDougal and Magladery in 1950, and was so named because it was originally recorded from foot muscles. The F wave is a motor response often recorded from a muscle belly after stimulation of the peripheral nerve trunk innervating the muscle. It is thought to arise from the "backfiring" of motor neurons as impulses arrive antidromically from a peripheral site of nerve trunk stimulation. The F wave occurs after the CMAP, but as the point of nerve trunk stimulation is moved more proximally, the CMAP latency lengthens and the F-wave latency shortens, indicating that the impulse eliciting the F wave travels away from the recording electrodes toward the spinal cord before returning to activate distal muscles. Traditionally, the shortest latency of at least eight consecutive discharges is measured. The absence of an F-wave response from stimulation of the median, ulnar, or tibial nerve in the presence of normal evoked CMAPs from the same muscle suggests conduction block or very recent (<5–8 days) axon loss somewhere along the nerve trunk proximal to the point of nerve stimulation. This is most often encountered in the setting of acute demyelinating polyneuropathy, but could conceivably be a feature of isolated radiculopathy when occurring in a single myotomal distribution. Peroneal F responses are not reliably recorded in normal individuals. A shortest F-wave latency of 25 milliseconds is identified with stimulation of the ulnar nerve at the wrist in **Fig. 2.**

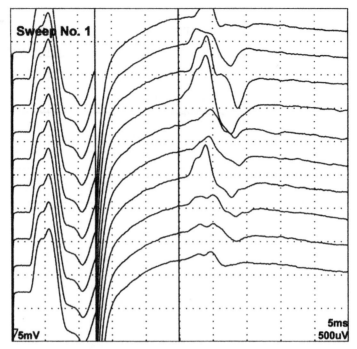

Fig. 2. F waves elicited with ulnar nerve stimulation at the wrist.

Several studies have suggested that other F-wave measurements may be more sensitive than shortest latency, including F-wave duration, mean F latency, and chronodispersion, which measures the interval between the shortest and longest F latency in a consecutive series of stimuli.[13] Several studies suggest that using these methods increases the sensitivity of F-wave analysis in L5-S1 radiculopathy to a level close to the sensitivity of the NEE.[14,15] One study reported that F-wave chronodispersion increased in patients with lumbar canal stenosis and L5-S1 root lesions after 3 minutes of standing.[16] However, F-wave changes may be seen in several different peripheral neuropathic disorders, and cannot support radiculopathy by themselves. An evidence-based review concluded that peroneal and tibial F waves have low sensitivity in the diagnosis of lumbosacral radiculopathy (class II–III evidence, possibly effective in diagnosis).[17]

H Reflex

The H reflex was first described by Hoffmann in 1918. Traditionally, this response has been considered the electrophysiologic equivalent of the Achilles tendon (ankle) muscle stretch reflex. Although the contention that the H reflex represents conduction through a monosynaptic pathway is likely to be overly simplistic, it is clear that the electrical stimulus travels orthodromically along Ia afferents to the spinal cord, where the motor neuron in the same segment is activated, producing a motor response peripherally.[18,19] When elicited from the tibial nerve with stimulation at the popliteal fossa, a motor response in the soleus–gastronemius muscle occurs. In some normal individuals there is discordance between the ability to elicit the H reflex and the presence of the ankle muscle stretch reflex.[20] An H reflex with a latency of 33 milliseconds and amplitude of 3 mV is identified with tibial nerve stimulation in **Fig. 3**.

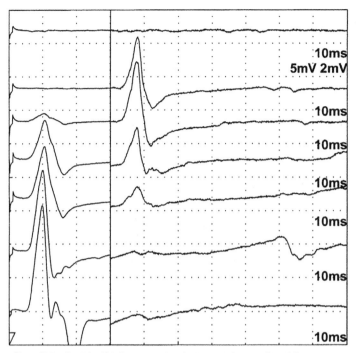

Fig. 3. H reflex elicited with tibial nerve stimulation at the popliteal fossa.

The H reflex can be elicited from other nerve trunks. In the presence of corticospinal tract disease, they can be elicited from many nerve trunks, as a result of loss of the normal central inhibitory influences on motor neuron pools. Under normal circumstances, aside from the tibial H reflex, the H reflex can be elicited reliably only from the median nerve, recording over the flexor carpi radialis. Abnormalities of the median H reflex have been found in patients with C6-7 radiculopathy. One study identified 11 of 25 patients with absence of the median H reflex, whereas 6 of the remaining 14 had a prolonged H-reflex latency.[21] The upper limit for the median H reflex has been reported as 20 milliseconds, but nomograms taking into account the effect of arm length allow more precision in diagnosis.[21]

Only the tibial H reflex is routinely used in clinical practice, where it is an extremely sensitive test for the assessment of the integrity of the tibial–S1 sensory pathway, including the intraspinal course of the S1 root. In one study, the H reflex was absent or low in amplitude in more than 80% of surgically proved cases of S1 radiculopathy.[22] It is markedly reduced in amplitude or absent in axon loss lesions affecting the S1 root, the tibial division of the sciatic nerve, and the posterior tibial nerve at or proximal to the popliteal fossa. Reports have explored the sensitivity of the H-reflex latency compared with the H-reflex amplitude.[23] The upper limit of normal for the tibial H-reflex latency is often described as 34 to 35 milliseconds, but normal latency values vary depending on age, limb length, and height. Use of nomograms can narrow the normal range and potentially improve diagnostic precision.[24] Still, the most direct and reliable measurement seems to be the assessment of the side-to-side difference in H amplitude. A report of side-to-side differences in normal individuals suggested that an H-amplitude ratio (abnormal H amplitude divided by the contralateral H amplitude) of less than 0.4 is likely to be abnormal, although 1 of the 47 normal individuals had a ratio of 0.33.[25] In the author's laboratory, an additional criterion for abnormality is amplitude of less than 1 mV in individuals less than 60 years of age. An evidence-based review concluded that the H reflex probably aids in the diagnosis of S1 radiculopathy (class II–III evidence).[17]

The H reflex is likely to show an abnormality with any disturbance of conduction through the tibial–S1 pathway. Although sensitive, the H reflex has reduced specificity, resulting in several clinical limitations. First, the response is not reliably present in normal subjects after the age of 60 years, although normal responses have been identified at all ages. Second, although unilateral absence of the H reflex is clearly abnormal at any age, bilateral absence of H responses is often of uncertain clinical significance. Technical factors and generalized neuropathic processes can affect the H reflex. Possible causes include obesity and inadequate penetration of the stimulus in the popliteal fossa; prior lumbar spine surgery; and peripheral polyneuropathy, especially in the setting of diabetes. Bilateral absence of the H reflex may be the earliest electrodiagnostic feature of acute demyelinating peripheral polyneuropathy (Guillain-Barré syndrome). Finally, abnormalities anywhere along the tibial–S1 sensory or motor pathway alter the H response, including posterior tibial mononeuropathies proximal to the branch point of the nerve to the soleus and gastrocnemius muscles. Thus, an H-reflex abnormality is insufficient by itself to confirm the presence of an S1 radiculopathy.

Somatosensory Evoked Responses

Theoretically, somatosensory evoked potentials (SEPs) should be a valuable tool in the assessment of conduction abnormalities along sensory fibers at the root level. Electrical stimuli are delivered on the skin surface to a mixed sensory and motor nerve trunk, a sensory nerve trunk, or the skin in a specific dermatomal distribution. Responses are recorded over the spine and scalp, and latencies are measured to assess the conduction time along large-diameter sensory fibers across various segments of the peripheral and central conduction pathways primarily subserving proprioception and vibratory sense.

Unfortunately, a number of limitations diminish the value of this technique. First, amplitude measurements are too variable in normal individuals to have clinical significance, thus the assessment of partial axon loss lesions and partial conduction block is not reliable. Second, focal slowing in the root segment is diluted by normal conduction along the rest of the sensory pathway. Third, nerve trunk stimulation often simultaneously activates nerve fibers belonging to more than one root segment, masking the abnormality in the abnormal root in question.[26] SEPs assess conduction along primarily large-fiber sensory pathways that subserve proprioceptive and vibratory perception functions, not the pain and cutaneous sensation pathways that are more likely to be affected in radiculopathy. Finally, the procedure is time consuming and subject to technical artifacts.

Given these limitations, SEPs obtained from nerve trunk stimulation have been shown to add little diagnostic value.[27,28] Likewise, SEPs derived from L5-S1 dermatomal stimulation have not been found to be as useful as standard electrodiagnostic techniques.[28,29] An evidence-based review concluded that there is inadequate evidence to reach a decision on the use of dermatomal or segmental SEP of the L5 and S1 dermatomes in the diagnosis of lumbosacral radiculopathy (class III evidence).[17]

Cutaneous sensory nerves have more specific and isolated root innervations, and thus SEPs derived from cutaneous nerve stimulation have a potential diagnostic advantage. Studies have been performed on the saphenous, sural, and superficial peroneal sensory nerves. Scalp recorded cutaneous SEPs were abnormal in 57% of

28 cases of cervical and lumbosacral radiculopathy in one report, based on findings of abnormal amplitude and waveform configuration.[30] Using the same technique Seyal and colleagues[31] found only 20% of their patients had abnormal scalp recordings, although the number of abnormal cases increased to about 50% when spine recorded SEP latency or response size was measured. Despite these results, the overall correlation was poor between the SEP abnormality and the clinical localization of the sensory radicular symptoms.[32]

SEPs do not seem to have either the specificity or sensitivity of other electrodiagnostic techniques, such as the NEE, to recommend them at this time for the routine diagnosis of radiculopathy.

Other Conduction Studies

Several studies have explored the value of spinal nerve root stimulation, performed at the level of the vertebral lamina. Studies assessed latency and amplitude asymmetry, and seemed to have greater reliability at the cervical levels than at the lumbosacral levels.[33,34] Several factors decrease the potential value of this technique. First, it is not clear at what site the root is being stimulated. Stimulation of the root at or distal to the neural foramen does not include the likely site of nerve compression for most cases of radiculopathy. Second, the procedure is uncomfortable because it produces contraction of paraspinal muscles and proximal muscles in the shoulder or hip girdles.

Studies have also explored the value of magnetic stimulation at the spinal root level. Opinions differ regarding whether the exact site of root stimulation occurs at or distal to the neural foramen.[35,36] Measuring latency and conduction times at cortical and spinal stimulation sites, reports have suggested a correlation with clinical patterns of weakness and the ability to discriminate medially versus laterally located disk herniations producing nerve root compression.[37,38]

THE NEEDLE ELECTRODE EXAMINATION
General Concepts

Although the NEE assesses only the motor component of radiculopathy, it is the most specific and sensitive electrodiagnostic test for the identification of axon loss radiculopathy. In many cases the NEE can provide information regarding the root level of involvement, the degree of axon loss present, the degree of ongoing motor axon loss, and the chronicity of the process. Several general comments can be made. In most laboratories, patients with arm or leg pain receive a general NEE survey that samples all major root and nerve trunk distributions in the limb in question. If abnormalities are identified, the examination is modified to focus on the cause for the abnormality. If there is a symptom in a specific region of the limb, such as the shoulder girdle or posterior thigh, muscles in that region are also examined. **Tables 3** and **4** outline the screening NEE for nonspecific arm and leg symptoms, respectively.

The localization of a nerve root lesion requires the identification of neurogenic abnormalities in a distribution of muscles that shares the same root innervation, but involves more than one peripheral nerve distribution. The abnormalities may include one or more of the following: increased insertional activity in the form of positive waves or sharp spikes; abnormal spontaneous activity in the form of fibrillation potentials; reduced (neurogenic) recruitment of motor unit firing; and features of chronic motor unit action potential (MUAP) reinnervation, such as increased duration, increased amplitude, and polyphasia.

The timing of the NEE is important. In acute radiculopathy, fibrillation potentials are the abnormality most likely to confirm the presence of a motor radiculopathy.

Table 3
Screening needle electrode survey for arm pain

Muscle	Root Level	Nerve Trunk
First dorsal interosseus	C8	Ulnar
Flexor pollicis longus	C8	Anterior interosseus (median)
Extensor indicis proprius	C8	Posterior interosseus (radial)
Pronator teres	C6-7	Median
Triceps	C6-7	Radial
Biceps	C5-6	Musculocutaneous
Deltoid	C5-6	Axillary
C7 paraspinal	Overlap	

Fibrillation potentials seldom develop before 2 weeks have elapsed from the onset of weakness, and in some patients may not appear for 4 to 6 weeks. The most efficient use of the EMG is to delay the performance of the NEE for at least 3 weeks after the onset of motor symptoms.

Root Localization by NEE

The choice of muscles for the NEE must be tailored to the clinical question and specific symptoms, but must be comprehensive enough to maximize diagnostic certainty. The particular muscles showing neurogenic changes in the myotome in question vary from case to case because most root lesions are partial, and not all muscles in the myotome are affected equally. During the NEE, the more muscles identified as abnormal in the myotome, the more secure the electrodiagnosis. To make a reliable diagnosis of a single-root lesion, at least two muscles in that myotome should be found with neurogenic changes, and they should not share the same peripheral nerve innervation. In myotomes where it is possible, involvement of proximal and distal muscles should be sought to increase the certainty of the diagnosis and exclude peripheral mononeuropathy as the cause for the abnormalities. To complete the NEE in an individual with an identified single-root lesion, muscles in the myotomes framing the involved root level should be examined to verify that those myotomes are normal. For example, the biceps and first dorsal interosseus muscles should be normal in a patient with a C7 radiculopathy.

Paraspinal muscle involvement should always be sought, because it adds important support for the diagnosis of an intraspinal lesion, and rules out plexopathy and

Table 4
Screening needle electrode survey for leg pain

Muscle	Root Level	Nerve Trunk
Abductor hallucis	S1	Posterior tibial
Medial gastrocnemius	S1	Posterior tibial
Biceps femoris (short head)	S1	Peroneal
Extensor digitorum brevis	L5 (S1)	Peroneal
Tibialis anterior	(L4) L5 (S1)	Peroneal
Tibialis posterior	L5	Posterior tibial
Gluteus medius	L5 (S1)	Superior Gluteal
Rectus femoris	L2-4	Femoral
S1 paraspinal	Overlap	

peripheral mononeuropathy as the cause of extremity muscle involvement. However, several factors reduce their value. First, paraspinal muscle fibrillation can be seen not only in disorders of the root, but also in processes affecting anterior horn cells and in muscle disorders, such as necrotizing myopathy. Second, paraspinal muscle involvement cannot precisely localize the segmental level of root damage because the segmental innervation of paraspinal muscles can overlap by as much as four to six segments.[39] Third, clear evidence of paraspinal denervation with cervical and lumbosacral radiculopathies is seen only in approximately 50% of cases.[22,40] Likely causes include the overlapping segmental innervation of paraspinal muscles and the tendency for muscles close to the site of the nerve lesion to reinnervate sooner and more completely than muscles at greater distance from the point where nerve regeneration must begin. Finally, in paraspinal muscles that are close to a prior laminectomy site, fibrillation may persist indefinitely because of iatrogenic denervation. In routine practice paraspinal muscles in areas of prior surgery are not examined.

Anatomic, clinical, and electromyographic myotomal charts are used to correlate the pattern of EMG abnormalities in a limb with a specific root level. Anatomic charts have been derived by tracing root and peripheral nerve innervations of muscles from cadaver studies. Clinical charts have been derived by correlating the distribution of clinical muscle weakness in patients with specific traumatic lesions. Although these charts are useful, they are not entirely applicable to the NEE. Muscles are chosen for the NEE because of specific attributes of root innervation and accessibility. Some muscles, such as the anconeus, pronator teres, and brachioradialis, are not easily isolated in the clinical examination, but are easily isolated by the NEE, and are important in root localization. Thus, electromyographically derived myotomal charts are useful in the electrodiagnosis of radiculopathy.[22,40,41] **Figs. 4** and **5** are electromyographically derived myotomal charts.

Defining an Acute Radiculopathy

In an axon loss radiculopathy, determining the age of the lesion requires combining information about the duration of the symptoms with NEE attributes of active and chronic motor axon loss. When motor unit potentials are of normal configuration and size, the presence of abnormal insertional or spontaneous activity in the form of trains of brief sharp spikes or positive waves indicates recent motor axon loss. Abnormal insertional activity alone suggests that the process may be only several weeks old. The presence of spontaneous activity in the form of fibrillation potentials indicates a process at least 3 weeks of age.

Although electrodiagnostic testing for radiculopathy is most valuable when significant axon loss has occurred, testing may also uncover evidence of a prominent conduction block lesion at the root level as the cause for weakness. When examining a muscle whose CMAP is of normal amplitude, the presence of a reduced recruitment pattern of motor unit potential activation in the absence of fibrillation potentials suggests conduction block. If this pattern is seen in multiple muscles of a specific myotome, a diagnosis of radiculopathy can be made. This strategy is not reliable for the diagnosis of conduction block if the onset of weakness is less than 4 weeks before the electrodiagnostic study, because an acute axon loss lesion may not clearly manifest fibrillation potentials for 3 or more weeks after onset of symptoms.

Defining a Chronic Radiculopathy

The diagnosis of a chronic-active or a chronic-remote root lesion is based on the observation of neurogenic MUAP changes, in the presence or absence of evidence of fibrillation potentials, respectively. In the early stages of reinnervation of denervated

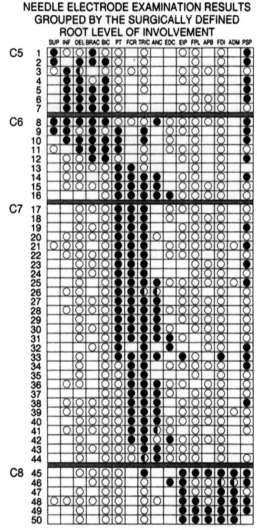

Fig. 4. NEE results grouped by the surgically defined root level of involvement. *Shaded circle*, positive waves or fibrillation potentials, with or without neurogenic recruitment and motor unit changes. *Half-shaded circle*, neurogenic recruitment changes only. *Open circle*, normal examination. ADM, abductor digiti minimi; ANC, anconeus; APB, abductor pollicis brevis; BIC, biceps; BRAC, brachioradialis; DEL, deltoid; EDC, extensor digitorum communis; EIP, extensor indicis proprius; FCR, flexor carpi radialis; FDI, first dorsal interosseus; FPL, flexor pollicis longus; INF, infraspinatus; PSP, paraspinal muscle; PT, pronator teres; SUP, supraspinatus; TRIC, triceps. (*From* Levin KH, Maggiano HJ, Wilbourn AJ. Cervical radiculopathies: comparison of surgical and EMG localization of single-root lesions. Neurology 1996;46:1022–5; with permission.)

muscle fibers, between 6 and 26 weeks after nerve root injury, collateral sprouting from surviving nerve fiber terminals gives rise to MUAPs of increased serration or polyphasia. These MUAPs may also demonstrate instability (moment-to-moment variation in configuration). As more time elapses and reinnervation becomes more complete,

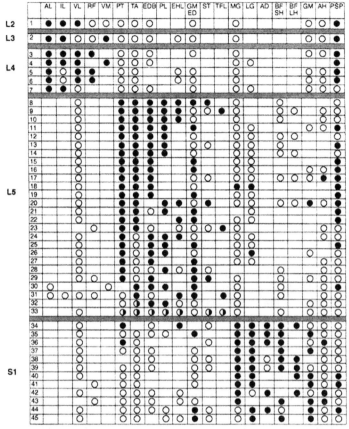

- ● Fibrillation potentials
- ◑ Neurogenic recruitment changes only
- ○ Normal examination

Fig. 5. NEE results grouped by the surgically defined root level of involvement. *Shaded circle,* positive waves or fibrillation potentials, with or without neurogenic recruitment and motor unit changes. *Half-shaded circle,* neurogenic recruitment changes only. *Open circle,* normal examination. AD, abductor digiti quinti; AH, abductor hallucis; AL, adductor longus; BFLH, biceps femoris (long head); BFSH, biceps femoris (short head); EDB, extensor digitorum brevis; EHL, extensor hallucis longus; GM, gluteus medius; GMX, gluteus maximus; H, H reflex; IL, iliacus; LG, lateral gastrocnemius; MG, medial gastrocnemius; PL, peroneus longus; PSP, paraspinal; PT, posterior tibialis/flexor digitroum longus; RF, rectus femoris; ST, semitendinosus; TA, tibialis anterior; TFL, tensor fascia lata; VL, vastus lateralis; VM, vastus medialis. (*From* Tsao B, Levin KH. Comparison of surgical and electrodiagnostic findings in single root lumbosacral radiculopathies. Muscle Nerve 2003;27:60–4; with permission.)

MUAPs lose their instability and develop the characteristic features of a chronic lesion, increased duration and amplitude. A NEE demonstrating chronic neurogenic MUAP changes without fibrillation potentials indicates the residuals of a remote lesion. These MUAP changes are permanent, reflecting the histopathologic changes in the reinnervated muscle, and remain unchanged unless the motor unit is injured again. After a significant motor axon loss process has occurred MUAPs never return to their pre-injury morphology.

Chronic lesions can be classified into a chronic-active category if there are fibrillation potentials and chronic neurogenic MUAPs. In root distributions where the myotome includes muscles in distal and proximal regions of a limb (especially the L5 and S1, and perhaps the C5-6 root distributions), the presence of a chronic and ongoing axon loss process can be even more clearly defined when fibrillation potentials are seen in distal and proximal muscles in the root distribution. In lesions where fibrillation potentials are seen in distal muscles only, the presence of an ongoing axon loss process is less certain. Some inactive but severe axon loss processes never fully reinnervate, especially in muscles farthest from the injury site, leaving some muscle fibers denervated indefinitely. The NEE findings at progressive stages of axon loss radiculopathy are summarized in **Table 5**, and are schematically represented in **Fig. 6**.

Defining the Severity of a Radiculopathy

The severity of an axon loss process can be assessed during the NEE by the degree of motor unit loss in the root distribution. This is determined by a subjective measurement of the degree of reduced recruitment of motor unit potential activation. Although there is a correlation between the degree of reduced recruitment of motor units in a neurogenic process and the degree of weakness, reduced recruitment is not necessarily caused by axon loss unless the CMAP elicited from the same muscle is also reduced in amplitude. Thus, defining the severity of an axon loss radiculopathy requires evaluation of the CMAPs in the myotome in question (when possible) and the degree of reduced recruitment of MUAP activation. Measuring the number of fibrillation potentials present in a muscle is highly subjective and does not correlate as well with the degree of axon loss.

Cervical Radiculopathies

The most complete clinical study of specific cervical root lesions was performed by Yoss and colleagues.[42] According to that study clinical and radiographic evidence of radiculopathy occurs at the C7, C6, C8, and C5 levels 70%, 19% to 25%, 4% to 10%, and 2% of the time, respectively. The following NEE data on individual cervical radiculopathies come from a study of isolated single-root lesions based on confirmed surgical localization (see **Fig. 4**).[40]

C5 radiculopathy produces a stereotyped pattern of muscle involvement, affecting the spinati, biceps, deltoid, and brachioradialis with about equal frequency, but not

Table 5
Findings in the needle electrode examination at progressive stages of axon loss radiculopathy

	RECRUIT	INSERTION	PSP	FIB	POLY/VAR	NEUR	MTP/CRD
<3 wk	++	+/++	+	...	...	...	...
3–6 wk	++	++	++	+++	...	...	...
6–26 wk	++	+	±	++	+++	...	...
Chronic/active	++	...	±	+	++	++	...
Chronic/remote	+/++	...	...	...	...	+++	+

Abbreviations: FIB, fibrillation potentials in myotomal muscles; INSERTION, abnormal insertional activity in myotomal muscles; MTP/CRD, myotonic discharges/complex repetitive discharges; NEUR, neurogenic motor unit potential changes (increased duration and amplitude); POLY/VAR, polyphasic motor unit potential changes/motor unit potential variation; PSP, paraspinal fibrillation; RECRUIT, neurogenic recruitment of myotomal motor units; ±, equivocal amount; +, mild amount; ++, moderate amount; +++, greatest amount.

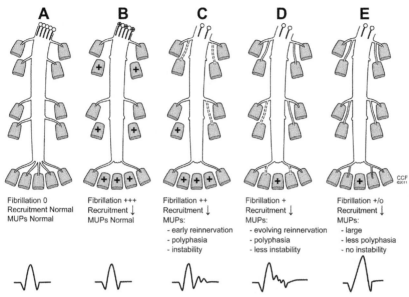

Fig. 6. Diagram demonstrating the evolution of reinnervation of muscle fibers after an acute axon loss injury at the root or anterior horn cell level. (*A*) Normal state. (*B*) Fibrillation potentials developing in muscle fibers whose motor axons have been lost. (*C*) Early regeneration of nerve branches to denervated muscle fibers closest to the site of nerve injury, with MUAPs showing newly acquired satellite potentials. (*D*, *E*) Evolving reinnervation to more distal sites and maturation of reinnervating nerve branches at proximal sites, with associated maturation of MUAPs reflecting increased motor unit territories.

all of them together in any patient. The pronator teres was never involved in C5 radiculopathy. Because the rhomboid major muscle is said to have prominent C5 innervation, it should be examined in unclear cases. The upper trapezius, with its prominent C4 innervation, was spared in C5 radiculopathy. NCS are not likely to be helpful, although severe lesions may be associated with axillary and musculocutaneous CMAP amplitude loss.

C7 radiculopathy produces a stereotyped pattern of muscle involvement, affecting particularly the triceps, but also the anconeus, flexor carpi radialis, and pronator teres. The triceps muscle was affected in essentially all cases of C7 radiculopathy. Because the extensor carpi radialis is not reliably affected in most C7 radiculopathies, it is not usually part of the routine NEE survey for radiculopathy. An important part of the clinical diagnosis of C7 radiculopathy rests on the finding of a diminished triceps deep tendon reflex, but several studies have shown that the reflex is abnormal in less than 70% of patients.[40,42] There are no reliably performed motor NCS that can be used to generate CMAPs from C7 innervated muscles.

With C6 radiculopathy there is no single characteristic pattern of muscle involvement. Rather, two patterns are discernible: the first very similar to the C5 pattern, with additional involvement of triceps and pronator teres in some; and the second similar to the C7 pattern. The pronator teres was abnormal in 80% of patients with C6 radiculopathy, but was also abnormal in 60% of the cases of C7 radiculopathy. The triceps was abnormal in more than half the cases of C6 radiculopathy. Thus, significant electromyographic overlap occurs between C5 and C6 radiculopathy, and between C6 and C7 radiculopathy. There are no reliably performed motor NCS that can be used to generate CMAPs from C6 innervated muscles.

C8 radiculopathy produces a stereotyped pattern of muscle involvement, including the ulnar innervated muscles, extensor indicis proprius, and flexor pollicis longus. Abductor pollicis brevis was involved less often, and to a lesser degree than other muscles. Of all the root lesions, C8 radiculopathy was the most clearly identified by NEE because of the limited myotomal overlap. NCS are not likely to be helpful, although severe lesions may be associated with ulnar (recording from the abductor digiti minimi or first dorsal interosseus) CMAP amplitude loss.

T1 radiculopathy is the most uncommon isolated root lesion affecting the arm. Although all C8 muscles of the hand are said to have T1 contributions, the abductor pollicis brevis muscle seems to be the only muscle with predominately T1 innervation.[43,44] A single case of T1 radiculopathy with neuroimaging and intraoperative confirmation has been reported. The EMG picture showed chronic and active denervation limited to the abductor pollicis brevis.[44]

Lumbosacral Radiculopathies

According to one large study, lumbar disk herniation leading to electromyographically determined motor radiculopathy occurs at the L4-5, L5-S1, and L3-4 levels 55%, 43%, and 2% of the time, respectively.[45] At lumbosacral levels the anatomic localization of the site of root injury, the identification of single root lesions, and the accuracy of electrodiagnosis are less successful than at the cervical levels. First, there is the issue of the longer intraspinal course of most lumbosacral roots. All lumbar and sacral spinal nerve roots are constituted at the T12-L1 vertebral level, where the spinal cord ends as the conus medullaris. The roots then course down the canal as the cauda equina, until they exit at their respective neural foramina. Depending on the nature and location of intraspinal compression, roots may be injured at any disk level, from the L1-2 level to the level of their exit into the neural foramen. For example, the L5 root can be compressed by a central disk protrusion at the L2-3 or L3-4 level, a lateral disk protrusion at the L4-5 level, or foraminal stenosis at the L5-S1 level. Thus, the electrodiagnostic localization of a specific root lesion does not specify the vertebral level of damage. Second, because of the presence of multiple spinal nerve roots in the cauda equina, the likelihood of multiple, bilateral radiculopathies increases. This occurrence reduces electrodiagnostic accuracy and introduces possible confusion with other disorders, such as peripheral polyneuropathy and motor neuron disease. Thus, the identification of a lumbosacral radiculopathy requires at least a limited evaluation of the contralateral side for evidence of concurrent lesions. The following NEE data on individual lumbosacral radiculopathies comes from a study of isolated single-root lesions with active axon loss, confirmed by surgical localization (see **Fig. 5**).[22]

With S1 radiculopathy there is a stereotyped pattern of muscle involvement, including the gastrocnemius muscles, the short and long heads of the biceps femoris, and the abductor hallucis. The biceps femoris short head, biceps femoris long head, and medial gastrocnemius were all found to be exclusively innervated by the S1 root, although other studies have described significant L5 root innervation of these muscles.[46–48] Muscles involved in over 80% of these patients included the gastrocnemius (medial and lateral heads) and the biceps femoris (short and long heads). Paraspinal denervation was seen in only 25% of patients, because of the significant overlap of paraspinal segmental innervation. The gastrocnemius muscles are often difficult to voluntarily activate, making the assessment of motor unit potential recruitment and morphologic changes incomplete. The identification of abnormalities in proximal muscles, such as the biceps femoris short head and long head, and the gluteus maximus is crucial for the confirmation of an S1 radiculopathy, eliminating the possibility of more distal peripheral mononeuropathies. The biceps femoris short head was not involved in any L5 root lesions, although some reports have described significant L5 innervation of that muscle.[46]

With L5 radiculopathy the NEE showed involvement of the peroneus longus and tensor fascia lata in essentially all patients, and in the flexor digitorum longus and posterior tibialis, and tibialis anterior muscles in more than 75%. In this study the tibialis anterior was exclusively innervated by the L5 root, although other studies have described significant L4 root innervation of that muscle.[1,49–51] A total of 50% of patients with L5 radiculopathy demonstrated paraspinal fibrillation potentials. NEE of the posterior tibialis or flexor digitorum longus is critical, because they are the only L5 innervated muscles below the knee not innervated by the peroneal nerve. Abnormalities in either of these muscles exclude the diagnosis of peroneal mononeuropathy. To verify the presence of an L5 radiculopathy abnormalities should be sought in proximal L5 muscles, such as the tensor fascia lata and gluteus medius, to eliminate the diagnoses of sciatic and peroneal mononeuropathies. This is especially true in elderly individuals whose superficial peroneal sensory responses are absent because of age, and in whom peroneal and sciatic mononeuropathy may not be as easily excluded.

L2, L3, and L4 root lesions cannot be reliably distinguished from each other because of the overlap of innervation of the anterior thigh muscles. The problem in reliable localization is compounded by the absence of proximal and distal muscles to examine, and the low incidence of L2, L3, and L4 radiculopathies, which has prevented definitive analysis. The author routinely examines the rectus femoris, vastus lateralis, iliacus, and adductor longus in patients with a clinical question of upper lumbar radiculopathy. All these muscles seem to be equally likely to be involved at these levels, but they are seldom all involved in any one root lesion. Because the adductor longus is the only muscle not innervated by the femoral nerve, its evaluation is critical for the differentiation of femoral mononeuropathy and L2, L3, and L4 radiculopathy. Paraspinal fibrillation potentials are very commonly seen in patients with active axon loss radiculopathies at these segmental levels, but the paraspinal fibrillation potentials are often seen at the L5, S1, or S2 vertebral levels.

Value of EMG in the Diagnosis of Radiculopathy

The lack of an established reference standard for the diagnosis of radiculopathy, other than the observation of nerve compression at surgery for structural radiculopathy, and the subjective nature of EMG data collection and analysis, make a comparison of sensitivity and specificity of various diagnostic tests studied in the scientific literature difficult. As a result few electrodiagnostic scientific studies have been able to meet the traditional standards set for class I or II evidence of effectiveness. Those studies that do meet evidence-based guidelines in systematic literature reviews often do not directly answer the question of clinical use that is important to have in daily clinical care of patients.

For cervical radiculopathy, a systematic evidence-based literature review concluded that needle EMG examination provided confirmatory evidence of cervical root pathology in 30% to 72% of patients presenting with appropriate symptoms or signs. Needle EMG abnormalities were highly correlated with weakness. Good agreement between imaging studies and needle EMG was seen in 65% to 85% of cases.[51] For lumbosacral radiculopathy, an evidence-based review concluded that needle EMG of the limb is probably effective in clinical diagnosis (class II evidence).[17]

One study retrospectively analyzed 47 patients with a clinical history compatible with either cervical or lumbosacral radiculopathy who were evaluated with an EMG and a spine MRI. Among these patients, 55% had an EMG abnormality and 57%

had an MRI abnormality that correlated with the clinically estimated level of radiculopathy. The two studies agreed in 60% of patients, with normal in 11 and abnormal in 17; however, only one study was abnormal in a significant minority (40%), suggesting that the two studies were complementary diagnostic modalities. The agreement was higher in patients with abnormal findings on neurologic examination.[50]

OTHER RADICULAR DISORDERS
Extraspinal Radiculopathies

Extraspinal radiculopathy (focal damage to anterior primary rami) constitutes an unusual group of disorders that is difficult to diagnose. In the lumbosacral region this involves a unilevel anterior primary ramus proximal to its connection with other rami to form elements of the lumbar or sacral plexus.[10,11]

In the cervical region two such disorders have traditionally been categorized as types of brachial plexopathy, but electrodiagnostic evidence suggests that they are more likely to represent damage to extraspinal root fibers traveling in the anterior primary rami. First, neurogenic thoracic outlet syndrome, long considered a type of lower trunk brachial plexopathy, produces most severe axon loss in the abductor pollicis brevis muscle and the medial antebrachial cutaneous SNAP, both sharing principally T1 root innervation.[43] In most cases lower trunk and C8 structures are affected to a much lesser extent. Second, median sternotomy brachial plexopathy, an iatrogenic disorder that can result from rib cage retraction during open heart surgery, is manifested by most severe axon loss in the ulnar SNAP and C8 root distribution, with little involvement of T1 innervated structures.

These two lesions show distributions of involvement that, in their purest forms, may be mutually exclusive: the abductor pollicis brevis and the medial antebrachial cutaneous response with neurogenic thoracic outlet syndrome, and C8 muscles and the ulnar sensory response with median sternotomy brachial plexopathy. However, the nerve fibers innervating all these structures travel together in the lower trunk of the brachial plexus. Neurogenic thoracic outlet syndrome and median sternotomy brachial plexopathy more likely represent, respectively, extraspinal T1 and C8 root lesions proximal to the formation of the lower trunk, as diagrammed in **Figs. 7** and **8**.

Polyradiculopathies

The term "polyradiculopathy" indicates damage to multiple root segments simultaneously or in progressive order, occurring in a single limb, or more frequently bilaterally, and sometimes diffusely. The causes are diverse, and at times unclear. In some neurologic disorders polyradiculopathy coexists with lesions in distal peripheral nerves, lesions in the central nervous system, or both. A brief description of the most prominent causes of polyradiculopathy follows, and **Table 6** lists causes of polyradiculopathy and their differential diagnosis.

Compressive Polyradiculopathies

Spondylosis of the spine is often multifocal, and multiple roots may suffer compressive damage concurrently. This is especially true at the lumbosacral level, where spondylosis causes lumbar canal stenosis and multilevel neural foraminal stenoses. In the author's laboratory, few elderly patients are seen with single lumbosacral root lesions, but many more with multiple simultaneous radiculopathies, often showing a combination of active and more chronic features. Lumbar canal stenosis exerts compressive effects on the cauda equina resulting in the potential for multiple root involvement. It may present clinically with weakness in a single-root distribution, in several

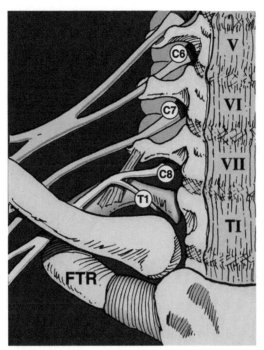

Fig. 7. Diagram depicting the likely anatomic relationship between the T1 and C8 nerve roots and the offending ligamentous band in neurogenic thoracic outlet syndrome, showing entrapment of the T1 and C8 nerve trunks. *Roman numerals*, vertebral body levels. *Circled numbers*, root levels. FTR, first thoracic rib.

distributions, or as chronic progressive weakness of the legs in a diffuse distribution. Alternatively, lumbar canal stenosis may present as intermittent progressive fatigability and aching of the legs elicited by walking or exercise, a symptom complex known as "intermittent neurogenic claudication." The EMG picture of lumbar canal stenosis is extremely variable, spanning the gamut from normal to multilevel, bilateral motor axon loss.

Regardless of the cause of the lumbosacral polyradiculopathy, electrodiagnostic specificity is hampered when the NEE abnormalities are bilateral and confluent. In the chronic state the NEE changes are usually most prominent in distal muscles of the myotome, shading to normal in more proximal muscles. When chronic motor axon loss spans the L5 and S1 distributions symmetrically, the electrical picture resembles the confluent changes seen in peripheral polyneuropathy. This is especially true in the elderly, when physiologic loss of sural and superficial peroneal sensory responses can prevent the clear distinction between axon loss peripheral polyneuropathy and a chronic or active pattern of bilateral L5 and S1 radiculopathies.

When the process is chronic and active, the EMG pattern may be difficult to distinguish from early to mid-stage progressive motor neuron disease (amyotrophic lateral sclerosis) or progressive necrotizing myelopathy. In amyotrophic lateral sclerosiscontiguous muscles of the same root or an adjoining root level are more likely to show a similar degree of neurogenic damage. Early to mid-stage amyotrophic lateral sclerosisis is also more likely to show a significant distal to proximal gradient of muscle involvement in a limb.

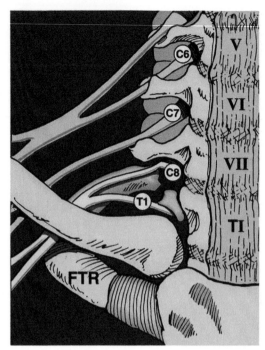

Fig. 8. Diagram depicting the anatomic relationship between the C8 nerve root and fracture of the first rib near the costotransverse articulation, in a patient who has undergone median sternotomy. *Roman numerals*, vertebral body levels. *Circled numbers*, root levels. FTR, first thoracic rib.

Diabetic Polyradiculopathies

Radiculopathies caused by diabetes can occur at the thoracic, lumbar, and sacral levels, and have been rarely reported at cervical levels.[52] Approximately 25% occur in the absence of underlying peripheral polyneuropathy.[53]

Thoracic radiculopathies occur either unilaterally or bilaterally. They are clinically characterized by cutaneous pain and dysesthesia in the posterior and anterior aspects of the torso in the distributions of the involved roots, and there may be weakness and bulging of the abdominal wall from denervation of rectus abdominus muscles. Thoracic radiculopathies can be confused clinically with intra-abdominal disorders. The NEE shows evidence of denervation in thoracic paraspinal muscles and in associated rectus abdominis muscles.

Diabetic lumbosacral radiculopathies may occur at any segmental level, but the L3-4 levels are especially vulnerable. In one study, 15 of 16 cases of diabetic lumbosacral radiculopathy included the L3-4 level, and 5 of the 15 were limited to that distribution.[54] L5 root involvement occurred in 10 cases. S1 root involvement occurred in seven cases, all but one of which in the presence of L5 root involvement. In only one case did L5 and S1 root involvement occur in the absence of L3-4 root involvement. Bilateral involvement occurred in 11 cases. These data support the clinical observation that diabetic lumbosacral radiculopathy usually begins at the L3-4 level, and often spreads over weeks and months to involve contiguous root levels, and eventually the contralateral side.

Table 6
Differential diagnosis of polyradiculopathies

	Polyradiculopathy	Polyneuropathy	Myelopathy
Disorders with true root involvement			
Arachnoiditis	+	...	...
Inflammatory polyneuropathy	+	+	...
Diabetes	+	+	...
HNPP	+	+	...
Adrenal insufficiency	+	+	...
Procainamide polyradiculoneuropathy[55]	+	+	...
Spondylosis	+	...	+
Radiation	+	...	+
Vascular malformation (conus medullaris)	+ +	+	+ +
Malignant invasion	+	+	+
Sarcoidosis	+	+	+
Lyme disease	+	+	+
Viral infection (HZ, CMV, HSV, EBV)	+	+	+
Mycoplasma infection	+	+	+
Vasculitis	+	+	+
Angiotropic lymphoma	...	...	...
Disorders mimicking root involvement			
Porphyric polyneuropathy	...	+	...
α-Lipoprotein deficiency	...	+	+
X-linked bulbospinal neuronopathy	...	+	+
Motor neuron disease	...	...	+
Juvenile monomelic amyotrophy	...	...	+
Spinal cord infarction	...	...	+
Multiple sclerosis	...	...	+
Syringomyelia	...	...	+

Abbreviations: CMV, cytomegalovirus; EBV, Epstein-Barr virus; HNPP, hereditary neuropathy with tendency to pressure palsy; HSV, herpes simplex virus; HZ, herpes zoster.

SUMMARY

Electrodiagnostic testing provides an objective assessment of radiculopathy. Although electrodiagnostic testing is not a stand-alone tool for the diagnosis of radiculopathy, it provides unique information regarding the physiologic damage of the disorder, and is complementary to other diagnostic tools, such as MRI, especially in the presence of axon loss. Electrodiagnostic testing is also valuable as a tool to rule out other neuromuscular disorders that can mimic radiculopathy.

REFERENCES

1. Johnson EW, Melvin JL. Value of electromyography in lumbar radiculopathy. Arch Phys Med Rehabil 1971;52:239–43.

2. LaJoie WJ. Nerve root compression: correlation of electromyographic, myelographic, and surgical findings. Arch Phys Med Rehabil 1972;53:390–2.
3. Tullberg T, Svanborg E, Isacsson J, et al. A preoperative and postoperative study of the accuracy and value of electrodiagnosis in patients with lumbosacral disc herniation. Spine 1993;18:837–42.
4. Kaar GF, Fraher JP. The vascularisation of central-peripheral transitional zone of rat lumbar ventral rootlets: a morphological and morphometric study. J Anat 1987;150:145–54.
5. Kozu H, Tamura E, Parry GJ. Endoneurial blood supply to peripheral nerves is not uniform. J Neurol Sci 1992;111:204–8.
6. Hamanishi C, Tanaka S. Dorsal root ganglia in the lumbosacral region observed from the axial views of MRI. Spine 1993;18:1753–6.
7. Kikuchi S, Sato K, Konno S, et al. Anatomic and radiographic study of dorsal root ganglia. Spine 1994;19:6–11.
8. Yabuki S, Kikuchi S. Positions of dorsal root ganglia in the cervical spine: an anatomic and clinical study. Spine 1996;21:1513–7.
9. Spencer DL, Irwin GS, Miller JA. Anatomy and significance of fixation of the lumbosacral nerve roots in sciatica. Spine 1983;8:672–9.
10. Levin KH. L5 radiculopathy with reduced superficial peroneal sensory responses: intraspinal and extraspinal causes. Muscle Nerve 1998;21:3–7.
11. Wiltse LL, Guyer RD, Spencer CW, et al. Alar transverse process impingement of the L5 spinal nerve: the far-out syndrome. Spine 1984;9:31–41.
12. Berger AR, Sharma K, Lipton RB. Comparison of motor conduction abnormalities in lumbosacral radiculopathy and axonal polyneuropathy. Muscle Nerve 1999;22:1053–7.
13. Panayiotopoulos CP, Chroni E. F-waves in clinical neurophysiology: a review, methodological issues and overall value in peripheral neuropathies. Electroencephalogr Clin Neurophysiol 1996;101:365–74.
14. Bischoff C, Meyer BU, Machetanz J, et al. The value of magnetic stimulation in the diagnosis of radiculopathies. Muscle Nerve 1993;16:154–61.
15. Toyokura M, Murakami K. F-wave study in patients with lumbosacral radiculoathies. Electromyogr Clin Neurophysiol 1997;37:19–26.
16. Tang LM, Schwartz MS, Swash M. Postural effects on F wave parameters in lumbosacral root compression and canal stenosis. Brain 1988;111:207–13.
17. Cho SC, Ferrante MA, Levin KH, et al. Utility of electrodiagnostic testing in evaluating patients with lumbosacral radiculopathy: an evidence-based review. Muscle Nerve 2010;42:276–82.
18. Burke D, Gandevia SC, McKeon B. Monosynaptic and oligosynaptic contributions to human ankle jerk and H-reflex. J Neurophysiol 1985;52:435–48.
19. Fisher MA. H reflexes and F waves: physiology and clinical indications. Muscle Nerve 1992;15:1223–33.
20. Katirji B, Weissman JD. The ankle jerk and the tibial H-reflex: a clinical and electrophysiological correlation. Electromyogr Clin Neurophysiol 1994;34:331–4.
21. Schimsheimer RJ, Ongerboer de Visser BW, Kemp B. The flexor carpi radialis H-reflex in lesions of the sixth and seventh cervical nerve roots. J Neurol Neurosurg Psychiatry 1985;48:445–9.
22. Tsao B, Levin KH. Comparison of surgical and electrodiagnostic findings in single root lumbosacral radiculopathies. Muscle Nerve 2003;27:60–4.
23. Shahani BT. Late responses and the silent period. In: Aminoff M, editor. Electrodiagnosis in clinical neurology. 2nd edition. New York: Churchill-Livingstone; 1986. p. 333–45.

24. Bromberg M, Jaros L. Symmetry of normal motor and sensory nerve conduction measurements. Muscle Nerve 1998;21:498–503.
25. Jankus WR, Robinson LR, Little JW. Normal limits of side-to-side H-reflex amplitude variability. Arch Phys Med Rehabil 1994;75:3–6.
26. Wilbourn AJ, Aminoff MJ. Radiculopathies. In: Brown WF, Bolton CF, editors. Clinical electromyography. 2nd edition. Boston: Butterworth-Heinemann; 1993. p. 177–209.
27. Yiannikas C, Shahani BT, Young RR. Short-latency somatosensory-evoked potentials from radial, median, ulnar, and peroneal nerve stimulation in the assessment of cervical spondylosis. Comparison with conventional electromyography. Arch Neurol 1986;43:1264–71.
28. Aminoff MJ, Goodin DS, Parry GJ, et al. Electrophysiological evaluation of lumbosacral radiculopathy; electromyography, late responses and somatosensory evoked potentials. Neurology 1985;35:1514–8.
29. Aminoff MJ, Goodin DS, Barbaro NM, et al. Dermatomal somatosensory evoked potentials in unilateral lumbosacral radiculopathy. Ann Neurol 1985;17:171–6.
30. Eisen A, Hoirch M, Moll A. Evaluation of radiculopathies by segmental stimulation and somtosensory evoked potentials. Can J Neurol Sci 1983;10:178–82.
31. Seyal M, Sandhu LS, Mack YP. Spinal segmental somatosensory evoked potentials in lumbosacral radiculopathies. Neurology 1989;39:801–5.
32. Dumitru D, Dreyfuss P. Dermatomal/segmental somatosensory evoked potential evaluation of L5/S1 unilateral/unilevel radiculopathies. Muscle Nerve 1996;19:442–9.
33. Berger AR, Busis NA, Logigian EL, et al. Cervical root stimulation in the diagnosis of radiculopathy. Neurology 1987;37:329–32.
34. MacDonnell RA, Cros D, Shahani BT. Lumbosacral nerve root stimulation comparing electrical with surface magnetic stimulation techniques. Muscle Nerve 1992;15:885–90.
35. Epstein CM, Fernandez-Beer E, Weissman JD, et al. Cervical magnetic stimulation: the role of the neural foramen. Neurology 1991;41:677–80.
36. Schmid UD, Walker G, Schmid-Sigron J, et al. Transcutaneous magnetic and electrical stimulation over the cervical spine: excitation of plexus roots rather than spinal roots. Electroencephalogr Clin Neurophysiol Suppl 1991;43:369–84.
37. Braddom RI, Johnson EW. Standardization of H reflex and diagnostic use in S1 radiculopathy. Arch Phys Med Rehabil 1974;55:161–6.
38. Linden D, Berlit P. Comparison of late responses, EMG studies, and motor evoked potentials (MEPs) in acute lumbosacral radiculopathies. Muscle Nerve 1995;18:1205–7.
39. Gough J, Koepke G. Electromyographic determination of motor root levels in erector spinae muscles. Arch Phys Med Rehabil 1966;47:9–11.
40. Levin KH, Maggiano HJ, Wilbourn AJ. Cervical radiculopathies: comparison of surgical and EMG localization of single-root lesions. Neurology 1996;46:1022–5.
41. Phillips LH, Park TS. Electrophysiologic mapping of the segmental anatomy of the muscles of the lower extremity. Muscle Nerve 1991;14:1213–8.
42. Yoss RE, Corbin KB, MacCarty CS, et al. Significance of symptoms and signs in localization of involved root in cervical disk protrusion. Neurology 1957;7:673–83.
43. Levin KH, Wilbourn AJ, Maggiano HJ. Cervical rib and median sternotomy related brachial plexopathies: a reassessment. Neurology 1998;50:1407–13.
44. Levin KH. Neurological manifestations of compressive radiculopathy of the first thoracic root. Neurology 1999;53:1149–51.

45. Knuttson B. Comparative value of electromyographic, myelographic, and clinical neurological examination in the diagnosis of lumbar root compression syndrome. Acta Orthop Scand Suppl 1961;49:1–135.
46. Liguori R, Krarup C, Trojaborg W. Determination of the segmental sensory and motor innervation of the lumbosacral spinal nerves. Brain 1992;115:915–34.
47. Thage O. The myotomes L2-S2 in man. Acta Neurol Scand 1965;41(Suppl 13): 241–3.
48. Young A, Getty J, Jackson A, et al. Variations in the pattern of muscle innervation by the L5 and S1 nerve roots. Spine 1983;8:616–24.
49. Johnson E, Fletcher FR. Lumbosacral radiculopathy: review of 100 consecutive cases. Arch Phys Med Rehabil 1981;62:321–3.
50. Nardin RA, Patel MR, Gudas TF, et al. Electromyography and magnetic resonance imaging in the evaluation of radiculopathy. Muscle Nerve 1999;22:151–5.
51. So YT. Guidelines in electrodiagnostic medicine. Practice parameter for needle electromyography evaluation of patients with suspected cervical radiculopathy. Muscle Nerve 1999;8(Suppl):S209–21.
52. Riley D, Shields RW. Diabetic amyotrophy with upper extremity involvement [abstract]. Neurology 1984;34(Suppl 1):216.
53. Bastron JA, Thomas JE. Diabetic polyradiculopathy, clinical and electromyographic findings in 105 patients. Mayo Clin Proc 1981;56:725–32.
54. Levin KH, Wilbourn AJ. Diabetic radiculopathy without peripheral neuropathy [abstract]. Muscle Nerve 1991;14:889.
55. Sahenk Z, Mendell JR, Rossio JL, et al. Polyradiculopathy accompanying procainamide-induced lupus erythematosus: evidence for drug-induced enhanced sensitization to peripheral nerve myelin. Ann Neurol 1977;1:378–84.

The Electrophysiology of the Motor Neuron Diseases

Eric J. Sorenson, MD

KEYWORDS

- Amyotrophic lateral sclerosis • Spinal muscular atrophy
- Primary lateral sclerosis • El Escorial criteria
- Progressive muscular atrophy • Multifocal motor neuropathy

Charcot is credited with the first descriptions of amyotrophic lateral sclerosis (ALS) in the 1860s.[1] He named the disease based on the pathologic features of muscle atrophy (amyotrophy) and sclerosis of the cortical spinal tracts (or lateral columns) in the spinal cord. In the early British literature the disease came to be known as *motor neuron disease*, and since that time the two terms are generally considered synonymous. The illness gained particular notoriety in the United States around 1940 when Lou Gehrig, the famous baseball player for the New York Yankees, was diagnosed with and died of the disease. In the United States, the disease soon became widely known in the lay literature eponymously as Lou Gehrig's disease.

Lou Gehrig offers a unique perspective in ALS that is not possible in most other cases. His baseball statistics offer a nearly daily assessment of his physical abilities. In analyzing these, one can observe when his physical decline began. A review of his batting average indicates that in 1939, his last full year of baseball, a steady and continuous decline occurred in his batting average[2]; this was a full year before the onset of his symptoms in 1940. This fact highlights the difficulty facing experimental treatment trials in ALS; the disease is already well established and advanced before presentation, limiting the potential impact of any disease-modifying therapy.

Also interesting historically was Lou Gehrig's participation in a clinical trial studying the effects of vitamin E in the treatment of ALS. Lou Gehrig was a patient of Dr Wechsler's in New York and appears as index case #4 in Wechsler's publication of this clinical trial.[3] In his case description, Wechsler identifies the classic features of ALS, including the upper motor neuron features of spasticity, slowness of movements, and hyperreflexia, and the lower motor neuron features of atrophy, weakness, and fasciculations. The only missing clinical feature from his description is the asymmetric focal onset that is characteristic of the disease.

Department of Neurology, Mayo Clinic, 200 1st Street SW, Rochester, MN 55905, USA
E-mail address: sorenson.eric@mayo.edu

Neurol Clin 30 (2012) 605–620
doi:10.1016/j.ncl.2011.12.006
0733-8619/12/$ – see front matter © 2012 Elsevier Inc. All rights reserved.

Over time, the motor neuron syndromes have been further classified into ALS and other much less common forms, including primary lateral sclerosis (PLS), progressive muscular atrophy (PMA), spinal muscular atrophy (SMA), and X-linked spinobulbar atrophy (SBMA; also known by its eponym, Kennedy disease). The clinical features of each are reviewed in **Table 1**. The clinical syndrome of ALS is characteristic. The role of nerve conduction studies and needle electromyography (collectively referred to as *EMG*) is often straightforward. The objective of EMG is to confirm the clinical suspicion while excluding certain mimic syndromes. As with other ancillary tests, no pathognomonic findings are seen on EMG, but in the proper clinical context it can be diagnostic. Because of its ability to investigate alternative etiologies and provide supportive evidence, EMG is the single most important ancillary testing in evaluating ALS.

SUMMARY

1. Motor neuron disorders can be separated into ALS, PLS, PMA, SMA, and SBMA. Each has a unique phenotype and prognosis.
2. Motor neuron disease and ALS are considered synonymous terms.

ALS

ALS is the most common of all the motor neuron disorders. Pathologically it can be distinguished by the gliosis and neuronal loss within the motor cortex and the anterior horns of the spinal cord. More recently, pathologic aggregation of the proteins TAR DNA-binding protein 43 (TDP-43) and ubiquilin 2 has been identified in most sporadic cases of ALS.[4,5] This pathology is indistinguishable from that of ubiquitin-positive frontotemporal dementia (u-FTD), raising suspicion that these two disorders may represent separate phenotypes of a common underlying cause.

The incidence of ALS is 1.5 to 2.0 cases per 100,000 population per year.[6] The incidence rate increases with age up to approximately 80 years, followed by a sharp decline in the most senior years. The median survival from diagnosis is approximately 18 months. Age of onset is the most significant prognostic variable.[6] Patients who are younger when diagnosed have a better long-term survival than those who are older. A minority (5%–10%) of cases will live beyond 5 years after diagnosis. The only treatment currently approved by the U.S. Food and Drug Administration (FDA) is riluzole. Two randomized controlled studies showed a dose-dependent mean survival benefit

Table 1
Clinical features of the motor neuron disorders

	Onset	Bulbar Involvement	Fasciculations	Lower Motor Neuron Features	Upper Motor Neuron Features
ALS	Asymmetric and focal	Prominent	Prominent	Prominent	Prominent
PMA	Asymmetric and focal	Less prominent	Prominent	Prominent	Absent
PLS	Symmetrically usually in lower limbs	Prominent in later stages	None	Absent	Prominent
SMA	Symmetrically in proximal limbs	Less prominent	Variable	Prominent	Absent
SBMA	Symmetrically in proximal limbs	Prominent	Very prominent	Prominent	Absent

of approximately 4 months that did reach significance.[7,8] Approximately 5% to 10% of cases are familial, with most being autosomal dominant. A variety of mutations are now known to be associated with this disorder, the most common of which are mutations with the *SOD* (Cu/Zn) gene.

EMG IN ALS

ALS most commonly presents with a classic phenotype of focal onset weakness. Typically it will begin in one hand, one leg, or with dysarthria. In a small minority of cases it may begin with dyspnea (pulmonary onset) or in a generalized fashion. The disease generally evolves into contiguous body regions as it progresses, resulting in the classic lower motor neuron signs (weakness, atrophy, and fasciculations) in combination with the upper motor neuron signs (spasticity, hyperreflexia, and slowness of movements) within the same body region. These symptoms occur while sparing the sensory modalities and other neurologic systems. In these classical cases, EMG serves as an extension of the neurologic examination and is used to confirm the distribution of the lower motor neuron involvement. In less classical cases, EMG is valuable for excluding other mimic syndromes, such as the other motor neuron diseases, other peripheral neuropathies, and neuromuscular disorders.

ALS is a disorder that begins focally and spreads contiguously, and EMG findings will reflect that evolution. In classic cases, nerve conduction studies provide little supportive evidence for the diagnosis. The sensory nerve action potentials are normal for age and the compound muscle action potentials (CAMPs) may be reduced in amplitude, reflective of the loss of motor axons from the death of the anterior horn cells. Because of the loss of motor axons, the motor nerve conduction velocities and distal latencies may be mildly delayed, but only modestly. No evidence should be present of motor conduction block. Sensory conduction velocities and distal latencies should remain normal.

In established cases, needle EMG will identify the classic features of fibrillation potentials, fasciculation potentials, and large, complex, unstable motor unit potentials with reduced recruitment diffusely in all body regions. Early in the disease, however, these abnormalities may be identified only in the affected regions, begging the question of how diffuse the abnormalities need to be on EMG to confirm a diagnosis.

In 1998, a consensus conference was held in El Escorial, Spain, to establish standard inclusion criteria for ALS clinical trials.[9] These criteria are known as the *El Escorial criteria* and have become the standard on which the diagnosis of ALS is based. These criteria allow for a level of diagnostic certainty (from possible to definite) based on the number of regions clinically involved. The body is divided into four regions: bulbar, cervical, thoracic, and lumbar. Involvement of each region on EMG requires the presence of fibrillation and fasciculation potentials and neurogenic motor unit potentials in at least two muscles innervated by separate nerves and myotomes. In the proper clinical setting, one region of involvement is classified as possible ALS; two regions, probable; and three or four regions, definite ALS. The El Escorial criteria were subsequently revised to allow for EMG data alone to support the diagnosis, with the additional diagnostic category of "probable ALS–laboratory-supported." The EMG components of the El Escorial criteria are summarized in **Table 2**.

In 2006, a follow-up consensus conference held in Awaji, Japan, resulted in further revision of the diagnostic criteria.[10] These criteria are known as the *Awaji criteria* and differ from the revised El Escorial criteria in the equating fasciculation potentials with fibrillation potentials. In the Awaji criteria, a region can be included as affected in the presence of either fasciculation or fibrillation potentials (in contrast to the revised El

Table 2	
EMG features of the revised El Escorial criteria	
Level of Certainty	**Regions Involved**
Possible ALS	1 region
Probable ALS	2 regions
Probable ALS–laboratory-supported	1 region clinically; 1 electrodiagnostically
Definite ALS	3 or 4 regions

Regions include bulbar, cervical, thoracic, and lumbar.
Involvement requires two muscles affected innervated by two separate nerves in two separate myotomes.

Escorial criteria, which require the presence of both). The Awaji criteria remain under investigation and have not yet replaced the revised El Escorial criteria as the standard for diagnosis. A concern regarding the Awaji criteria is an unacceptable loss of specificity if they are adopted for general use, although studies have not yet found the drop in specificity to be problematic.[11]

EARLIEST CHANGES ON EMG IN ALS

In advanced cases of ALS, the EMG findings of fibrillation and fasciculation potentials and large complex motor unit potentials are found diffusely. In these circumstances, the diagnosis can be easily confirmed. However, in earlier cases, when the process is just beginning, the findings are much more subtle. To address the earliest abnormalities on needle EMG, data from the animal models can be reviewed. Animal studies have shown that the earliest detectable morphologic changes of the motor unit occur while the anterior horn cell is still viable. At this stage, a dying back of the terminal motor axons occurs, followed by reinnervation through axonal sprouting.[12] This remodeling of the terminal motor unit results in a series of immature terminal axon sprouts that do not conduct the nerve action potential reliably. This process results in instability of the motor unit potential and blocking of the action potential to individual muscle fibers, creating the visual and auditory appearance of significant motor unit instability and blocking, even in motor units of normal amplitude and duration (**Fig. 1**). As the motor unit remodeling becomes more established, the fiber density begins to increase (**Fig. 2**). Fiber density is the electrophysiological equivalent of fiber type grouping on muscle pathology, and is the hallmark of reinnervation within the muscle. As the disease progresses and the anterior horn cells are lost, the more typical changes in motor unit potentials that are associated with ALS will appear, including long duration, increased complexity, and reduced recruitment. Motor unit instability remains a prominent feature, and motor unit variability remains highly visible and audible throughout the course of ALS. The nerve conduction and needle EMG findings in ALS and other mimic syndromes are summarized in **Table 3**.

Fasciculations

Fasciculations are commonly associated with ALS and other motor neuron disorders. Fasciculations represent random action potentials of a single, isolated motor unit potential. They are involuntary and spontaneous, and occur in widely distributed within the muscle. Fasciculations are not specific for ALS; they occur in other disorders, and occasionally in people of normal health. One study that followed more than 100

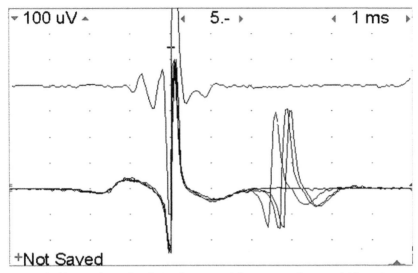

Fig. 1. Single-fiber analysis of early involvement of the motor unit potential in ALS. Note the significant jitter and blocking in an otherwise normal motor unit potential.

subjects with clinical and electromyographic fasciculations but no other signs of denervation failed to identify any cases of ALS at a mean follow-up of 5 years.[13]

However, ALS clearly has a strong association with fasciculations, and these play an important role in the diagnosis of ALS. Nearly all patients with ALS will have clinical and electromyographic fasciculations during the course of their illness. When examining for fasciculations, the muscle must be completely at rest. Muscle twitches that occur

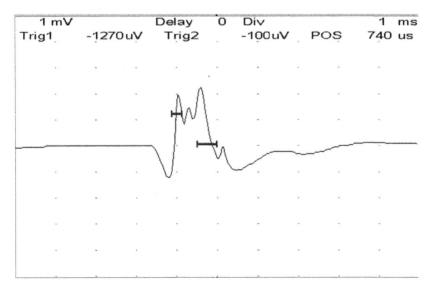

Fig. 2. Single motor unit potential by a single fiber, indicating four muscle fibers in this muscle region. Normal fiber density ranges from one to three in most motor unit potentials. The gain of the image is set at 1 mV per division with a sweep speed of 1 msec per division.

Table 3
Nerve conduction and needle EMG findings in ALS and the mimic syndromes

	Motor NCS	Sensory NCS	Fibrillation	Fasciculation	MUP
ALS	Normal to low amplitude	Normal	Prominent	Prominent	Large and unstable
PMA	Normal to low amplitude	Normal	Prominent	Prominent	Large and unstable
SBMA	Usually normal, may be low amplitude	May be reduced in amplitude	Present	Prominent	Large and stable
SMA	Usually normal, may be low amplitude	Normal	Present	Present	Large and stable
PLS	Normal	Normal	Absent	Absent	Normal but may have poor activation
IBM	Usually normal, may be low amplitude	Normal	Prominent	Absent	Mixed large and small
MFMN	Conduction block present	Normal	Present	Present	Large and stable
Hirayama disease	Normal to low amplitude	Normal	Present	Present	Large and stable

Abbreviations: IBM, inclusion body myositis; MFMN, multifocal motor neuropathy; MUP, motor unit potential; NCS, nerve conduction study.

without relaxation (so-called contraction fasciculations) do not impart the same pathologic implications that resting fasciculations do. Also, on needle EMG, fasciculations that occur with needle movement lose their specificity. When examining for fasciculations, either clinically or with EMG, the muscle should be relaxed and observed for a minimum of 30 seconds. During this time the needle should not be moved and should remain at rest. The density and frequency of fasciculation potentials do not impart any known prognostic significance, however; merely their presence in the proper clinical situation, along with other findings of acute denervation, is strongly supportive of an ALS diagnosis.

Why fasciculations are so prominent in ALS is not well-known. Evolving evidence shows that within the neuron, one of the earliest metabolic derangements to occur is dysfunction of the mitochondria.[14] The mitochondria has three key functions that are relevant to the pathogenesis of ALS: calcium buffering and calcium-related excitotoxicity; apoptosis regulation; and energy metabolism. Energy failure is now known to occur early in ALS.[15] The motor neuron consumes a considerable amount of energy to maintain the neuron's resting membrane potential and to maintain normal excitability for the transmission of the nerve action potential. Maintaining this resting membrane potential is an energy-dependent process. In the setting of a compromised energy supply, the resting membrane potential will drift. During this drift, the resting potential may reach threshold and spontaneously activate the voltage-gated sodium channels, thus trigging an action potential of that motor axon. This action potential will then cause activation of the entire motor unit, resulting in a single isolated motor unit potential or fasciculation. Because the energy state and resting membrane potential vary, these action potentials occur randomly and spontaneously.

SUMMARY

1. ALS presents as a focal disorder, with mixed upper and lower motor neurons, and spreads contiguously.
2. The diagnosis of ALS has been standardized through the El Escorial criteria.

OTHER MOTOR NEURON DISORDERS
PLS

PLS is an uncommon variant of motor neuron disease. It occurs with pathologic loss of the cortical motor neurons only, sparing the anterior horn cells of the spinal cord. Whether PLS represents a disorder unique from ALS or is simply a phenotypic variant remains a matter of debate.[16] The strongest argument favoring a phenotypic variant is from the familial forms of ALS. The PLS phenotype is now well described in familial forms of ALS.[17] The coexistence of these two phenotypes from the same genetic mutation strongly favors separate phenotypes of a common origin. Regardless, patients with PLS are known to have a much more indolent progression with a much longer survival than those with ALS. PLS should be distinguished from upper motor neuron–onset ALS, in which evolution to lower motor neuron involvement typically occurs in the first year. Some clinical features help make this distinction. First, a very high proportion of PLS begins symmetrically in the lower extremities, with the onset of a spastic gait, and then ascends. Conversely, upper motor neuron–predominate ALS begins in a focal asymmetric manner and can occur in any region of the body. PLS will progress indolently, whereas upper motor neuron–predominate ALS typically progresses more rapidly. Fasciculations are notably absent in PLS, whereas they are present in upper motor neuron–predominate ALS.

PLS tends to evolve very slowly over several years, and is overall associated with much better survival than ALS. After years of involvement, a small proportion of patients with PLS may develop lower motor neuron involvement and convert to an ALS phenotype, but this is uncommon. More commonly, after years of indolent progression, the disease tends to plateau, followed by years of relative stability. The timing of this is variable, and in some patients with PLS the neurologic deficits remain modest, whereas in others severe quadriplegia and spastic bulbar palsy may develop.

Neurophysiology testing is an important ancillary test for all patients who present with progressive spastic paraparesis. In PLS, the nerve conduction studies and needle EMG are generally normal or merely indicate poor voluntary activation. Changes consistent with denervation early in the disease are concerning for upper motor neuron–predominate ALS, and patients should be counseled appropriately. Given the prognostic significance, follow-up studies at a later date, including serial electrodiagnostic testing, should be performed to make this distinction definitively.

Early PLS may be difficult to distinguish from hereditary spastic paraparesis (HSP). Most patients with PLS have no family history, and a family history consistent with HSP should prompt genetic counseling and testing. In contrast to PLS, most forms of HSP do not evolve to include the upper limbs or bulbar regions.

PMA

PMA is a lower motor neuron disorder that is otherwise phenotypically indistinguishable from ALS. Like ALS, it starts in a focal region and spreads to contiguous regions. Muscle atrophy, weakness, and fasciculations are prominent, but upper motor neuron signs are absent. As with PLS, it remains debated whether PMA is a distinct disorder from ALS or merely a phenotypic variant. Independent autopsy studies support a common origin for PMA and ALS. Postmortem studies in PMA have consistently shown subclinical loss of cortical motor neurons and sclerosis of the lateral columns.[18] Recent pathology studies have confirmed a common TDP-43 pathology in PMA and ALS.[19] Because PMA is a lower motor neuron disorder, nerve conduction studies and needle EMG in PMA are indistinguishable from those in ALS. Classical ALS and PMA are differentiated through clinical examination and the lack of upper motor neuron signs.

SMA

SMA is a hereditary lower motor neuron disorder. It is now known to be caused by a deletion in the survival motor neuron gene (*SMN1*) on chromosome 5q.[20] Genetic testing is now commercially available for this genetic mutation. Onset ranges from infancy to early adulthood. SMA type 1, also known by its eponym Werdnig-Hoffmann disease, is the most common form, with infantile onset, and is usually fatal within the first year of life. SMA type 2 has its onset in toddlers, usually before 2 years of age. The overall prognosis is better than that for type 1, but these children typically never achieve the ability to walk. SMA type 3 (Kugelberg-Welander syndrome) has its onset later in childhood and has a more indolent course generally thought to be compatible with a normal life expectancy. SMA type 4 is the rarest form and has its onset in young adulthood. The distinction between the four types is somewhat arbitrary. It is now known that the age of onset and the severity of the phenotype is associated with the number of copies present for the modifier gene *SMN2*; the larger the copy number of the *SMN2* gene, the later the onset of disease and the more benign the clinical course.[21] Phenotypically, all four types share several common clinical features. All four have symmetric proximal-predominate weakness. Bulbar weakness is common in SMA type 1 but is not a prominent feature in the other types. Loss of reflexes early in the disease is typical.

Electrodiagnostic testing in SMA will reveal the underlying pathology and distribution of disease. As with the other motor neuron disorders, fibrillation and fasciculation potentials are noted. Motor unit potentials are large but tend to be less complex and more stable because of the more indolent and chronic nature of the disorder. The distribution of findings follows the clinical distribution of weakness. The changes are greatest in the proximal limbs and paraspinal muscles, with less-prominent changes distally. The EMG findings also tend to be symmetric. On nerve conduction studies, the sensory nerve action potentials remain unaffected and normal for age. The CMAPs appear similar to those in other motor neuron disorders. The CMAPs may be reduced in amplitude, reflective of the loss of motor axons from the death of the anterior horn cells. Because of the loss of motor axons, the motor nerve conduction velocities and distal latencies may be mildly delayed, but only modestly. No evidence should be present of motor conduction block.

SBMA

SBMA is an X-linked inherited disorder that occurs almost exclusively in men. Rarely, female carriers may have mild clinical manifestations. The responsible mutation is a trinucleotide repeat within the androgen receptor gene on the X-chromosome.[22] This genetic mutation is also commercially available for testing. How a mutation in the androgen receptor results in degeneration of the lower motor neurons is unknown. Other clinical manifestations include partial androgen insensitivity with gynecomastia and testicular atrophy in many affected men. The neurologic manifestations result from slow degeneration of the anterior horn cells and the bulbar motor neurons. This degeneration results in the clinical manifestations of a flaccid bulbar palsy and symmetric weakness of the proximal limb muscles.

Fasciculations are prominent, particularly around the facial muscles. In contrast to ALS, no upper motor neuron signs are present. The age of onset is variable and can occur at any time during adulthood.[23,24] Survival in SBMA is only modestly reduced.[24]

On electrodiagnostic testing, the needle EMG shows the fibrillation and fasciculation potentials. As with SMA, the motor unit potentials are large and may have some increased complexity. In contrast to ALS, the motor unit potentials are stable, indicative of the chronic indolent nature of the disease. As with SMA, the needle examination findings are most prominent in the proximal limb muscles, symmetrically. On nerve conduction studies, the CMAPs may be reduced in amplitude, reflective of the loss of motor axons from the death of the anterior horn cells. Because of the loss of motor axons, the motor nerve conduction velocities and distal latencies may be mildly delayed, but only modestly. No evidence should be present of motor conduction block. Although these patients do not report any sensory symptoms, sensory nerve action potentials on nerve conduction studies often show a loss of amplitude (**Fig. 3**). This feature is unique among the motor neuron disorders.

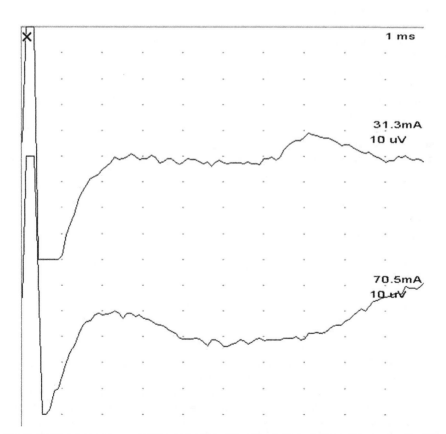

Fig. 3. Sural sensory nerve action potential with stimulation at the ankle and calf while recording posterior to the lateral malleolus. In this young patient with SBMA, no elicitable nerve action potential is seen from either site.

SUMMARY

1. PLS and PMA are currently considered phenotypic variants of ALS, both with a more benign prognosis.
2. SMA is a unique genetic disorder associated with deletions in the survival motor neuron gene and a variable age of onset and prognosis.
3. SBMA is a unique genetic disorder associated with a trinucleotide repeat in the androgen receptor gene, a variable age of onset, and only modestly reduced survival.
4. Unique features of the clinical examination and electrodiagnostic testing help differentiate the motor neuron disorders.

OTHER MIMIC SYNDROMES
Multifocal Motor Neuropathy

Multifocal motor neuropathy is a rare peripheral neuropathy that affects the motor axons exclusively. The disorder is characterized by focal or multifocal regions of conduction block along the length of the axon. The pathology at these sites is indeterminate, and whether this is caused by focal demyelination or an ion channel disorder is unclear. In either case, a blocking of the action potential results clinically in weakness and conduction block on motor nerve conduction studies. The disorder is believed to be immune-mediated, and a proportion of these cases are associated with a marked titer of antiganglioside antibodies, which can be clinically tested. This syndrome typically begins unilaterally with hand weakness. Early in the course little muscle atrophy occurs, but in established cases the muscle atrophy will appear because of secondary axonal loss from the local inflammatory attack of the nerve. Fasciculations are common, which contributes to the misdiagnosis of motor neuron disease in many patients. This syndrome has a particular predilection for the radial motor nerve, and prominent finger extensor or wrist extensor weakness should raise suspicion for this disorder. Uncommonly, the disorder may begin distally in a lower extremity. The disorder rarely affects proximal muscles and almost never has bulbar involvement. In contrast to ALS, no upper motor neuron signs are apparent. The natural history is for periods of slow, indolently progressive weakness that occurs over years. Although inflammatory, it is believed to be resistant to most immunotherapies, except intravenous gammaglobulin (IV Ig), which is the mainstay of therapy. With IV Ig, patients may experience prolonged periods of stability, but many patients become IV Ig–dependent,[25] and eventually many experience slow indolent progression despite the treatment.[25]

Electrodiagnostic testing is critical to the diagnosis of this disorder. The needle EMG findings may be similar to those of the motor neuron disorders, with fibrillation and fasciculation potentials and large complex motor unit potentials. The nerve conduction studies, however, are the key to diagnosing this disorder. In multifocal motor neuropathy, the motor nerve conduction studies are critical. The identification of areas of motor conduction block is the hallmark of this disorder and these must be examined for carefully. Often the areas of conduction block are in the proximal nerve segments, which may not be identified on routine conduction studies. Therefore, motor nerve conduction studies should be performed proximally through the plexus or even the root, with needle stimulation, if this disorder is suspected. Routine conduction studies at distant sites may miss the area of conduction block that is critical to the diagnosis (**Fig. 4**). Given the predilection of this disorder for the radial nerve, a radial motor conduction study should also be considered when investigating for areas of conduction block.

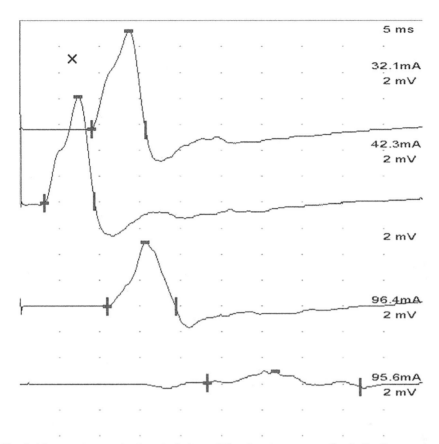

Fig. 4. Ulnar motor conduction study in multifocal motor neuropathy, indicating conduction block in the proximal segment. Routine nerve conduction studies at the wrist and elbow would have missed this area of conduction block.

Inclusion Body Myositis

Inclusion body myositis (IBM) is an adult-onset inflammatory myopathy that is commonly mistaken for a motor neuron disease. This mistake arises from the needle EMG of IBM, which shows a mixed pattern of small and large complex motor unit potentials. The larger neurogenic-appearing motor unit potentials deceptively suggest a primary neurogenic process, and the clinical disorder is often mistakenly interpreted as motor neuron disease. Despite the neurogenic-appearing motor unit potentials, whether IBM has a neurogenic component is of debate. Currently, researchers believe the larger motor unit potentials seen are merely reflective of the chronic nature of the illness, but this remains speculative. Despite the presence of an inflammatory exudate on muscle biopsy, the disorder does not seem to be immunoresponsive, and no effective treatment is known.

Clinically, IBM has a rather classic presentation. Patients typically report slowly progressive weakness of either the proximal lower extremities (most notable on stairs or rising from low seated positions) or reduction of hand grip strength. Often the process is so indolent that patients cannot date the onset of the illness accurately. When questioned in retrospect, often subtle problems can be identified many years before the weakness was first noted. The weakness tends to be symmetric, although it may be asymmetric in a minority. On examination, weakness and atrophy are notable primarily in the quadriceps muscles and the deep finger flexors of the hands, and is most prominent in the flexor pollicis longus and flexor digitorum profundus. Fasciculations are absent and no upper motor neuron signs are present.

A high clinical suspicion is critical for interpreting the electrodiagnostic testing. The nerve conduction studies will seem similar to those of the motor neuron diseases, with sparing of the sensory nerve action potentials and normal- to reduced-amplitude CAMPs. The needle examination is most challenging. Mixed populations of large and small complex and unstable motor unit potentials are seen in this disorder. If IBM is suspected, the examiner must look carefully throughout the muscle to properly identify this pattern of involvement. Fibrillation potentials tend to be diffuse and prominent, and fasciculation potentials should be absent.

Hirayama disease

Hirayama disease is a rare disorder that was initially described in the Japanese literature[26] and subsequently has been described in non-Asian populations. It has also been referred to as *Sobue's neuropathy*, *juvenile focal amyotrophy*, and *monomelic motor neuron disease*. Clinically it presents with unilateral (or at least markedly asymmetric) weakness and atrophy within the C8 and T1 myotomes, with preservation of sensation and absence of pain. It occurs almost exclusively in young, athletic patients, and has a very strong male predominance. The weakness tends to progress for several years before stabilizing. Recent literature suggests that flexion MRI scans of the cervical spine will show an expanded dorsal epidural space.[27] How this translates into anterior horn cell loss and why it is so specific to the lower cervical myotomes is unknown. Hypotheses include venous congestion and secondary ischemia to the anterior horn cells, and compression from the dilated epidural space.[28–31] However, neither is fully adequate in explaining the clinical presentation. This disorder lacks upper motor neuron features, but fasciculations may be prominent. Throughout its course, it tends to remain asymmetric, and complete plegia of the hands is uncommon. Fortunately, patients can be reassured that it does not spread to other regions. Cervical decompression has been reported with mixed results.[31–33]

SUMMARY

1. Multifocal motor neuropathy is an important disorder to distinguish from ALS given its more benign prognosis and treatable nature.
2. IBM is commonly mistaken for ALS given the unique needle EMG features. The clinical pattern of weakness should suggest this disorder and should be examined for carefully on needle EMG.

Other Neurophysiology Techniques

Motor unit number estimates

Motor unit number estimates (MUNEs) represent an attempt to quantitate the number of motor units innervating a muscle or muscle group. A variety of techniques been developed to accomplish this estimation. However, all techniques share a common formula for calculating the MUNE. The supramaximal CMAP for a muscle or muscle group is divided by average size of the individual motor unit potentials as recorded from the surface electrodes. This calculation results in a unitless number that estimates the number of motor axons innervating that muscle group. The difference between the techniques is how the size of the average motor unit potential is calculated. Quantitating the number of motor units in the motor neuron diseases has obvious advantages. Studies have shown that a decrease in the MUNE counts correlates well with disease progression, and the MUNE has been used as an outcome measure in several ALS clinical trials.[34] Its value in following patients with ALS is its rate of change over time, requiring sequential measurements. Currently, the MUNE techniques are time-consuming, and whether MUNE as a prognosticating factor adds information beyond other clinical measures in ALS is unclear. Furthermore, MUNE is only informative for the muscle examined, providing no information for other regions of the body that may not be evolving at the same rate.

Central motor conduction time

Electrodiagnostic testing is very effective at interrogating the lower motor neuron involvement in ALS. However, a paucity of ancillary testing has been performed for the upper motor neurons. In some patients, imaging will show abnormal signal in the corticospinal tracts. However, this only occurs in a minority of patients in whom the upper motor neuron signs are obvious clinically, limiting its diagnostic value. Stimulation of the motor cortex, either magnetically or electrically, and observing the CMAP responses in the periphery is one method described to interrogate the upper motor neurons.[35] The central motor conduction time is reportedly delayed in ALS with loss of the upper motor neurons. The central motor conduction time is obtained through determining the CMAP latency with cortical stimulation. Because this latency incorporates both central and peripheral conduction times, the peripheral conduction time must be subtracted away to obtain the central conduction time. The peripheral conduction time can either be estimated from the F-wave latency or from root stimulation. From the F-wave latency, the peripheral conduction latency can be derived from the following formula[36]:

Peripheral conduction latency = (CMAP distal latency + F-wave latency − 1)/2

The central conduction time then represents the motor evoked potential latency with the peripheral conduction latency subtracted away:

Central conduction time = motor evoked potential latency − peripheral conduction latency

In ALS with upper motor neuron involvement, a delay has been shown in the central conduction time. Magnetic stimulation motor evoked potentials are not FDA-approved in the United States, and motor evoked potentials induced by electrical stimulation require sedation, increasing the risk and complexity of the procedure. As with imaging, abnormalities in the central motor conduction time are typically present in patients with readily apparent upper motor neuron signs on clinical examination, causing the technique to be of little clinical use. Therefore, this technique is not widely used in general clinical practice.

Neurophysiology index

The neurophysiology index (NPI) was developed as a quantitative measure of disease severity in ALS. The initial intent was as a surrogate outcome measure to be used in ALS clinical trials.[37] It is derived from the CMAP amplitude, distal latency, and F-wave frequency. The formula for calculating the index is:

NPI = (CMAP amplitude/distal latency) × F-wave frequency %)

One limitation of the NPI is that is does not represent a specific biologic process, and change in the NPI has no inherent clinical significance. It is not useful as a diagnostic measure, and therefore is not widely used in general clinical practice.

Electrical impedance myography

Electrical impedance myography (EIM) is a novel and innovative technique being investigated in ALS.[38] This technique bears little resemblance to traditional neurophysiology testing. In EIM, a low-intensity, high-frequency alternative current (AC) is applied through a muscle while the voltage patterns are recorded with surface electrodes overlying the muscle of interest. In diseased muscle, changes are seen in the phases and impedance of the underlying muscle tissue. Currently this technique is not capable of distinguishing diseases diagnostically, but the results do change in a predictable manner with disease progression. A disadvantage of the technique is that it requires special equipment and cannot be performed with standard commercially available neurophysiology equipment. What role this technique will have in the evaluation of neuromuscular disorders is uncertain.

SUMMARY

1. MUNE refer to a group of methods to estimate the number of remaining motor units innervating a muscle group.
2. Loss of the MUNE over time correlates well with ALS progression.
3. Central motor conduction time is a neurophysiology parameter that can be used to interrogate for upper motor neuron involvement.
4. EIM is a new and novel neurophysiology technique currently being investigated in the evaluation of the motor neuron disorders.

REFERENCES

1. Charcot J-M. Amyotrophies spinales deuteropathiques sclérose latérale amyotrophique & Sclérose latérale amyotrophique. Bureaux du Progrès Médical 1874;2: 234–66.
2. Kasarskis EJ, Winslow M. When did Lou Gehrig's personal illness begin? Neurology 1989;39(9):1243–5.
3. Wechsler IA. The treatment of amyotrophic lateral sclerosis with vitamin E (tocopherols). Am J Med Sci 1940;200:765–78.
4. Deng H, Chen W, Hong S, et al. Mutations in UBQLN2 cause dominant X-linked juvenile and adult-onset ALS and ALS/dementia. Nature 2011;477(7363):211–5.
5. Sreedharan J, Blair IP, Tripathi VB, et al. TDP-43 mutations in familial and sporadic amyotrophic lateral sclerosis. Science 2008;319(5870):1668–72.
6. Sorenson EJ, Stalker AP, Kurland LT, et al. Amyotrophic lateral sclerosis in Olmsted County, Minnesota, 1925 to 1998. Neurology 2002;59(2):280–2.
7. Bensimon G, Lacomblez L, Meininger V. A controlled trial of riluzole in amyotrophic lateral sclerosis. ALS/Riluzole Study Group. N Engl J Med 1994;330(9): 585–91.
8. Miller RG, Bouchard JP, Duquette P, et al. Clinical trials of riluzole in patients with ALS. ALS/Riluzole Study Group-II. Neurology 1996;47(4 Suppl 2):S86–90 [discussion: S90–2].
9. Brooks BR. El Escorial World Federation of Neurology criteria for the diagnosis of amyotrophic lateral sclerosis. Subcommittee on Motor Neuron Diseases/Amyotrophic Lateral Sclerosis of the World Federation of Neurology Research Group on

Neuromuscular Diseases and the El Escorial "Clinical limits of amyotrophic lateral sclerosis" workshop contributors. J Neurol Sci 1994;124(Suppl):96–107.

10. Carvalho MD, Swash M. Awaji diagnostic algorithm increases sensitivity of El Escorial criteria for ALS diagnosis. Amyotroph Lateral Scler 2009;10(1): 53–7.

11. Boekestein WA, Kleine BU, Hageman G, et al. Sensitivity and specificity of the 'Awaji' electrodiagnostic criteria for amyotrophic lateral sclerosis: retrospective comparison of the Awaji and revised El Escorial criteria for ALS. Amyotroph Lateral Scler 2010;11(6):497–501.

12. Schaefer AM, Sanes JR, Lichtman JW. A compensatory subpopulation of motor neurons in a mouse model of amyotrophic lateral sclerosis. J Comp Neurol 2005;490(3):209–19.

13. Blexrud MD, Windebank AJ, Daube JR. Long-term follow-up of 121 patients with benign fasciculations. Ann Neurol 1993;34(4):622–5.

14. Pasquali L, Longone P, Isidoro C, et al. Autophagy, lithium, and amyotrophic lateral sclerosis. Muscle Nerve 2009;40(2):173–94.

15. Coussee E, De Smet P, Bogaert E, et al. G37R SOD1 mutant alters mitochondrial complex I activity, Ca(2+) uptake and ATP production. Cell Calcium 2011;49(4): 217–25.

16. Singer MA, Statland JM, Wolfe GI, et al. Primary lateral sclerosis. Muscle Nerve 2007;35(3):291–302.

17. Praline J, Guennoc AM, Vourc'h P, et al. Primary lateral sclerosis may occur within familial amyotrophic lateral sclerosis pedigrees. Amyotroph Lateral Scler 2010; 11(1–2):154–6.

18. Ince PG, Evans J, Knopp M, et al. Corticospinal tract degeneration in the progressive muscular atrophy variant of ALS. Neurology 2003;60(8):1252–8.

19. Geser F, Stein B, Partain M, et al. Motor neuron disease clinically limited to the lower motor neuron is a diffuse TDP-43 proteinopathy. Acta Neuropathol 2011; 121(4):509–17.

20. Lefebvre S, Burglen L, Reboullet S, et al. Identification and characterization of a spinal muscular atrophy-determining gene. Cell 1995;80(1):155–65.

21. Feldkotter M, Schwarzer V, Wirth R, et al. Quantitative analyses of SMN1 and SMN2 based on real-time lightCycler PCR: fast and highly reliable carrier testing and prediction of severity of spinal muscular atrophy. Am J Hum Genet 2002; 70(2):358–68.

22. La Spada AR, Wilson EM, Lubahn DB, et al. Androgen receptor gene mutations in X-linked spinal and bulbar muscular atrophy. Nature 1991;352(6330):77–9.

23. Finsterer J. Bulbar and spinal muscular atrophy (Kennedy's disease): a review. Eur J Neurol 2009;16(5):556–61.

24. Chahin N, Klein CJ, Sorenson E. Natural history of spinal and bulbar muscular atrophy. Neurology 2008;70:1967–71.

25. Taylor BV, Wright RA, Harper CM, et al. Natural history of 46 patients with multifocal motor neuropathy with conduction block. Muscle Nerve 2000;23(6): 900–8.

26. Hirayama K, Tsubaki T, Toyokura Y, et al. Juvenile muscular atrophy of unilateral upper extremity. Neurology 1963;13:373–80.

27. Yin B, Liu L, Geng DY. Features of Hirayama disease on fully flexed position cervical MRI. J Int Med Res 2011;39(1):222–8.

28. Ciceri EF, Chiapparini L, Erbetta A, et al. Angiographically proven cervical venous engorgement: a possible concurrent cause in the pathophysiology of Hirayama's myelopathy. Neurol Sci 2010;31(6):845–8.

29. Yoshiyama Y, Tokumaru Y, Arai K. Flexion-induced cervical myelopathy associated with fewer elastic fibers and thickening in the posterior dura mater. J Neurol 2010;257(1):149–51.

30. Ibanez Sanz L, de Vega VM, Arranz JC, et al. [MRI in flexed and extended positions for the diagnosis of cervical myelopathy in Hirayama's disease]. Radiologia 2009;51(5):516–9 [in Spanish].

31. Kwon O, Kim M, Lee KW. A Korean case of juvenile muscular atrophy of distal upper extremity (Hirayama disease) with dynamic cervical cord compression. J Korean Med Sci 2004;19(5):768–71.

32. Arrese I, Rivas JJ, Esteban J, et al. A case of Hirayama disease treated with laminectomy and duraplasty without spinal fusion. Neurocirugia (Asturias, Spain) 2009;20(6):555–8 [discussion: 558].

33. Chiba S, Yonekura K, Nonaka M, et al. Advanced Hirayama disease with successful improvement of activities of daily living by operative reconstruction. Intern Med 2004;43(1):79–81.

34. Shefner JM, Cudkowicz ME, Zhang H, et al. Northeast ALSC. The use of statistical MUNE in a multicenter clinical trial. Muscle Nerve 2004;30(4):463–9.

35. Floyd AG, Yu QP, Piboolnurak P, et al. Transcranial magnetic stimulation in ALS: utility of central motor conduction tests. Neurology 2009;72(6):498–504.

36. Kimura J. Principles and pitfalls of nerve conduction studies. Ann Neurol 1984; 16(4):415–29.

37. Swash M, de Carvalho M. The Neurophysiological Index in ALS. Amyotroph Lateral Scler Other Motor Neuron Disord 2004;5(Suppl 1):108–10.

38. Tarulli AW, Garmirian LP, Fogerson PM, et al. Localized muscle impedance abnormalities in amyotrophic lateral sclerosis. J Clin Neuromuscular Dis 2009;10(3): 90–6.

Evaluation of Neuromuscular Junction Disorders in the Electromyography Laboratory

Vern C. Juel, MD[a,b],*

KEYWORDS

- Neuromuscular junction • Repetitive nerve stimulation
- Single-fiber electromyography • Jitter • Myasthenia gravis
- Lambert-Eaton myasthenic syndrome

Although neuromuscular junction (NMJ) disorders are rare, patients are often referred to electrodiagnostic (EDx) medicine laboratories for evaluation of a suspected or known NMJ disorder. Patients with NMJ disorders typically experience painless and fatigable weakness that increases with exercise. In acquired myasthenia gravis (MG), postjunctional immunologic attack on the acetylcholine (ACh) receptor and associated proteins results in variable weakness in ocular, bulbar, and extremity muscles. Lambert-Eaton myasthenic syndrome (LEMS) typically involves prominent proximal lower limb weakness, fatigue, and autonomic dysfunction as a consequence of antibodies directed against voltage-gated calcium channels (VGCC). In botulism, patients experience prominent craniobulbar weakness with descending paralysis and autonomic dysfunction related to interruption of the exocytotic release of ACh by clostridial neurotoxins. Congenital myasthenic syndromes (CMS) present with weakness generally beginning around the time of birth and caused by several genetically determined presynaptic and postsynaptic defects. Repetitive nerve stimulation (RNS) testing and single-fiber electromyography (SFEMG) are specific EDx techniques that may confirm the presence, type, and severity of NMJ disorders.

The author has nothing to disclose.
[a] Duke University School of Medicine, Durham, NC, USA
[b] Electromyography Laboratory, Duke University Medical Center, DUMC 3403, Trent Drive, Clinic 1L, Room 1255, Durham, NC 27710, USA
* Duke University Medical Center, DUMC 3403, Trent Drive, Clinic 1L, Room 1255, Durham, NC 27710.
E-mail address: vern.juel@duke.edu

THE NEUROMUSCULAR JUNCTION

The neuromuscular junction is the specialized region where motor nerve synapses with muscle. It includes the motor nerve terminal, the synaptic space or cleft, and the highly folded muscle endplate region. The neurotransmitter ACh is synthesized in the motor nerve terminal and stored in vesicles. Each vesicle contains 1 quantum of ACh, or about 6000 to 10,000 ACh molecules.[1] Motor nerve action potentials propagated distally to motor nerve terminals elicit presynaptic calcium influx through VGCC in the active or release zones of the nerve terminal. The calcium influx initiates the docking and fusion of ACh vesicles with the presynaptic membrane via soluble N-ethylmaleimide-sensitive fusion attachment protein receptor (SNARE) proteins with exocytotic release of ACh into the synaptic space.[2] ACh rapidly diffuses across the 50-nm synaptic cleft and binds to ACh receptors (AChR) located on the tips of the end plate folds.[1] This interaction results in opening of sodium channels with movement of sodium into the adjacent end plate region. The resulting potential is called the *end plate potential* (EPP). If the EPP amplitude exceeds the threshold level for generating a muscle fiber action potential (MFAP), a wave of depolarization spreads from the end plate region throughout the muscle fiber. The process of excitation-contraction coupling is thereby initiated, and the muscle fiber contracts. The effects of ACh on the end plate are terminated by acetylcholinesterase (AChE) that is bound to the end plate basal lamina and hydrolyzes ACh to choline and acetate. Choline undergoes reuptake by the presynaptic neuron for resynthesis to ACh.

After synthesis, ACh is stored in vesicles. There are several pools of stored ACh potentially available for release. A primary or immediate store of ACh in the nerve terminal is readily available for release. A secondary or mobilization store is available in the distal motor axon, and a tertiary or reserve store is located in the motor nerve axon and cell body.

EPP amplitude is determined by the amount of ACh released and by the number and density of functional AChRs on the end plate. EPP amplitude is variable and, because of this variability, EPPs reach threshold at slightly different times to generate MFAPs. This variability represents the major source of neuromuscular *jitter*, or the latency variability in MFAPs derived from motor nerve impulses.[3]

With normal physiology, each nerve impulse causes release of more ACh than necessary to generate an EPP that exceeds threshold for MFAP generation. The *safety factor* is the ratio between the EPP and the threshold for initiating an MFAP, and represents the extra amount of ACh released beyond the minimum necessary for the EPP to reach threshold. The safety factor ensures that each motor nerve action potential (NAP) results in muscle fiber contraction. In NMJ disorders, the EPP may be delayed or may fail to reach threshold in response to an NAP, and neuromuscular transmission is impaired or blocked.

Each nerve impulse elicits release of about 20% of the primary or immediate store of ACh.[4] With motor nerve firing rates greater than 0.1 Hz, the number of quanta released declines for the first 4 to 5 nerve impulses, and then stabilizes with mobilization of the secondary ACh stores with corresponding changes in EPP amplitude (**Table 1**).[5,6] Normally, this reduction in EPP amplitude has no impact on NMT because of the safety factor. However, if there is a disorder of NMT, the EPP may take longer to reach threshold (increased jitter) or may fail to reach threshold (impulse blocking).

Quantal release of ACh is calcium dependent, and each NAP opens VGCC in active zones on the motor nerve terminal. After entry, calcium is removed from the motor nerve terminal over 100 to 200 milliseconds.[7] When motor nerve firing rates exceed

Table 1
Quantal mobilization of ACh and EPP amplitude in normal individuals and patients with postsynaptic disorders with 3-Hz motor nerve stimulation

Stimulus Number	Available ACh (Quanta)	ACh Released (Quanta)	EPP Amplitude (mV)
1	1000	200	40
2	800	160	32
3	640	128	26
4	512	102	20
5	640	128	26

Data from Howard JF. Repetitive nerve stimulation. Workshop 3SW.001, Advanced EMG techniques. American Academy of Neurology Annual Meeting. San Francisco, CA, April 26, 2004.

10 Hz with NAPs more frequent than every 100 milliseconds, there is a net increase in presynaptic calcium concentration with increased quantal ACh release for each nerve impulse. This potentiated ACh release persists for 30 to 60 seconds and is followed about 2 to 5 minutes later by reduced release of ACh with each nerve impulse or post-activation exhaustion.[4,8]

The amount of ACh released with each nerve impulse and resulting EPPs reflect the interaction between the depletion of immediate ACh stores and the presynaptic calcium concentration. NMJ disorders reduce the safety factor through a reduction of quantal release and/or by postsynaptic dysfunction of ACh receptors.

REPETITIVE NERVE STIMULATION TESTING

In an early predecessor of RNS, Friedrich Jolly[9] used a direct motor point electrical stimulation technique to elicit lower limb muscle contraction in patients with MG. The size of muscle contractions became progressively reduced following repeated muscle stimulation in patients with MG, and was termed the "myasthenic reaction."[9] Harvey and Masland[10,11] subsequently described decrementing muscle electrical responses to repetitive motor nerve stimulation in patients with MG and proposed that the technique could be used diagnostically. Since that time, RNS testing has served as a standard test in EDx laboratories for assessment of NMT.

RNS exploit the depletion of immediate ACh stores with low stimulation frequencies to unmask the reduced safety factor common to all NMJ disorders. The reduced number of EPP that successfully elicit MFAPs is reflected by a reduction of CMAP amplitudes or decrement. In presynaptic disorders, the augmentation of presynaptic calcium concentration with high stimulation frequencies or following brief exercise increases EPP amplitudes, and may unblock MFAPs with increased CMAP amplitude or facilitation.

Technique: General Concepts

The general technique for performing RNS is similar to that for motor nerve conduction studies (NCS). A motor or mixed nerve is stimulated supramaximally (10%–25% more than the level needed to activate all muscle fibers) and surface CMAP recordings are made with a recording electrode placed over the corresponding muscle belly with a reference over the distal tendon. The negative peak amplitude of each CMAP represents the summation of MFAPs responding to motor nerve stimulation and serves as an index of successful neuromuscular transmission.

Stimulation

Nerve stimulation is typically performed with surface stimulating electrodes. A near-nerve stimulating electrode is required for some RNS (eg, mandibular RNS recording in the masseter) or may permit the use of shorter duration and lower intensity stimulus that is less painful (eg, musculocutaneous RNS recording in the biceps brachii). Low-frequency RNS at stimulation rates of 2 to 3 Hz are optimal to elicit decremental responses in MG.[12] In low-frequency RNS, a rate of 2 to 3 Hz is preferred, and no more than 5 to 10 stimuli are needed to show significant decrement. Stimulation rates greater than 5 Hz should be avoided because of pseudofacilitation, a phenomenon in which the CMAP negative peak amplitude increases with reduced duration and no change in CMAP negative peak area (**Fig. 1**). With high-frequency RNS, CMAP amplitude may increase by up to 50%.[13] Pseudofacilitation likely results from synchronization of MFAP propagation velocities or from muscle fiber shortening.[14]

High-frequency (greater than 10 Hz) RNS should be reserved for evaluation of suspected presynaptic NMT disorders when a patient cannot perform isometric exercise against an examiner's resistance with maximum voluntary contraction (MVC), as in infants, adults with impaired cognition or consciousness, or with severe paralysis related to possible botulism or LEMS. In such patients, the optimal frequency is 20 to 50 Hz for 2 to 10 seconds. In other situations, 10 seconds of MVC serves as the equivalent of high-frequency RNS and is more comfortable for patients.[15]

Temperature

Reduced limb temperature augments NMT and renders RNS testing less sensitive. Muscles should therefore be warmed to 34 to 37°C, and this temperature should be maintained during RNS testing.[16] Proximal muscles such as the trapezius and craniobulbar muscles do not require warming.

Immobilization

Securing the stimulating and recording electrodes and immobilizing the joint moved by the muscle undergoing testing is important to reduce recording artifact. Artifact from electrode movement or limb movement appears as an abrupt change in CMAP

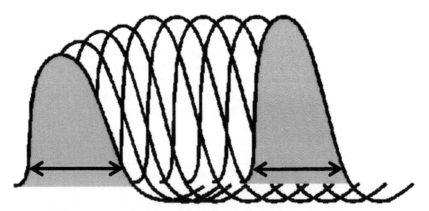

Fig. 1. Pseudofacilitation with RNS. Although the compound muscle action potential (CMAP) amplitude increases with several stimuli, the duration (*arrows*) shortens with no net change in CMAP area. (*Adapted from* Sanders DB. Electrophysiologic study of disorders of neuromuscular transmission. In: Aminoff M, ed. Electrodiagnosis in clinical neurology. 5th edition. New York: Churchill Livingstone; 2005. p. 335–55; with permission.)

waveform during a train of stimuli. Movement of the stimulating electrodes may result in submaximal nerve stimulation and generate a pseudodecrement.[17] Immobilization of intrinsic hand muscles is not difficult, but immobilization of larger, more proximal limb muscles is challenging.

Activation Methods

Activation methods may be used to increase the sensitivity of RNS in NMJ disorders, and exercise may unmask an NMJ defect that is not otherwise detectable. Isometric exercise is performed with MVC against resistance provided by the examiner. Postactivation exhaustion or postexercise exhaustion (PAE) that elicits a significant or increased CMAP amplitude decrement may be observed 2 to 5 minutes following exercise periods of 30 to 60 seconds. Patients with normal responses to initial RNS trains may exhibit PAE with abnormal decremental responses.[18] However, the degree of increased sensitivity that results from assessing PAE may be small.[19] In patients with low-amplitude CMAPs or decremental responses at baseline, postactivation facilitation or postexercise facilitation (PAF) may reflect the unblocking of MFAPs caused by increased quantal release. PAF is best elicited following a brief, 10-second exercise period. PAF may be significant in presynaptic NMT disorders, and generally exceeds 100% in LEMS (**Fig. 2**).

Ischemia to enhance PAE has been used to increase the sensitivity of RNS. This "double-step" technique involves prolonged low-frequency RNS before and after placement of a blood pressure cuff on the arm inflated to more than systolic pressure while recording median or ulnar RNS in hand muscles.[20] In patients with MG with normal RNS in hand muscles, the technique was only slightly more sensitive than spinal accessory RNS recorded in trapezius, and only 60% as sensitive as SFEMG in the extensor digitorum communis (EDC).[21] Regional curare infusions have also been used to increase sensitivity of RNS by producing competitive, nondepolarizing neuromuscular blockade.[22] Given the inherent risk for excessive paralysis, regional curarization methods using low doses in an ischemic forearm have been suggested,[23] although they may elicit abnormal findings in nonprimary NMJ disorders (eg, motor neuron disease), require intensive care monitoring, and do not achieve diagnostic sensitivity superior to SFEMG in MG.[3]

Muscle Selection

Whenever feasible, RNS testing should be performed in clinically weak muscles. Although the easiest muscles for performing RNS are the intrinsic hand muscles, the distribution of weakness in MG generally involves proximal and bulbar muscles. Therefore, RNS testing for MG should include proximal limb or bulbar muscles as well as intrinsic hand muscles. In the hand, the abductor digiti quinti manis (ADM) is studied with ulnar nerve stimulation at the wrist. Although it is easily accessible, well tolerated, and readily immobilized by taping fingers together or with folded cloth padding or towels, it is rarely abnormal in MG. RNS in the abductor pollicis brevis (APB) has similar attributes as in the ADM, although it is sometimes more difficult to immobilize. The trapezius is the most straightforward shoulder muscle for RNS testing and is studied with spinal accessory nerve stimulation at the posterior border of the sternocleidomastoid muscle recording along the superior border of the muscle. Trapezius RNS testing is frequently abnormal in generalized MG involving limb muscles (**Fig. 3**).[24] Although the trapezius cannot be immobilized, movement artifact is minimized by placing the patient in a seated position with the arms extended and grasping a chair back or bar, with the arms adducted grasping the chair seat, or in a recumbent, semireclined position. In the lower limb, RNS testing of both the extensor digitorum

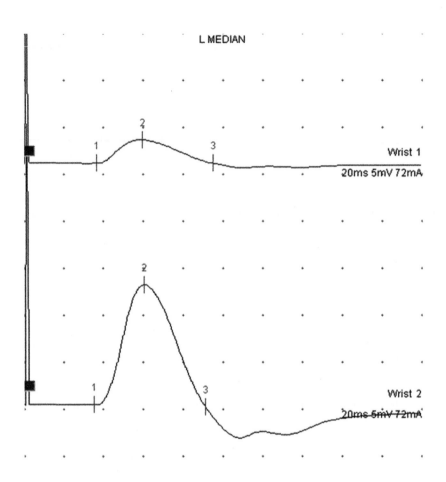

Fig. 2. CMAPs recorded in the abductor pollicis brevis muscle in a patient with LEMS at rest (upper trace) and after 10 seconds of MVC (lower trace). The resting CMAP amplitude is less than half of normal, and there is more than 500% PAF. (Copyright © 2010, VC Juel.)

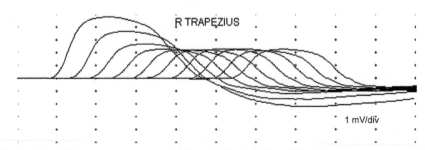

Fig. 3. 3-Hz RNS testing in trapezius in a patient with moderate generalized MG with predominant limb weakness. The testing was performed before exercise. The amplitude decrement is 53% between the first and fourth CMAPs in the series. (Copyright © 2010, VC Juel.)

brevis (EDB) and tibialis anterior are straightforward and well tolerated with surface stimulation of the deep fibular (peroneal) nerve at the ankle, and the common fibular (peroneal) nerve at the knee.

Proximal upper limb muscles are often clinically weak in MG and exhibit significant decremental responses with RNS testing, although technical issues limit the usefulness of RNS testing in this region. Deltoid RNS studies are performed with axillary nerve stimulation at the Erb's point with a surface electrode held firmly behind the clavicle. This study is frequently confounded by costimulation of the brachial plexus and is often uncomfortable. Immobilization is difficult and is best achieved by patients placing the forearm over the abdomen and grasping the wrist with the other hand to minimize movement artifact. Biceps brachii RNS testing is performed with stimulation of the musculocutaneous nerve in the axilla. As with deltoid studies, immobilization can be difficult, and patient discomfort can be significant. Surface stimulating electrodes are placed posterior to the medial head of the muscle, about 2.5 cm (1 inch) inferior to the axillary fold.[3] Near-nerve needle stimulation is more comfortable with less displacement of the stimulating electrodes compared with the surface stimulation technique.[3]

Facial RNS testing is performed with surface stimulation anterior to the stylomastoid foramen. The reference electrode is placed over the bridge of the nose. Although recordings can be made from the orbicularis oculi and several facial muscles, nasalis recordings are associated with the least movement and stimulus artifact. Facial muscles frequently show abnormal RNS testing in MG, but the testing is uncomfortable and poorly tolerated. Trigeminal RNS testing recorded in the masseter muscle uses a near-nerve technique to stimulate the masseteric branch of the trigeminal nerve at the mandibular notch. Although not as sensitive as facial RNS testing, it is better tolerated by patients.[25]

Data Analysis

Decrement

Decrement is a calculation of the percentage of amplitude reduction between the initial CMAP generated by a train of nerve stimulation ($CMAP_1$) and the lowest amplitude CMAP generated ($CMAP_n$), and is computed from the formula: % $Decrement_n$ = $[(CMAP_n - CMAP_1)/CMAP_1] \times 100\%$. With appropriate technique and quality control, the fourth or fifth CMAP amplitude should represent the lowest CMAP amplitude and reflect the depletion of primary ACh stores. Mobilization of secondary ACh stores occurs after the fourth or fifth stimulation, and accordingly, CMAP amplitudes increase slightly giving rise to a characteristic saddle-shaped or U-shaped series of CMAP waveforms (**Fig. 4**). Decrement is therefore typically calculated based on the amplitude of the first CMAP and the fourth or fifth CMAP in an RNS train of 2 to 3 Hz. Normal patients exhibit less than 8% decrement, and greater than 10% decrement is considered abnormal.[26]

Facilitation

In presynaptic NMJ disorders, the percentage of amplitude facilitation with high-frequency nerve stimulation is calculated from the formula: % $Facilitation_n$ = $[(CMAP_n - CMAP_1)/CMAP_1] \times 100\%$, where $CMAP_n$ is the highest CMAP amplitude generated by a train of nerve stimulation. When high-frequency RNS testing must be performed, it is important to assess for pseudofacilitation by comparing the amplitude facilitation with area facilitation. These values should be comparable in the absence of pseudofacilitation (**Fig. 5**). Whenever possible, facilitation is best assessed following 10 seconds of MVC of the tested muscle to avoid patient discomfort and pseudofacilitation associated with high-frequency RNS. The percentage of

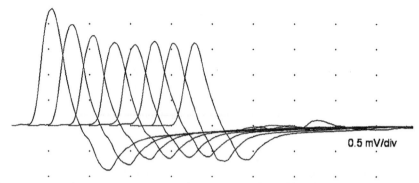

Fig. 4. 3-Hz RNS in ADM in a patient with LEMS. Note the saddle-shaped or U-shaped series of CMAP waveforms with a nadir in CMAP amplitude with the fourth and fifth CMAPs of the series (34% amplitude decrement). The subsequent 3 CMAP amplitudes are slightly higher, reflecting mobilization of secondary ACh stores. (Copyright © 2010, VC Juel.)

facilitation following MVC is calculated from the same formula: % Facilitation = $[(CMAP_{Post} - CMAP_{Pre})/CMAP_{Pre}] \times 100\%$, where $CMAP_{Post}$ is the first postexercise CMAP elicited after the 10-second exercise period, and $CMAP_{Pre}$ is the first CMAP in the baseline, preexercise RNS train.

Quality Control Issues

Quality control to eliminate technical error is essential when performing RNS testing. Each CMAP waveform train should be inspected. Quality assessment limited to the stylized or stick renderings displayed by contemporary electromyography (EMG)

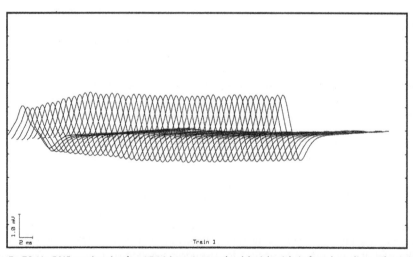

Fig. 5. 50-Hz RNS testing in the ADM in a 4-month-old girl with infant botulism. The initial CMAP amplitude is about 25% of normal and, over 1 second of tetanic stimulation, there is sustained 50% CMAP amplitude facilitation. Some of the CMAP amplitude facilitation is due to pseudofacilitation, because the CMAP duration diminishes by 15% during the stimulation, and the CMAP area facilitation is only 40%. (Copyright © 2010, VC Juel.)

machine software does not reveal critical CMAP changes that may influence data analysis. The baseline should be stable, and shifting of the baseline suggests movement artifact involving the recording electrodes and leads. Sudden changes in CMAP amplitude and morphology within trains suggests understimulation related to movement of the stimulating electrodes. Inadequate muscle warming renders RNS testing insensitive and may eliminate abnormal findings. Muscle shortening caused by poor immobilization, patient discomfort, or high-frequency RNS testing may elicit pseudofacilitation. With NMJ disease, a regular, orderly decline in CMAP amplitude is expected during the first 4 stimuli with an increase in CMAP amplitude after the fourth or fifth stimulus (see **Fig. 4**). Although the fourth or fifth CMAP amplitude is typically the lowest, the maximum amplitude decrement between stimuli is often observed between the first and second CMAPs. Findings should be reproducible after appropriate rest periods.

RNS Protocols

When performing RNS for possible NMJ disease, cholinesterase inhibitors and 3,4-diaminopyridine should be held for at least 12 hours before testing if medically safe to do so, because these agents may improve neuromuscular transmission and reduce the diagnostic sensitivity of the testing.[27] History, examination, and findings on standard EDx studies help to determine what type of NMJ disorder is likely prior to RNS testing.

If MG is suspected, RNS testing at 2 to 3 Hz should be performed in at least 1 hand and 1 proximal muscle. Responses from an initial train of 5 to 10 stimuli are inspected. If there is a decrement, an additional train of 5 to 10 stimuli is given after a 1-minute rest period to ensure that the findings are reproducible. The muscle is then exercised (MVC) for 30 to 60 seconds. A train of 5 stimuli is given immediately after the exercise, and additional stimulus trains are given at intervals of 30 to 60 seconds for 5 minutes to assess for PAE.

If LEMS is suspected or if CMAP amplitudes are reduced with standard motor NCS, at least 1 hand and foot muscle should be tested as follows. Baseline CMAP should be assessed in a hand muscle rested for several minutes. The patient should then activate the muscle with MVC for 10 seconds, relax completely, and receive a postactivation stimulus within 5 seconds. Delay in administering the postactivation stimulus may result in underestimating or missing PAF, and longer exercise periods may deplete ACh stores and mask facilitation. In LEMS, more than 100% PAF is typically observed. RNS of 2 to 3 Hz should be performed in the muscle after several minutes of additional rest with an initial train of 5 to 10 stimuli to establish a decremental response. After another 10 seconds of MVC, a train of 5 stimuli is given immediately after the exercise to confirm PAF, and additional stimulus trains are given at intervals of 30 to 60 seconds for 5 minutes to assess for PAE.

RNS FINDINGS IN DISEASE
Myasthenia Gravis

In autoimmune, acquired MG, decremental responses are most likely to be shown in proximal or craniobulbar muscles and with more severe disease (see **Fig. 3**). PAF may be observed after 30 to 60 seconds of MVC, but this is generally less than 20% and rarely greater than 50%. PAE may be observed 2 to 4 minutes after exercise. In a large series, RNS were abnormal in a hand or shoulder muscle in 76% of patients with MG with disease extending beyond the ocular muscles.[14] By comparison with RNS, SFEMG is a more sensitive test for showing abnormal NMT in MG, especially in ocular MG.[28]

Lambert-Eaton Myasthenic Syndrome

In LEMS, the most sensitive RNS finding is decrement to low-frequency RNS in at least 1 hand muscle virtually all patients. The decremental response has the characteristic saddle shape (see **Fig. 4**). Resting CMAP amplitude is usually reduced. Marked PAF greater than 100% after brief exercise or following high-frequency RNS is the most specific finding in LEMS (see **Fig. 2**). PAF may be shown in at least 1 hand or foot muscle in more than 80% of patients with LEMS.[29]

Hypermagnesemia

Hypermagnesemia may occur in pregnant women receiving magnesium for tocolysis or preeclampsia or in individuals with renal failure receiving supplementary magnesium.[30] As in LEMS, proximal limb weakness with depressed tendon reflexes is observed. RNS testing reveals decrement to low-frequency RNS, significant PAF, and low-amplitude resting CMAPs.[3]

Botulism

Infant intestinal botulism is the most common form of botulism. Within the first year of life, infants may ingest *Clostridium botulinum* spores that germinate in the intestine and produce botulinum toxin that is absorbed and distributed systemically. Wound botulism involves clostridial colonization and infection of devitalized, relatively anaerobic tissue from which botulinum toxin is absorbed and circulated systemically. Foodborne botulism involves ingestion of preformed toxin from contaminated foodstuffs. Botulism classically presents with a descending pattern of weakness with early oculobulbar findings with subsequent limb and respiratory paralysis. The characteristic findings on RNS testing in infant botulism include reduced resting CMAP amplitudes, more than 40% PAF, the striking persistence of PAF for several minutes with activation, and the absence of PAE (see **Fig. 5**).[31,32] RNS testing in clinically weak muscles is essential, because the disease may be restricted to these muscles.[33] Adults with mild disease may exhibit normal RNS findings with only a mild degree of PAF,[34] and only about 60% of adult cases exhibit significant PAF.[32]

Congenital Myasthenic Syndromes

In many CMS, RNS testing may exhibit decremental responses as in MG. In more mild cases of CMS with episodic apnea (CMS-EA) or end plate choline acetyltransferase (CHAT) deficiency, prolonged low-frequency RNS or exercise for 5 to 10 minutes may be needed to elicit significant decrement. A prolonged period of PAE is subsequently observed and may persist for 5 to 10 minutes.[33] CMS associated with increased EPP duration, such as slow channel syndrome and congenital AChE deficiency, may exhibit repetitive discharges with low-frequency RNS. These discharges are smaller than the initial CMAPs, and they arise as a result of prolonged end plate depolarization exceeding the absolute refractory period of the MFAP.[35,36] Such repetitive discharges may also be observed in patients with autoimmune, acquired MG treated with high doses of cholinesterase inhibitors or with organophosphate intoxication. Patients with muscle-specific tyrosine kinase (MuSK) MG may exhibit marked cholinergic hypersensitivity with numerous extra repetitive discharges when receiving low therapeutic doses of cholinesterase inhibitors.[37]

Other Motor Unit Disorders

Abnormal findings on RNS testing are not limited to primary NMJ disorders. Patients with progressive motor neuron disease[38,39] and myotonic disorders[40] may exhibit decremental responses to low-frequency RNS. It is therefore essential to interpret RNS findings in the context of clinical history, examination, and standard EDx studies including motor and sensory NCS and needle electrode examination.

NEEDLE EMG IN NEUROMUSCULAR JUNCTION DISORDERS

Conventional needle EMG is often unremarkable in NMJ disorders, and motor unit potential (MUP) morphology (amplitude, duration, complexity) and recruitment are often normal, particularly in MG. When an NMJ disorder is suspected, needle EMG serves largely to exclude other neuromuscular diseases such as a motor neuron disorder or myopathy in which MUP duration, morphology, and recruitment exhibit characteristic changes. However, moment-to-moment amplitude and/or configurational changes in the MUP, known as *jiggle* or instability, may be observed in NMJ disease as the number and synchronization of MFAPs composing the MUP varies with successive firings (**Fig. 6**).[41] Such instability may also be observed with immature

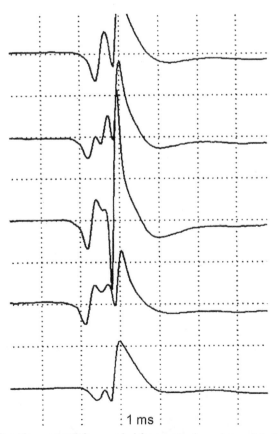

1 ms

Fig. 6. Motor unit action potentials recorded from a single motor unit in the biceps brachii in a patient with LEMS using a concentric needle electrode. Moment-to-moment configurational changes or jiggle is shown in the rastered responses. (*From* Sanders DB. Lambert-Eaton myasthenic syndrome: clinical diagnosis, immune-mediated mechanisms, and update of therapies. Ann Neurol 1995;37(S1):S63–73; with permission.)

reinnervation in peripheral nerve disease, especially in motor neuron disorders. When there is a high degree of impulse blocking, as in LEMS, MUP may appear small and complex and be misinterpreted as indicating myopathy. Spontaneous activity is usually absent, although fibrillation potentials may be seen in MG in bulbar and paraspinal muscles.[42]

SINGLE-FIBER ELECTROMYOGRAPHY

SFEMG is a technique that selectively assesses individual MFAPs. The ability to record individual MFAPs is achieved by the use of a specialized concentric needle electrode with a 25-μm recording surface on a side port about 3 mm from the needle tip (**Fig. 7**). By comparison, the recording surface of a standard concentric needle is about 120-μm in diameter. In addition, a low-frequency filter setting of 500 Hz rejects low-frequency signals that originate in distant muscle fibers and increases the selectivity of the technique.[14]

Jitter and Fiber Density

SFEMG is a sensitive and powerful technique for assessing neuromuscular transmission, because it facilitates simultaneous recording of individual MFAPs within the same motor unit. Essentially all of the temporal variability between firing of MFAPs innervated by the same motor neuron is related to neuromuscular transmission. This temporal variability or neuromuscular jitter reflects the fluctuations in the time needed for EPPs to reach the threshold to generate MFAPs. When processes affecting the NMJ reduce the safety factor, some EPPs take longer to reach threshold, MFAP generation is delayed, and jitter correspondingly increases. When EPPs fail to reach threshold following a nerve impulse, blocking occurs. Clinical weakness in a muscle occurs when a critical number of end plates are blocked in that muscle. Along with

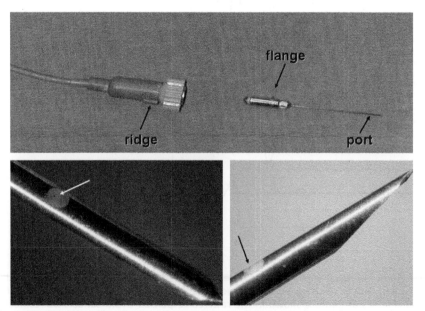

Fig. 7. The SFEMG electrode. The selectivity of SFEMG is largely due to the 25-μm diameter recording surface at the side port (*arrows*). (Copyright © 2011, DB Sanders.)

jitter, SFEMG demonstrates fiber density (FD), the concentration of MFAPs within the small recording field of the SF electrode. FD may be increased with reinnervation and in some myopathies, and represents an electrophysiologic analog to histologic muscle fiber–type grouping.

Voluntary Activated SFEMG

In cooperative patients, jitter is most readily assessed with voluntary muscle activation. With the voluntary activation technique, the recording needle electrode is inserted in a muscle and positioned to record from a pair of muscle fibers innervated by the same motor neuron as the patient minimally contracts the muscle. The oscilloscope is triggered by one of the MFAPs, and that potential is displayed in a fixed position on the oscilloscope screen. MFAPs from the other muscle fiber are time-locked to the triggering potential, but exhibit some temporal variability or jitter with respect to the triggering potential. The normal amount of jitter depends on the muscle being tested and the age of the patient.[43,44] MFAPs that have a rise time less than 300 microseconds and amplitude greater than 200 μV are suitable for jitter analysis, and a minimum of 50 discharges of the triggering potential are recorded (**Fig. 8**). An increased degree of jitter is seen when neuromuscular transmission is abnormal and, when the abnormality is severe, impulse blocking may also be seen. Blocking must occur in order for RNS to elicit a decrement in a train of CMAPs. Blocking is only seen with jitter values greater than 100 microseconds.[14]

Stimulated SFEMG

In patients unable to cooperate with voluntary muscle activation procedures, such as very young children, patients with severe tremor, or patients with disturbed consciousness, stimulated SFEMG may facilitate jitter assessment. In this technique, axonal stimulation of an intramuscular motor nerve branch (eg, posterior interosseous nerve branch within the EDC muscle) or of a motor nerve proximal to a muscle (eg, facial nerve) is used to trigger the oscilloscope.[45] Jitter is then measured between the stimulus and a single MFAP. The technique is also useful to show rate-dependent

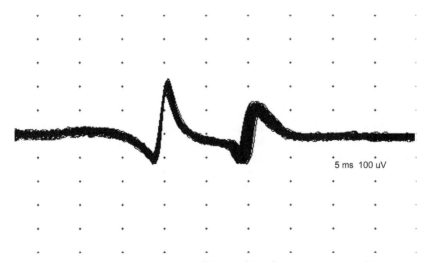

5 ms 100 uV

Fig. 8. Normal jitter (mean consecutive difference [MCD] = 31 microseconds) recorded in the EDC muscle. (Copyright © 2011, VC Juel.)

jitter in presynaptic NMJ disorders such as botulism and LEMS. A monopolar stimulating needle is placed just proximal to the end plate zone for intramuscular stimulation and just anterior to the tragus for facial nerve stimulation. A surface or second monopolar electrode serves as the anode. The nerve is stimulated between 2 and 10 Hz to elicit subtle twitches of the muscle, and the SFEMG needle is inserted for recording. Liminal or direct stimulation of muscle fibers and electrode movement related to muscle twitching are technical pitfalls, particularly with the intramuscular stimulating technique.[45] Stimulated SFEMG is therefore only recommended for electromyographers experienced with the voluntary activation technique that is subject to fewer technical issues.

Jitter Calculation

Jitter is calculated as the mean consecutive difference (MCD) between consecutive interpotential intervals (IPI):

$$MCD = \frac{|IPI_1 - IPI_2| + \cdots + |IPI_{n-1} - IPI_n|}{(n-1)}$$

For stimulated SFEMG, the mean difference between the stimulus and the single MFAP responses is calculated.

Influence of Firing Rate

With voluntary activation, differences in firing rates of MFAPs may influence the IPI variability because of changes in MFAP propagation. This influence can be minimized by sorting the IPI by the interdischarge interval (IDI), and then calculating the mean sorted-data difference (MSD) between interpotential intervals. MCD is normally reported for each pair of potentials, but when slow trends such as variable firing rate influence IPI and the MCD/MSD ratio is greater than 1.25, the MSD should be reported.[33] Fiber pairs with very long IPIs (>4 milliseconds) should not be analyzed, because MFAP propagation significantly influences IPI in such fiber pairs. In stimulated SFEMG, MFAP propagation issues are avoided with the use of a constant stimulation rate and exclusion of the initial 10 stimulated MFAP responses from analysis.[14,45]

Data Collection and Reporting

At least 20 different potential pairs are assessed from different areas of each muscle, which requires about 3 separate needle insertions in many cases. Results are reported as the mean jitter (MCD) for all fiber pairs tested, the percentage of pairs with normal jitter, the percentage of pairs with abnormal jitter, and the percentage of pairs with impulse blocking. The SFEMG study is abnormal when greater than 10% of fiber pairs (≥3) exhibit increased jitter for the muscle studied, or when the mean jitter exceeds the upper limit of normal. Any impulse blocking is abnormal. Abnormally low jitter (<5 microseconds) may be seen in myopathy with fiber splitting. This data should be excluded from analysis, because it does not reflect neuromuscular transmission. Jitter reference values for the voluntary activation technique and for axonal stimulation have been determined.[43,44,46,47]

SFEMG Findings in Disease

SFEMG is a sensitive technique, and normal jitter in a clinically weak muscle virtually excludes an NMJ disorder as a cause of the muscle weakness. However, abnormal jitter may be observed in disease of nerve and muscle as well as in primary NMJ disorders.[48] In motor neuropathic disorders, jitter and FD are both increased, whereas FD is normal in primary NMJ disease.

SFEMG is the most sensitive diagnostic test available for MG; it is abnormal in 99% of patients with generalized MG and in 97% of patients with ocular MG.[14] In MG, jitter is most abnormal in clinically weak muscles, and the fraction of normal and abnormal end plates is related to the severity of disease.[49] The EDC should be tested when generalized MG is suspected. It is easily activated in a controlled fashion by patients, and findings are frequently abnormal in MG (**Fig. 9**). If the EDC findings are normal, if isolated ocular MG is suspected, or if there is limb tremor, a facial muscle such as the frontalis or the orbicularis oculi should be studied.

In LEMS, SFEMG reveals increased jitter and marked impulse blocking, often with an unexpectedly increased amount of jitter for the degree of clinical weakness (**Fig. 10**). Typically, jitter is rate dependent and decreases with increased firing rate, although this is not uniformly observed at all end plates or in all patients.[50] In botulism, jitter is generally increased with impulse blocking in clinically weak muscles with rate-dependent jitter that also decreases with increased firing rate.[51]

SFEMG Using Concentric Needle Electrodes

There has been contemporary interest in identifying MFAPs from MUPs recorded with concentric needle electrodes. This is performed by increasing the low-frequency filter to 1 kHz and using the smallest concentric needle available to minimize the size of the recording surface.[52] Because the concentric needle recording surface remains larger than the SF electrode recording surface, it cannot be determined whether a single spike recorded with this technique represents a single MFAP or a composite of several MFAPs. These composite spikes are therefore referred to as apparent single-fiber action potentials (ASFAPs).[53,54] ASFAPs are lower in amplitude than MFAPs because of the effect of the additional low-frequency filtering. Because of the large recording area of monopolar electrodes, they cannot be used for jitter analysis. Jitter analysis with the concentric needle technique can show abnormal neuromuscular transmission, but mild increases in jitter are better shown with SF

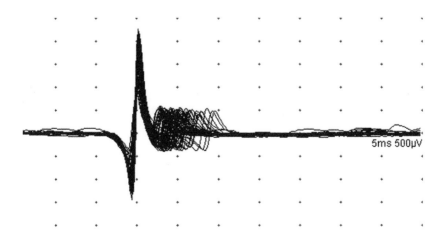

5ms 500μV

Fig. 9. SFEMG findings in the EDC muscle in a patient with moderate generalized MG. Jitter is increased (MCD = 118 microseconds) with impulse blocking. (Copyright © 2011, VC Juel.)

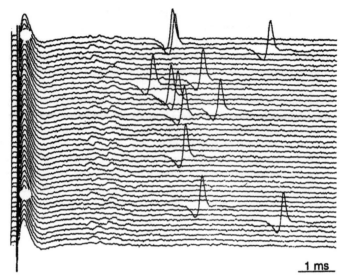

Fig. 10. Extremely large jitter (MCD = 1260 microseconds) with blocking elicited by stimulated SFEMG recordings in the orbicularis oculi muscle in a patient with LEMS. (*From* Stålberg EV, Trontelj JV, Sanders DB. Myasthenia gravis and other disorders of neuromuscular transmission. In: Single fiber EMG. 3rd edition. Fiskebäckskil (Sweden): Edshagen Publishing House; 2010; with permission.)

electrodes. Jitter measured with concentric needles is about 5 microseconds lower than with SF electrodes, and reference values derived for concentric needle electrodes should therefore be used.[52]

SUMMARY

When there is clinical suspicion for an NMJ disorder, RNS and SFEMG may demonstrate the presence, type, and severity of the neuromuscular transmission defect. RNS are widely available and straightforward to perform. Although they are sensitive when study of a clinically weak muscle is feasible, they are insensitive in ocular MG. SFEMG is sensitive for demonstrating abnormal neuromuscular transmission, but requires special equipment and training not available in all centers. Both RNS and SFEMG must be interpreted in the clinical context and in the context of standard NCS and needle EMG, because abnormal findings may be observed in other disorders of nerve and muscle as well as in primary NMJ diseases.

REFERENCES

1. Engel AG. The neuromuscular junction. In: Engel AG, Franzini-Armstrong C, editors. Myology. 3rd edition. New York: McGraw-Hill; 2004. p. 325–72.
2. Bajjalieh SM, Scheller RH. The biochemistry of neurotransmitter secretion. J Biol Chem 1995;270:1971–4.
3. Sanders DB. Clinical neurophysiology of disorders of the neuromuscular junction. J Clin Neurophysiol 1993;10:167–80.
4. Magleby KL. Neuromuscular transmission. In: Engel AG, Franzini-Armstrong C, editors. Myology. 3rd edition. New York: McGraw-Hill; 2004. p. 373–95.

5. Stålberg E, Sanders DB. Electrophysiological tests of neuromuscular transmission. In: Stålberg E, Young RR, editors. Clinical neurophysiology. London: Butterworths; 1981. p. 88–116.
6. Howard JF. Repetitive nerve stimulation. Workshop 3SW.001, Advanced EMG techniques. American Academy of Neurology Annual Meeting. San Francisco, CA, April 26, 2004.
7. Katz B, Miledi R. The role of calcium in neuromuscular facilitation. J Physiol 1968; 195:481–92.
8. Magleby KL. The effect of repetitive stimulation on facilitation of transmitter release at the frog neuromuscular junction. J Physiol 1976;257:449–70.
9. Jolly F. Ueber myasthenia gravis pseudoparalytica. Berliner Klinische Wochenschrift 1895;32:1–7 [in German].
10. Harvey AM, Masland RL. A method for the study of neuromuscular transmission in human subjects. Bull Johns Hopkins Hosp 1941;68:81–93.
11. Harvey AM, Masland RL. The electromyogram in myasthenia gravis. Bull Johns Hopkins Hosp 1941;69:1–13.
12. Desmedt JE. The neuromuscular disorder in myasthenia gravis. 1. Electrical and mechanical response to nerve stimulation in hand muscles. In: Desmedt JE, editor. New developments in electromyography and clinical neurophysiology. Basel: Karger; 1973. p. 241–304.
13. Oh SJ, Eslami N, Nichihira T, et al. Electrophysiological and clinical correlation in myasthenia gravis. Trans Am Neurol Assoc 1982;12:348–54.
14. Stålberg E, Trontelj JV, Sanders DB. Single fiber electromyography studies in healthy and diseased muscle. 3rd edition. Fiskebäckskil (Sweden): Edshagen Publishing House; 2010.
15. Katirji B, Kaminski HJ. Electrodiagnostic approach to the patient with suspected neuromuscular junction disorder. Neurol Clin North Am 2002;20:557–86.
16. Borenstein S, Desmedt JE. Local cooling in myasthenia. Improvement of neuromuscular failure. Arch Neurol 1975;32:152–7.
17. Borenstein S, Desmedt JE. New diagnostic procedures in myasthenia gravis. In: Desmedt JE, editor. New developments in electromyography and clinical neurophysiology. Basel: Karger; 1973. p. 350–74.
18. Lo YL, Dan YF, Leoh TH, et al. Effect of exercise on repetitive nerve stimulation studies: new appraisal of an old technique. J Clin Neurophysiol 2004;21:110–3.
19. Rubin DI, Hentshel K. Is exercise necessary with repetitive nerve stimulation in evaluating patients with suspected myasthenia gravis? Muscle Nerve 2007;35: 103–6.
20. Desmedt JE, Borenstein S. Double-step nerve stimulation test for myasthenic block: sensitization of postactivation exhaustion by ischemia. Ann Neurol 1977; 1:55–64.
21. Gilchrist JM, Sanders DB. The double-step technique of repetitive nerve stimulation. Muscle Nerve 1985;8:624.
22. Horowitz SH, Sivak M. The regional curare test and electrophysiologic diagnosis of myasthenia gravis: further studies. Muscle Nerve 1978;1:432–4.
23. Horowitz SH, Kraurp C. A new regional curare test of the elbow flexors in myasthenia gravis. Muscle Nerve 1979;2:478–90.
24. Costa J, Evangelista T, Conceição I, et al. Repetitive nerve stimulation in myasthenia gravis - relative sensitivity of different muscles. Clin Neurophys 2004; 115:2776–82.
25. Rubin DI, Harper CM, Auger RG. Trigeminal nerve repetitive stimulation in myasthenia gravis. Muscle Nerve 2004;29:591–6.

26. Slomic A, Rosenfalck A, Buchthal F. Electrical and mechanical responses of normal and myasthenic muscle. Brain Res 1968;10:1–78.
27. AAEM Quality Assurance Committee. Practice parameter for repetitive nerve stimulation and single fiber EMG evaluation of adults with suspected myasthenia gravis or Lambert-Eaton myasthenic syndrome: summary statement. Muscle Nerve 2001;24:1236–8.
28. AANEM Quality Assurance Committee. Literature review of the usefulness of repetitive nerve stimulation and single fiber EMG in the electrodiagnostic evaluation of patients with suspected myasthenia gravis or Lambert-Eaton myasthenic syndrome. Muscle Nerve 2001;24:1239–47.
29. Tim RW, Massey JM, Sanders DB. Lambert-Eaton myasthenic syndrome: electrodiagnostic findings and response to treatment. Neurology 2000;54:2176–8.
30. Howard JF, Sanders DB. Neurotoxicology of neuromuscular transmission. Handb Clin Neurol 2008;91:369–400.
31. Fakadej A, Gutmann L. Prolongation of post-tetanic facilitation in infant botulism. Muscle Nerve 1982;5:727–9.
32. Cornblath DR, Sladky JT, Sumner AJ. Clinical electrophysiology of infant botulism. Muscle Nerve 1983;6:448–52.
33. Meriggioli MN, Howard JF, Harper CM. Neuromuscular junction disorders: diagnosis and treatment. New York: Marcel Dekker; 2004.
34. Cherington M. Electrophysiologic methods as an aid in diagnosis of botulism: a review. Muscle Nerve 1982;5:528–9.
35. Engel AG, Ohno K, Sine S. Congenital myasthenic syndromes. In: Engel AG, editor. Myasthenia gravis and myasthenic disorders. New York: Oxford University Press; 1999. p. 251–97.
36. Engel AG. The investigation of congenital myasthenic syndromes. Ann N Y Acad Sci 1993;681:425–34.
37. Punga A, Flink R, Askmark H, et al. Cholinergic neuromuscular hyperactivity in patients with myasthenia gravis seropositive for MuSK antibody. Muscle Nerve 2006;34:111–5.
38. Denys EH, Norris FH. Amyotrophic lateral sclerosis. Impairment of neuromuscular transmission. Arch Neurol 1979;36:202–5.
39. Bernstein LP, Antel JP. Motor neuron disease: decremental responses to repetitive nerve stimulation. Neurology 1981;31:204–7.
40. Aminoff MJ, Layzer RB, Satya-Murti S, et al. The declining electrical response of muscle to repetitive nerve stimulation in myotonia. Neurology 1977;27:812–6.
41. Stålberg EV, Sonoo M. Assessment of the variability in the shape of the motor unit action potential, the "jiggle" at consecutive discharges. Muscle Nerve 1994;17:1135–44.
42. Barbieri S, Weiss GM, Daube JR. Fibrillation potentials in myasthenia gravis. Muscle Nerve 1982;5:S50.
43. Gilchrist JM, AAEM ad hoc committee. Single fiber EMG reference values: a collaborative effort. Muscle Nerve 1992;15:151–61.
44. Bromberg MB, Scott DM, AAEM ad hoc committee. Single fiber EMG reference values: reformatted in tabular form. Muscle Nerve 1994;17:820–1.
45. Trontelj JV, Stålberg EV. Jitter measurement by axonal micro-stimulation: guidelines and technical notes. Electroencephalogr Clin Neurophysiol 1992;85:30–7.
46. Trontelj JV, Khuraibet A, Mihelin M. The jitter in stimulated orbicularis oculi muscle: technique and normal values. J Neurol Neurosurg Psychiatry 1988;51:814–9.

47. Trontelj JV, Mihelin M, Fernandez JM, et al. Axonal stimulation for endplate jitter studies. J Neurol Neurosurg Psychiatry 1986;49:67–685.
48. Sanders DB, Howard JF. AAEE minimonograph #25: single-fiber electromyography in myasthenia gravis. Muscle Nerve 1986;9:809–19.
49. Sanders DB, Howard JF, Johns TR. Single-fiber electromyography in myasthenia gravis. Neurology 1979;29:68–76.
50. Sanders DB. The effect of firing rate on neuromuscular jitter in Lambert-Eaton myasthenic syndrome. Muscle Nerve 1992;15:256–8.
51. Schiller HH, Stålberg E. Human botulism studied with single fibre electromyography. Arch Neurol 1978;35:346–9.
52. Stålberg EV, Trontelj JV, Sanders DB. Measuring jitter with concentric electrodes. In: Single fiber electromyography studies in healthy and diseased muscle. 3rd edition. Fiskebäckskil (Sweden): Edshagen Publishing House; 2010. p. 267–83.
53. Ertas M, Baslo MB, Yildiz N, et al. Concentric needle electrode for neuromuscular jitter analysis. Muscle Nerve 2000;23:715–9.
54. Stålberg EV, Sanders DB. Jitter recordings with concentric needle electrodes. Muscle Nerve 2009;40:331–9.

Electrodiagnostic Approach to the Patient with Suspected Myopathy

David Lacomis, MD

KEYWORDS

- Electromyography • Myopathy • Neuromuscular disorders
- Electrodiagnostic testing

Electrodiagnostic testing is a key component of the evaluation of a patient with a suspected myopathy. Recognition of certain electrophysiologic patterns associated with acquired and inherited myopathies can help to guide appropriate use of laboratory studies, including genetic testing, and aid in determining the need for muscle biopsy and in selecting a biopsy site. This article emphasizes the electrodiagnostic approach to myopathies, but the clinical and laboratory features are also described because such knowledge is necessary for the electromyographer. This article is an update of a review published in *Neurologic Clinics*.[1]

CLINICAL FEATURES OF MYOPATHY

Whether a patient is being evaluated in the office or the electromyography (EMG) laboratory, the process begins with the history and neurologic examination. In the EMG laboratory, the findings such as the distribution of weakness and other associated clinical features obtained through a targeted history and examination help to direct the selection of the most appropriate nerves and muscles for study.

Weakness

The symptoms and signs of myopathy are listed in **Table 1**. The most typical symptoms are referable to proximal (limb-girdle) weakness, which is a manifestation of most myopathies and is usually symmetric. Patients may report difficulty arising from a chair (**Fig. 1**), climbing stairs, or performing tasks with their arms elevated. In most cases, the weakness is painless, but sometimes myalgias or cramps are present. Because of proximal as well as trunk muscle weakness, patients often experience

The author has nothing to disclose.

Division of Neuromuscular Diseases, University of Pittsburgh School of Medicine, UPMC-Presbyterian, F875, 200 Lothrop Street, Pittsburgh, PA 15213, USA

E-mail address: lacomisd@upmc.edu

Table 1
Symptoms and signs of myopathy

	Symptom	Sign
Most common	Proximal muscle weakness (eg, difficulty rising from a chair, climbing stairs, walking, or lifting and using the arms above the head)	Limb-girdle weakness Neck flexor weakness Waddling gait, hyperlordotic posture (chronic disorders) Trunk weakness (eg, difficulty with a sit-up maneuver)
Less common	Myalgias, cramps	Muscle tenderness
	Distal weakness (eg, foot-drop, hand weakness)	Foot-drop; forearm or intrinsic hand muscle weakness; pes cavus (chronic disorders)
	—	Scapular winging
	Diplopia	Extraocular muscle weakness
	Ptosis	Ptosis
	Dysphagia	Weak palate, tongue, or both
	Dysarthria	Dysarthria (eg, nasal speech)
	Fatigue	—
	Shortness of breath	Diaphragm weakness: tachypnea, use of accessory muscles, paradoxical respirations
	Impaired grip release	Grip or percussion myotonia
	Head drop	Neck extensor weakness Muscle atrophy (chronic) Muscle hypertrophy

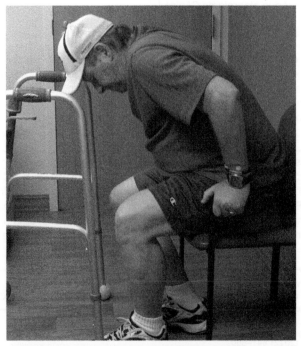

Fig. 1. A man with myotonic dystrophy type 2 has difficulty arising from a chair because of proximal weakness. He ambulates with a walker.

difficulty walking. Chronically, they may have a waddling gait, mainly because of gluteus medius weakness as well as a hyperlordotic posture because of hip extensor weakness and compensatory shifting of the center of gravity. Other patterns and distributions of weakness can occur in certain types of myopathies, including distal, scapulohumeral, scapuloperoneal, facial, oculopharyngeal, and isolated neck extensor weakness (**Table 2**).[2–8] These less typical patterns of involvement are important to recognize clinically to ensure that distal, facial, oropharyngeal, or neck extensor muscles are examined, in addition to proximal muscles, during EMG.

In addition, some patients with myopathy develop neuromuscular ventilatory failure. These patients may show shortness of breath, orthopnea, tachypnea, features of sleep apnea, use of accessory muscles of respiration, paradoxical chest movements, and morning headaches. Ventilatory weakness is common in acid maltase deficiency and critical illness myopathy (CIM), and it occurs in some inflammatory myopathies, muscular dystrophies, congenital myopathies, and rarely in mitochondrial myopathy.[9] Performing phrenic nerve conduction studies (NCSs) and needle EMG of the diaphragm may be useful in this setting.[10]

Myotonia and Muscle Pain

Patients with myotonic dystrophies, myotonia congenita, and some other channelopathies may subjectively report cramping or stiffness, rather than impaired muscle relaxation, as a manifestation of myotonia. Such patients should be queried as to events that may trigger cramping or weakness or lead to improvement in such symptoms.

Table 2
Myopathies without a typical limb-girdle distribution of weakness

Pattern of Weakness	Disorder
Distal (with or without proximal)	Inclusion body myositis (proximal and distal usually)[a] Myotonic dystrophy type 1 Congenital Distal dystrophies Myofibrillar myopathy Fascioscapulohumeral muscular dystrophy[a] Some LGMDs LGMD 2G (telethoninopathy) and 2B (dysferlinopathy) Neuromyopathies (eg, toxic)
Scapulohumeral/scapuloperoneal	Fascioscapulohumeral muscular dystrophy[a] Scapuloperoneal dystrophy Emery-Dreifuss dystrophy LGMD 1B (myotilinopathy) and 2A (calpainopathy)
Facial and oropharyngeal (with or without limb weakness)	Oculopharyngeal dystrophy Mitochondrial myopathy Myotonic dystrophy type 1 Congenital myopathy
Neck extensors (head drop)	Isolated neck extensor myopathy Myositis Myotonic dystrophy type 2 Carnitine deficiency Adult rod body myopathy Amyloidosis

Abbreviation: LGMD, limb-girdle muscular dystrophies.
[a] May be asymmetric.

Such triggers include rest, carbohydrate loading, exercise, medication, and cold.[2] Recognition of these symptoms and triggers may lead to more specialized electro-diagnostic testing for channelopathies, such as the short and long exercise tests, as well as specialized DNA studies.[11,12] The presence of myoglobinuria, cramping, or pain occurring during or after exercise may point toward a glycogen or lipid storage disorder or possibly a mitochondrial myopathy. Other nonmyopathic conditions can also manifest with muscle pain with activity, such as peripheral arterial disease and spinal stenosis, and should be considered in the differential diagnosis.

Muscle Atrophy and Pseudohypertrophy

Patients with myopathy usually do not have a substantial loss of muscle bulk early in the course, but atrophy may occur later in the course of the disease. On the other hand, pseudohypertrophy, especially of the calves, may be seen at the time of diagnosis of some muscular dystrophies. Also absent are fasciculations and sensory loss.

Fatigue and Neuromuscular Junction Mimics of Myopathy

Patients with myopathy, as well as most neuromuscular disorders, may experience fatigue. Muscle and nonspecific fatigue can occur later in the day, but this diurnal variation is usually not as prominent as is seen in neuromuscular junction disorders, such as myasthenia gravis. However, the electromyographer must keep neuromuscular junction disorders in mind when evaluating patients with suspected myopathy, especially those with predominantly proximal weakness. Some patients with myasthenia gravis may have a limb-girdle presentation[13]; however, such a presentation is common with Lambert-Eaton myasthenic syndrome (LEMS). In addition to proximal weakness, patients with LEMS often have hyporeflexia and features of dysautonomia, such as dry mouth, impotence, or orthostatic intolerance (findings that are not typically present with myopathy).[14]

ASSOCIATED NONMUSCLE FEATURES AND FAMILY HISTORY

In addition to muscle-related symptoms, patients should be asked about other clinical features or symptoms that may be associated with certain types of myopathies. Non-muscle symptoms may include frontal baldness and cataracts in myotonic dystrophy, cardiomyopathy in muscular dystrophies, impaired bowel motility in mitochondrial neurogastrointestinal encephalomyopathy, and dysmorphic features in patients with congenital myopathies. Patients should also be asked about systemic symptoms such as rash and about the presence of rheumatologic, infectious, endocrine, and neoplastic disorders that may be associated with myopathies.

Assessment of the family history is important when evaluating any patient with myopathy. Questioning about family members with myopathic symptoms or diagnoses, as well as the presence of nonmyopathic features mentioned earlier, may provide a clue to the underlying cause.

Some patients with suspected myopathy are asymptomatic but may be referred to the electromyographer because of an increased serum creatine kinase (CK) level (hyper-CK-emia). Sometimes these patients have a family member with myopathy, a personal or familial presence of the systemic features noted earlier, or features such as isolated restrictive lung disease as is seen in several myopathies with diaphragm involvement.[15] Some patients with hyper-CK-emia receive cholesterol-lowering agents or other medications that may cause myopathy.

LABORATORY TESTING

After the history and neurologic examination, laboratory testing is performed to assist in the myopathy evaluation (**Table 3**). Although the results may be available to the electromyographer, there is not necessarily a direct correlation between the laboratory and EMG findings and therefore electrodiagnostic testing is important to supplement other methods of evaluating the patients. The most useful laboratory test is measurement of the serum CK level. Almost the entire MM component and most of the total CK measurement is derived from skeletal muscle. The CK measurement is more specific to muscle than aldolase. However, aldolase level may be increased in some connective tissue diseases, whereas CK is not.[16] CK levels are usually increased when there is muscle necrosis or a leaky muscle membrane. Most patients with inflammatory myopathies,

Table 3	
Possible laboratory screening tests for myopathy	
Laboratory Screening Test	**Myopathies Associated with Test Abnormality**
CK (increase)	Inflammatory myopathies, most (moderate to high) Some toxic myopathies (eg, cholesterol-lowering agents, colchicine) CIM (at least 50%) Hypothyroid myopathy Many dystrophies Some glycogen storage myopathies Carnitine deficiency Congenital myopathy (occasional, mild increase)
Aldolase (increase)	As above, and Perimysial connective tissue inflammation
Thyroid-stimulating hormone, other thyroid function tests	Hypothyroid myopathy Hyperthyroid myopathy
24-h urinary free cortisol	Cushing syndrome
Serum protein electrophoresis	Rod body myopathy (monoclonal gammopathy) Inflammatory myopathy (hypergammaglobulinemia)
Myositis associated antibodies (eg, antisynthetases such as Jo-1, signal recognition particle, Mi-2)	Antisynthetase syndrome Immune-mediated necrotizing myopathy Dermatomyositis
HIV antibody (Ab)	HIV
Alkaline phosphatase, calcium, phosphorus 25-OH-vitamin D, parathyroid hormone	Osteomalacia, hypovitaminosis D, parathyroid disorders (primary and secondary)
Vitamin E	Vitamin E deficiency
Serum and urine carnitine levels	Carnitine deficiency (primary and secondary)
GAA (acid maltase) assay	Pompe disease
ESR, CRP, antinuclear Ab, Sjögren Abs, Complement components C3, C4	Associated connective tissue disease
Serum lactate, pyruvate	Mitochondrial myopathy

Abbreviations: CIM, critical illness myopathy; CRP, C-reactive peptide; ESR, erythrocyte sedimentation rate; HIV, human immunodeficiency virus.

many muscular dystrophies, rhabdomyolysis, and some toxic and inherited metabolic myopathies (eg, acid maltase, debrancher, phosphorylase, and carnitine deficiencies) as well as hypothyroid myopathy typically show increased CK levels. The autosomal-recessive limb-girdle muscular dystrophies (LGMDs) typically have higher CK levels than the autosomal-dominant forms. The highest levels may be seen with Duchenne muscular dystrophy, Miyoshi myopathy, rhabdomyolysis, and polymyositis (PM).[17]

Increases in CK level are typically associated with electromyographic patterns that include fibrillation potentials, but there are exceptions. In addition, some disorders associated with fibrillation potentials, such as adult rod body myopathy, may be associated with a normal CK level.[7] The observations that CK levels are normal in chronic corticosteroid myopathy and that they may also be normal in treated myositis are important. However, EMG may be more useful than measurement of CK levels in differentiating active myositis from corticosteroid myopathy: fibrillation potentials are seen with active myositis but not corticosteroid myopathy.

Serum CK level should not be measured soon after EMG because the level may be transiently increased; however, such increases are usually of low magnitude (up to 1.5-fold more than baseline) and not consistently observed.[18,19] An increased CK level is not specific for myopathies and has many other nonmyopathic causes, including neurogenic disorders, exercise, trauma, and malignant hyperthermia.[17] In normal persons without myopathy, CK values are generally higher in men, especially African American men.[17,20]

Other laboratory studies performed in patients with suspected myopathy may include genetic testing for dystrophies or other inherited myopathies. Positive results may obviate additional studies including EMG, although EMG can provide information about the degree and distribution of muscle involvement that genetic testing cannot. In suspected acquired myopathies, other laboratory studies are used to screen for systemic disorders associated with myopathy (see **Table 3**). Ischemic exercise testing, when performed in patients with exercise-induced myalgias or contractures, may suggest some glycogen storage myopathies when there is an insufficient lactate increase. However, the findings are nonspecific, and additional testing may still be required to confirm the diagnosis.

For most patients, a specific cause is not found with clinical evaluation and laboratory testing, and electrodiagnostic testing becomes a helpful next step in the evaluation. In many instances, EMG is performed coincidentally with laboratory or genetic testing. In some patients, musculoskeletal imaging is also performed in addition to EMG. The pattern of findings on electrodiagnostic testing, in conjunction with clinical and other ancillary studies, helps to define the potential cause of the disorder.

ELECTRODIAGNOSTIC TESTING

Electrodiagnostic testing provides important information that can supplement clinical and laboratory testing in suspected myopathies. Information that can be obtained includes confirmation of a myopathy and exclusion of other mimicking disorders, assessment of the degree of muscle fiber destruction, determination of the distribution of muscle involvement, guidance in selection of a muscle for potential biopsy, and assessment of progression of disease or response to therapy. For example, patients with inflammatory myopathies treated with corticosteroids may show worsening weakness, and electromyographic testing can help to determine whether the progression is caused by active myositis or corticosteroid therapy.[15] Several different components of an electrodiagnostic study are important in the assessment of suspected myopathies.

NCSs

NCSs are usually normal in patients with myopathies. The typical electrodiagnostic workup of a suspected myopathy should include at least 1 motor and 1 sensory nerve from an arm and a leg.[21] Motor NCSs are normal in most myopathies because the motor recordings are typically performed over distal muscles, whereas muscle weakness and myofiber loss is usually most predominant in proximal muscles. Myopathies that are severe and more generalized, have a distal distribution, or affect muscle membrane depolarization, may be associated with low compound muscle action potential (CMAP) amplitudes. For example, CIM is typically associated with a low CMAP with increased CMAP duration as a result of slow conduction through the less excitable muscle membrane (**Fig. 2**).

Finding diffusely low CMAP amplitudes in a patient with suspected myopathic weakness should raise the possibility of a neuromuscular junction disorder, especially LEMS. In such patients, the motor nerve eliciting the low CMAP should be restimulated with a supramaximal single shock immediately after 10 seconds of exercise to look for an incremental response or facilitation (LEMS test). Two to 3 Hz repetitive stimulation should also be performed primarily to screen for a decrement in the CMAP amplitude and area, which typically occurs in a presynpatic or postsynaptic neuromuscular junction disorder. If there is no baseline decrement, postexercise testing may be performed to evaluate for postexercise exhaustion, which may increase the yield of identifying a mild neuromuscular junction disorder. Motor neuron diseases and motor axonopathies can also cause low CMAP amplitudes in the setting of normal sensory responses. The needle electrode examination is necessary to distinguish between a neurogenic and myopathic disorder.

Sensory NCSs are always normal in pure myopathies. However, the presence of abnormal sensory responses in a patient with a myopathy raises the possibility of a disorder that may involve both muscle and nerve (**Table 4**).

Needle Electrode Examination

In myopathies, when abnormalities are found on needle EMG, the weakest muscles typically show the most significant abnormalities. Therefore, a manual muscle strength

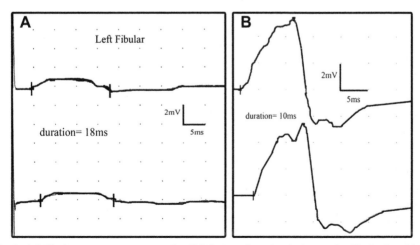

Fig. 2. (A) Fibular motor response to the tibialis anterior stimulating at the fibular head (*top recording*) and popliteal fossa (*bottom*) from a patient with CIM. The amplitudes are low and the durations are prolonged. (B) Normal study for comparison.

Table 4	
Disorders that cause myopathy and neuropathy	
Category	**Example**
Inflammatory disorders	Vasculitis
	Sarcoidosis
	Paraneoplastic
Infectious	Human immunodeficiency virus
Toxic	Colchicine, amiodarone, hydroxychloroquine
	Alcohol
Endocrine	Thyroid disease (neuropathy is rare)
Malabsorption syndromes with vitamin deficiencies	Celiac sprue
	Osteomalacia
	Postgastric bypass
Critical illness	CIM and polyneuropathy
Inherited	Mitochondrial disorders
Other	Amyloid

examination should always be performed before the needle examination to help guide selection of muscles to study. In general, we perform the needle examination in multiple proximal and distal arm and leg muscles as well as paraspinal muscles in all patients referred for myopathy, and modify the study based on the pattern of weakness. For example, in many individuals, it may be more useful to examine a weaker iliopsoas, hamstring, or a thigh adductor muscle rather than a stronger quadriceps. When no or minimal findings are seen in the limb muscles, paraspinal muscles are important to examine. A low thoracic rather than lumbar paraspinal is a preferable choice for the paraspinal muscle examination, because thoracic paraspinals are less likely to show fibrillation potentials from radiculopathy, a common finding in lumbosacral paraspinals with aging, which could confound interpretation of paraspinal fibrillations. Occasionally, paraspinal muscles may be the only muscles showing abnormal spontaneous activity or myopathic motor unit action potential (MUP) features (described later) as is seen in some inflammatory myopathies, glycogen storage diseases, myotonic disorders, and neck extensor myopathy.[22,23]

All 4 components of the needle electrode examination provide important information in patients with suspected myopathy. These components are: (1) insertional activity, (2) spontaneous activity, (3) MUP morphology, and (4) recruitment.

Insertional and spontaneous activity
Increased insertional and abnormal spontaneous activity may occur as part of a continuum of muscle fiber irritability. Insertional activity, which results from needle irritation of muscle fibers, is usually prolonged if there is a disturbance in the muscle membrane or motor axolemma or if there is a functional disconnection between muscle and motor nerve terminal, as in denervation or muscle necrosis, fiber splitting, or separation of a segment of fibers because of a vacuolar disturbance. In some channelopathies and toxic myopathies, insertional activity is prolonged in the form of myotonic discharges (**Figs. 3** and **4**). Diffusely prolonged insertional activity in most muscles examined, particularly in younger muscular men, may be a normal variant; however, this finding is sometimes a subtle sign of a mild myotonic disorder such as myotonic dystrophy type 2 (DM2).

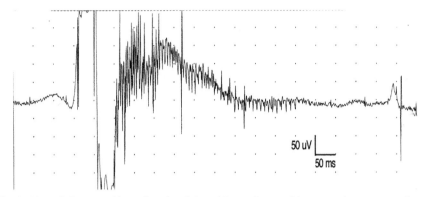

Fig. 3. There is increased insertional activity with waning positive wave form myotonia and some spikes in this patient with statin-induced myopathy.

In contrast to prolonged insertional activity, insertional activity may be decreased when there is marked loss of muscle with adipose replacement or if the muscle membrane cannot be depolarized. Decreased insertional activity can occur in end-stage muscles that have been replaced by fatty or connective tissue, such as in end-stage muscular dystrophies, in a periodic paralysis attack, or in McArdle disease during a contracture.[24]

Abnormal spontaneous activity in the form of positive waves or fibrillation potentials is caused by the abnormal spontaneous generation of action potentials from single muscle fibers that have lost their innervation, because of either structural or metabolic disturbances. Insertional activity is almost always increased when fibrillation potentials or positive waves are present. Myopathies associated with fibrillation potentials usually have components of inflammation, necrosis, or sarcolemmal membrane instability.[15,25] Fibrillation potentials alone are not specific for myopathies because they occur in neurogenic disorders as well as in neuromuscular junction disorders,

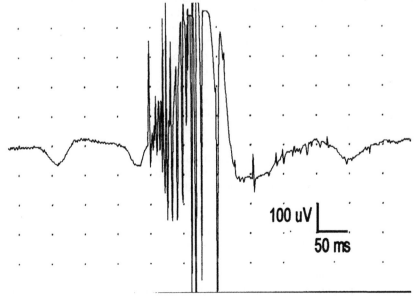

Fig. 4. Normal insertional activity.

including botulism, severe myasthenia gravis, and LEMS, as well as with muscle trauma.[24]

Myotonic discharges emanate spontaneously from single muscle fibers and fire repetitively over a prolonged period, usually because of a defect in sarcolemmal membrane depolarization. They usually wax and wane in amplitude and firing rate, and sound like a revving motorcycle engine. The waveforms have positive or spikelike morphology and may be elicited by needle movement or muscle contraction.[24]

Complex repetitive discharges (CRDs) consist of machinerylike, regular, polyphasic discharges of action potentials that generally begin and end abruptly. They are caused by ephaptic activation and discharge of groups of muscle fibers. They may also be considered a form of increased insertional activity and occur in myopathic as well as neurogenic conditions. They tend to be more common in chronic neuromuscular disorders, but there is evidence that they occur within 3 months of onset at a frequency similar to more chronic states.[26]

MUPs

Myopathic MUPs typically refer to short-duration, low-amplitude, and polyphasic MUPs, which are classically seen in myopathies. These myopathic MUPs are not specific for myopathy and may also be seen with neuromuscular junction disorders or during early reinnervation after a severe neurogenic process. Accurate assessment for abnormal MUPs is performed by semiquantitative or formal quantitative measures. Semiquantitative or qualitative evaluation of MUPs requires familiarity with the normal morphologies of MUPs from various muscles throughout the aging process.

Patients are initially asked to activate the muscle being examined at a low level of voluntary activity in which 1 or a few MUPs can be analyzed. It is important to assess the first recruited MUPs, which are generally smaller in amplitude and shorter in duration than MUPs that are recruited later and during stronger contraction. At least 20 MUPs with a rapid rise time should be examined in each muscle studied. The MUPs represent the summation of action potentials from a population of myofibers in a single motor unit. In myopathies, the duration is shortened because of loss, atrophy, or dysfunction of myofibers. Polyphasia is commonly seen as a result of loss of synchrony in depolarization caused by myofiber loss. Amplitudes are often, but not always, low for reasons similar to those described for shortening duration, but amplitude is more dependent on the size of the myofibers closest to the recording needle and may be normal in the context of short durations.[27]

In patients with chronic myopathies, such as inclusion body myositis (IBM), other forms of chronic myositis, and some dystrophies, a mixture of normal or long-duration, in addition to short-duration, MUPs may be seen. In these chronic conditions, polyphasia is usually present, and satellite potentials may occur after fiber splitting or local reinnervation. This so-called mixed pattern of MUP morphologies may be seen in patients with neuromyopathies as well. More typically, patients with neuromyopathies have longer-duration, high-amplitude MUPs in reinnervated distal muscles and short-duration, low-amplitude MUPs in proximal muscles (**Fig. 5**).

MUP recruitment

Compared with the normal state, recruitment tends to be rapid (early or increased) in myopathies, because relatively more motor units must be activated to generate the required degree of force. With rapid recruitment, the firing rates of the MUP are normal, and assessment of rapid recruitment requires assessment of the degree of effort that the patient is making during muscle contraction. Rapid recruitment may be relatively subtle and detection may require considerable experience.

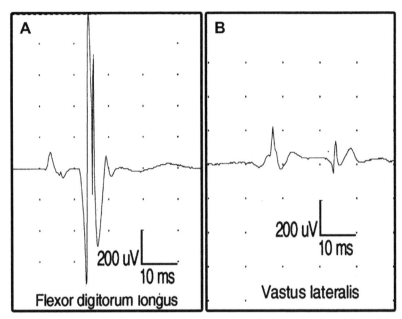

Fig. 5. A patient with human immunodeficiency virus infection/AIDS was referred for EMG for proximal weakness. She also had chronic numbness in both feet. Nerve conductions of an arm and leg revealed low sural and fibular sensory responses, a mildly reduced fibular motor amplitude, and mild slowing of fibular and tibial conduction velocities. (A) A long-duration MUP from a distal leg muscle (flexor digitorum longus) is shown. (B) Low-amplitude, short-duration MUPs were present in some proximal muscles (vastus lateralis MUP is shown). The findings were consistent with neuromyopathy.

With more severe or long-standing myopathies in which there is substantial myo-fiber loss, recruitment may be reduced.[24] Reduced recruitment is more characteristic of evolving neurogenic disorders, including the stage of early reinnervation after a severe neurogenic process when MUPs may be small and unstable (nascent) and mimic myopathic MUPs in morphology.

Quantitative EMG

Because some patients have only subtle or borderline findings on qualitative assessment of MUPs, some electromyographers perform formal quantitative methods to try to more accurately assess MUP changes. Many EMG machines come equipped with software for performing quantitative EMG (QEMG). However, most electromyographers do not routinely use QEMG in practice. QEMG can assess the morphology (duration, amplitude, and phases or turns) of MUPs as well as recruitment patterns. Duration is the most useful parameter to assess. With formal QEMG, at least 20 MUPs are recorded, and the EMG machine calculates the mean of the different MUP parameters, allowing the electromyographer to obtain a numerical value to compare with normative data. With QEMG, it is important to avoid selection bias when recording MUPs. The electro-myographer should not select only apparently short-duration MUPs for analysis. QEMG may be used to augment qualitative or semiquantitative EMG to improve accuracy and consistency, and QEMG may also be used in research. QEMG can be performed on multiple individual MUPs or groups of MUPs extracted from a composite EMG signal using triggering or decomposition techniques.[28]

Decomposition-based methods can be used with higher levels of contraction, and larger numbers of MUPs can be assessed at once.[28] Myopathies tend to have high turns per second and low amplitudes. Decomposition evaluation methods include (1) mean MUP amplitude as a function of number of turns assessed at both low and high contraction (cloud analysis) and (2) the maximum value of the ratio of turns per second to mean amplitude per turn (peak ratio).[29]

Fuglsang-Frederiksen[29] provided a comprehensive review of these and other EMG methods in evaluating myopathy. There are no evidence-based guidelines regarding which techniques should be used in practice. When using QEMG, the data must be compared with normative data and evaluated statistically, and QEMG should be assessed at several locations within a given muscle.

Single-fiber EMG

Single-fiber EMG is usually not performed in patients with suspected myopathy. However, it may be useful in patients in whom neuromuscular junction disorders or myopathy are being considered in a patient with weakness, and in whom routine needle EMG is normal. Abnormal findings on single-fiber EMG are nonspecific; although abnormal jitter and blocking is characteristic of neuromuscular junction disorders, these findings may also be identified in some myopathic processes, including inflammatory myopathies and muscular dystrophies. Fiber density can be normal or increased in myopathies.[30]

Electrical Impedance Myography

Electrical impedance myography is an emerging technique for evaluating neuromuscular disorders by assessment of current flow along muscle fibers.[31] There is some evidence that this technique may be useful in discriminating myopathic from neurogenic conditions but substantially more study is required to determine diagnostic sensitivity and specificity.[32]

PATTERNS OF EMG FINDINGS IN MYOPATHIES

The possible findings on needle electrode examination described in the previous section can be present to variable degrees in different types of myopathies. Although there are no EMG findings that are pathognomonic for a specific disorder or cause, the combined pattern of findings may be characteristic of certain types of myopathies, thereby narrowing the differential diagnosis and assisting the clinician by directing further evaluation with laboratory testing or identification of a suitable muscle for biopsy. The presence of myopathic EMG findings increases the yield of muscle biopsy in patients with suspected myopathy. There is a high concordance, up to 70% to 95%, in EMG and muscle biopsy findings of myopathy. In a study of 188 patients with myopathy who underwent QEMG studies, 87% had EMG features of myopathy, whereas 79% had histopathologic features of myopathy.[33] Another study using histopathologic features as the gold standard identified the clinical accuracy of myopathy diagnosis in elderly patients as about 50%; however, more than 68% of patients with EMG findings of myopathy or increases in CK level had myopathic histologic features.[34] Similarly, Lai and colleagues[35] noted a 43% diagnostic yield from 248 muscle biopsies for suspected myopathy. A specific diagnosis was more likely (odds ratio 2.75, 95% confidence interval) with EMG findings consistent with an irritable myopathy.

When selecting a site for muscle biopsy, it is important to choose a muscle that is significantly affected, but is not end-stage, which is more likely to be fibrotic and infiltrated by substantial amounts of adipose tissue. Muscles that feel gritty or like passing a knife through butter during needle examination should be avoided because they are likely to be end-stage. Similarly, muscles showing MUP findings consistent with a chronic or end-stage myopathy such as decreased insertional activity, reduced recruitment of a mixed population of MUPs, or long-duration, polyphasic MUPs should also be avoided for the same reason unless there is no other option. Ideally, the site should have the most fibrillation potential activity, if present, along with the characteristic MUP changes of myopathy. When the biopsy does not immediately follow the needle examination, a contralateral muscle is selected. It has been the author's impression that the quadriceps is often not the best leg muscle to biopsy because many patients with myopathy have more substantial weakness and electrodiagnostic abnormalities in hip flexors and other muscles aside from the quadriceps. Sometimes, it may be more appropriate to take a biopsy of an accessible proximal arm muscle that is more affected electrically even if the patient complains of leg weakness primarily.

In the following sections, the types of myopathic disorders that are associated with certain EMG features or patterns are discussed. These patterns are not distinctly specific for individual types of myopathies and some disorders show multiple patterns. The general patterns of abnormalities include:

Pattern 1: myopathic MUPs with fibrillation potentials
Pattern 2: myopathic MUPs without fibrillation potentials
Pattern 3: prominent myotonic discharges
Pattern 4: myopathic MUPs with CRDs
Pattern 5: myopathy with a normal EMG.

Pattern 1: Myopathic MUPs with Fibrillation Potentials

Inflammatory myopathies
This pattern is commonly seen in inflammatory and necrotizing myopathies (**Table 5**). Essentially all patients with IBM and 45% to 74% of patients with PM and

Table 5
EMG pattern 1: myopathic MUPs with prominent fibrillation potentials

Category of Myopathies	Examples
Inflammatory	PM
	Dermatomyositis
	IBM
	Sarcoid myopathy
Infiltrative	Amyloid myopathy
Toxic	Cholesterol-lowering agents
	CIM
	Penicillamine
Endocrine	Hypothyroid myopathy
Dystrophies	Dystrophinopathies
	Some LGMDs
	Myofibrillar myopathies (some with prominent CRDs also)
	Distal dystrophies
	Some LGMDs
	Emery-Dreifuss muscular dystrophy
	FSHD
Congenital	Centronuclear and myotubular
Metabolic	carnitine deficiency
	Acid maltase and debrancher deficiencies (patterns 2 and 4 also)
	Mitochondrial (some)

dermatomyositis (DM) show this pattern. Paraspinal muscles have the highest yield for fibrillation potential activity and should be examined in patients with suspected inflammatory myopathies in which abnormalities are not found in limb muscles.[36,37] In IBM, the quadriceps is usually substantially affected and forearm flexors are often involved. Occasionally, patients with PM and DM do not have fibrillation potentials and show only myopathic MUPs. Chronic myositis, especially IBM, can also show a mixed pattern of normal-duration and short-duration or long-duration and short-duration MUPs that are typically polyphasic. Polyphasia is more likely to occur during myofiber regeneration in conjunction with more variation in myofiber sizes that occurs over time.[38,39] Even with chronic myositis, recruitment is rapid until end-stage disease, which is an important finding that helps in differentiating chronic myositis from a subacute motor axon loss process. Myotonic discharges and CRDs may also occur in 1 or a few muscles in chronic myositis.[36] Treated myositis can be associated with or without fibrillation potentials, but fibrillation potentials are not seen in steroid myopathy. Other inflammatory myopathies including sarcoidosis (granulomatous myositis) and viral myositis may show this pattern but also may not show fibrillation potentials.

Infiltrative, toxic, or endocrine myopathies

Infiltrative disorders such as amyloid may mimic PM, including on EMG.[40] Some toxic myopathies, including cholesterol-lowering agent myopathies, may or may not be associated with fibrillation potentials. In addition, myotonic discharges and sometimes CRDs are noted. In some of these disorders, the myotonic discharges may be brief, poorly formed, and wane (**Fig. 3**). Hypothyroid myopathy shows a spectrum of EMG changes that includes fibrillation potentials.[41] Patients with CIM may manifest patterns 1 or 2.[42] In CIM, there is no clear correlation between the presence of fibrillation potentials and muscle necrosis but such correlation studies are limited.[42] The fibrillation potentials could also occur from muscle membrane dysfunction.

Dystrophies and congenital and metabolic myopathies

The more aggressive forms of muscular dystrophy such as Duchenne muscular dystrophy, certain LGMDs, and desminopathies may be associated with this pattern. However, extensive studies of EMG correlation with specific LGMD genotypes are not available. With desminopathy, CRDs are often present.[43] A mixed pattern of MUPs is also seen in long-standing muscular dystrophies, which may show reduced recruitment because of loss of muscle tissue and fatty replacement. CMAP amplitudes also decline over time.[15] More indolent dystrophies including fascioscapulohumeral muscular dystrophy (FSHD) are less commonly associated with pattern 1. Of the congenital myopathies, centronuclear or myotubular myopathies are the only ones commonly associated with pattern 1. Of the storage disorders, carnitine, acid maltase,[44] and occasionally phosphorylase deficiency (McArdle disease) may manifest pattern 1. Other inherited diseases that predispose to rhabdomyolysis may show pattern 1 during attacks. However, even during attacks, the EMG abnormalities may be minimal compared with the major increases in CK level.[45] Pattern 1 may also be seen in unusual conditions such as adult rod body myopathy.[7] In general, pattern 1 is the most common pattern associated with a diagnostic histopathologic finding of myopathy.[34]

Pattern 2: Myopathic MUPs Without Fibrillation Potentials

This pattern is most commonly seen in noninflammatory, nonnecrotizing myopathies, including metabolic myopathies and treated myositis (**Table 6**). Most congenital, endocrine, and some toxic and mitochondrial myopathies may also show this pattern,

Table 6	
EMG pattern 2: myopathic MUPs without spontaneous activity	
Category of Myopathies	**Examples**
Inflammatory (treated)	PM (sometimes untreated too)
	DM (sometimes untreated too)
Infiltrative	Amyloid myopathy
Toxic	Corticiosteroid myopathy (pattern 5 also)
	CIM (pattern 1 also)
Endocrine	Cushing syndrome
	Hyperthyroidism
	Hypothyroidism (pattern 1 also)
Dystrophies	LGMD (eg, LGMD2B)
	Oculopharyngeal muscular dystrophy
	FSHD
	Bethlem myopathy
	Distal (pattern 1 also)
Congenital	Myofibrillar myopathy (pattern 4 also)
	Congenital myopathy (pattern 5 also; centronuclear
	and myotubular, pattern 1 also)
Metabolic	Mitochondrial myopathy (pattern 5 also)
	Glycogen storage diseases (lysosomal types, also
	patterns 1, 4; nonlysosomal types, pattern 5)
	Lipid storage diseases
	Carnitine deficiency (pattern 1 also)
	Carnitine palmityl transferase deficiency (pattern 5 also)

as may some muscular dystrophies. The more indolent dystrophies such as FSHD, oculopharyngeal dystrophy, Bethlem, and some distal dystrophies such as myotilin-opathy are more likely to show this pattern.[6] Other disorders, such as acid maltase deficiency, that often are associated with fibrillation potentials may show only myopathic MUPs.[44]

Pattern 3: Myotonic Discharges with or Without Myopathic MUPs

This pattern is most commonly seen in myotonic dystrophies, myotonia congenitas, and other muscle channelopathies (**Table 7**). In these disorders, sarcolemmal membrane depolarization defects are the cause of the myotonia. The myotonic dystrophies are more commonly associated with short-duration, low-amplitude MUPs, whereas some of the myotonia congenitas have normal MUPs. Myotonic discharges without short-duration MUPs are also seen in paramyotonia congenita and hyperkalemic periodic paralysis. Occasionally, the profuse nature of the myotonia makes it difficult to clearly evaluate MUPs.

Myotonic dystrophy type 1 and myotonia congenita are commonly associated with clinical myotonia, whereas clinical myotonia may be less evident in DM2. Other disorders in which myotonic discharges are common yet clinical myotonia is absent include acid maltase and debrancher deficiencies and some toxic myopathies, including statin-induced myopathy and colchicine neuromyopathy. In inflammatory myopathies, EMG myotonia may be focal and clinical myotonia is absent. Danon disease, caused by lysosome-associated membrane protein 2 deficiency, and X-linked myopathy with excessive autophagy (XEMA) may also cause prominent electrical myotonia without clinical myotonia.[46] In 1 patient with XEMA, MUPs had high amplitudes, normal

Table 7
EMG pattern 3: prominent myotonic discharges

With Myopathic MUPs	Comment
Myotonic dystrophy type 1[a]	Discharges typically wax and wane
DM2[a]	Discharges commonly wane
Acid maltase/debrancher deficiency	Usually with CRDs
Toxic myopathy	—
Cholesterol-lowering agents	—
Hydroxychloroquine	May have axonal neuropathy
Colchicine	Often with axonal sensorimotor neuropathy
X-linked myopathy with excessive autophagy (XEMA)	—
Danon disease	—

Without Myopathic MUPs	Comment
Myotonia congenita[a]	Widespread with sodium channel mutations; sometimes variable with chloride channelopathies (12)
Hyperkalemic periodic paralysis	Variable myotonia; sometimes triggered by percussion (11)
Paramyotonia congenita	Widespread, profuse myotonia

[a] Associated with clinical myotonia.

durations, and polyphasia.[47] In some of these conditions, CRDs are also present. The electrodiagnostic abnormalities may be more prominent in paraspinal muscles. Biopsy specimens from patients with acid maltase and debrancher deficiency as well as XEMA and Danon disease reveal vacuolar changes. Presumably the vacuolar changes and fiber splitting lead to CRDs and possibly myotonic discharges.

Pattern 4: Myopathic MUPs with CRDs

The pattern of myopathic MUP with CRDs, but without fibrillation potentials or myotonic discharges, is uncommon because most patients with CRDs also show other spontaneous discharges (**Table 8**). Although less common, occasionally CRDs are present without myotonic discharges or fibrillation potentials in patients with desmin-related myopathies[43] and acid maltase deficiency.[44]

Table 8
EMG pattern 4: myopathic MUPs with CRDs

Disorder	Comment
Chronic myositis	Focal or multifocal CRDs
Acid maltase/debrancher deficiency	Paraspinal-predominant CRDs
Myofibrillar myopathy	CRDs are common; may have myotonic discharges
Muscular dystrophies	Various types (eg, LGMD, dystrophinopathy)
Hypothyroid myopathy	Patterns 2 and 1 are more common
Centronuclear myopathy	Rarely with CRDs

Table 9
EMG pattern 5: myopathies with normal EMG

Disorder	Comment
Corticosteroid myopathy	Pattern 2 also
Storage myopathies	—
Carnitine palmityl transferase deficiency	—
Glycogen storage diseases between attacks	Nonlysosomal types
Congenital myopathies	Except centronuclear or myotubular
Mitochondrial myopathy	Patterns 1 and 2 also

Pattern 5: Normal EMG

Several myopathic disorders may be associated with an entirely normal EMG (**Table 9**). These are typically disorders not associated with muscle fiber necrosis or destruction, such as some metabolic, endocrine, or congenital myopathies. About 20% of patients with mitochondrial myopathy have a normal EMG.[48] Some corticosteroid myopathies are associated with a normal EMG, but most show short-duration MUPs.[49] Congenital myopathies may show subtle EMG abnormalities that are missed in the pediatric population given the difficulties in performing the studies. In those patients with persistent weakness, possible myopathy, and a normal EMG, careful clinical follow-up, appropriate laboratory testing, and potentially a repeat EMG or QEMG are indicated. In some patients, it is still prudent to obtain a muscle biopsy specimen despite a normal EMG, although the yield of biopsy is generally lower than in those showing the abnormal EMG patterns.

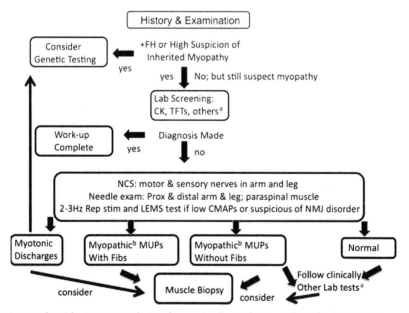

Fig. 6. An algorithmic approach to the evaluation of myopathy. The EMG patterns are described in the text. [a]Laboratory screening is tailored to the presentation. See **Table 3** for a list of possible screening tests. [b]Myopathic MUPs refers to short-duration, typically low-amplitude and polyphasic MUPs. FH, family history; Fibs, fibrillation potentials; Lab, laboratory; NMJ, neuromuscular junction; Rep stim, repetitive stimulation; TFTs, thyroid function tests.

SUMMARY

Electrodiagnostic testing is a useful component of the diagnostic approach to a patient with suspected myopathy. The workup begins with a history and neurologic examination, typically followed by laboratory and then electrodiagnostic testing (**Fig. 6**). Uncovering various electrodiagnostic patterns can lead to more targeted laboratory testing and histopathologic evaluations that can lead to a specific diagnosis.

REFERENCES

1. Lacomis D. Electrodiagnostic approach to the patient with suspected myopathy. Neurol Clin North Am 2002;20:587–603.
2. Barohn RJ, Watts GD, Amato AA. A case of late-onset proximal and distal weakness. Neurology 2009;73:1592–7.
3. Amato AA, Kagan-Hallet K, Jackson CE, et al. The wide spectrum of myofibrillar myopathy suggests a multifactorial etiology and pathogenesis. Neurology 1998; 51:646–55.
4. Cohn RD, Campbell KP. Molecular basis of muscular dystrophies. Muscle Nerve 2000;23:1456–74.
5. Moreira ES, Vainzof M, Marie SK, et al. The seventh form of autosomal recessive limb-girdle muscular dystrophy is mapped to 17q 11-12. Am J Hum Genet 1997; 61:151–9.
6. Berciano J, Gallardo E, Dominguez-Perles R, et al. Autosomal-dominant distal myopathy with a myotilin S55f mutation: sorting out the phenotype. J Neurol Neurosurg Psychiatry 2008;79:205–8.
7. Chahin N, Selcen D, Engel AG. Sporadic late onset nemaline myopathy. Neurology 2005;65:1158–64.
8. Chuquilin M, Al-Lozi M. Primary amyloidosis presenting as "dropped head syndrome". Muscle Nerve 2011;43:905–9.
9. Hutchinson D, Whyte K. Neuromuscular disease and respiratory failure. Pract Neurol 2008;8:229–37.
10. Bolton CF. AAEM minimonograph #40: clinical neurophysiology of the respiratory system. Muscle Nerve 1993;16:809–18.
11. Fournier E, Arzel M, Sternberg D, et al. Electromyography guides toward subgroups of mutations in muscle channelopathies. Ann Neurol 2004;56:650–61.
12. Tan SV, Matthews E, Barber M, et al. Refined exercise testing can aid DNA-based diagnosis in muscle channelopathies. Ann Neurol 2011;69:328–40.
13. Oh SJ, Kuruoglu R. Chronic limb-girdle myasthenia gravis. Neurology 1992;42: 1153–6.
14. Katirji B, Kaminski HJ. Electrodiagnostic approach to the patient with suspected neuromuscular junction disorder. Neurol Clin N Am 2002;20:557–86.
15. Gilchrist JM, Sachs SG. Electrodiagnostic studies in the management and prognosis of neuromuscular disorders. Muscle Nerve 2004;29:165–90.
16. Nozaki K, Pestronk A. High aldolase with normal creatine kinase in serum predicts a myopathy with perimysial pathology. J Neurol Neurosurg Psychiatry 2009;80:904–9.
17. Katirji B, Al-Jaberi M. Creatine kinase revisited. J Clin Neuromuscul Dis 2001;2: 158–63.
18. Chrissian SA, Stolov WC, Hongladarom T. Needle electromyography: its effect on serum creatine phosphokinase activity. Arch Phys Med Rehabil 1976;57: 114–9.

19. Maeyens E, Pitner SE. Effect of electromyography on CPK and aldolase levels. Arch Neurol 1968;19:538–9.
20. Nardin RA, Zarrin AR, Horowitz G, et al. Effect of newly proposed CK reference limits on neuromuscular diagnosis. Muscle Nerve 2009;39:494–7.
21. Katirji B. The clinical electromyography examination. Neurol Clin N Am 2002;20: 291–303.
22. Katz JS, Wolfe GF, Burns DK, et al. Isolated neck extensor myopathy: a common cause of the dropped head syndrome. Neurology 1996;46:917–21.
23. Streib EW, Wilbourn AJ, Mitsumoto H. Spontaneous electrical muscle fiber activity in polymyositis and dermatomyositis. Muscle Nerve 1979;2:14–8.
24. Daube JR, Rubin DI. Needle electromyography. Muscle Nerve 2009;39:244–70.
25. Desmedt JE, Bornestein S. Relationship of spontaneous fibrillation potentials to muscle fiber segmentation in human muscular dystrophies. Nature 1975; 258:531.
26. Fellows LK, Foster BJ, Chalk CH. Clinical significance of complex repetitive discharges: a case-control study. Muscle Nerve 2003;28:504–7.
27. Preston DC, Shaprio BE. Basic electromyography: analysis of motor unit action potentials. In: Preston DC, Shaprio BE, editors. Electromyography and Neuromuscular Disorders: Clinical-Electrophysiologic Correlations. 2nd edition. Boston: Butterworth-Heineman; 1998. p. 195.
28. Farkas C, Stashuk DW, Hamilton-Wright A, et al. A review of clinical quantitative electromyography. Crit Rev Biomed Eng 2010;38:467–85.
29. Fuglsang-Frederiksen A. The role of different EMG methods in evaluating myopathy. Clin Neurophysiol 2006;117:1173–89.
30. Bertorini T, Stalberg E, Yuson CP, et al. Single fiber electromyography in neuromuscular disorders: correlation of muscle histochemistry, single-fiber electromyography, and clinical findings. Muscle Nerve 1994;17:345–53.
31. Rutkove SB. Electrical impedance myography: background, current state, and future directions. Muscle Nerve 2009;40:936–46.
32. Garmirian LP, Chin AB, Rutkove SB. Discriminating neurogenic from myopathic disease via measurement of muscle anisotrophy. Muscle Nerve 2009;39:16–24.
33. Buchthal F, Kamieniecka Z. The diagnostic yield of quantified electromyography and quantified muscle biopsy in neuromuscular disorders. Muscle Nerve 1982;5: 265–80.
34. Lacomis D, Chad DA, Smith TW. Myopathy in the elderly: evaluation of the histopathologic spectrum and the accuracy of clinical diagnosis. Neurology 1993;43: 825–8.
35. Lai C, Melli G, Chang Y, et al. Open muscle biopsy in suspected myopathy: diagnostic yield and clinical utility. Eur J Neurol 2010;17:36–42.
36. Bohan A, Peter JB, Bowman RL, et al. A computer-assisted analysis of 153 patients with polymyositis and dermatomyositis. Medicine (Baltimore) 1977;56: 255–86.
37. Devere R, Bradley WG. Polymyositis: its presentation, morbidity, and mortality. Brain 1976;98:637–66.
38. Nandedkar SD, Sanders DB. Simulation of myopathic motor unit action potentials. Muscle Nerve 1989;12:197–202.
39. Stalberg E, Karlsson L. Simulation of EMG in pathological situations. Clin Neurophysiol 2001;112:869–78.
40. Rubin DI, Hermann RC. Electrophysiologic findings in amyloid myopathy. Muscle Nerve 1999;22:355–9.

41. Mastaglia FL, Sarnat HB, Ojeda VJ, et al. Myopathies associated with hypothyroidism. A review based upon 13 cases. Aust N Z J Med 1988;18:799–806.
42. Lacomis D, Giuliani MJ, Van Cott A, et al. Acute myopathy of intensive care: clinical, electromyographic, and pathological aspects. Ann Neurol 1996;40:645–54.
43. Olive M, Goldfarb L, Moreno D, et al. Desmin-related myopathy. Clinical, electrophysiological, radiological, neuropathological and genetic studies. J Neurol Sci 2004;219:125–37.
44. Muller-Felber W, Horvath R, Gempel K, et al. Late onset Pompe disease: clinical and neurophysiological spectrum of 38 patients including long-term follow-up of 18 patients. Neuromuscul Disord 2007;17:698–706.
45. Al-Shekhlee A, Hachwi R, Jaberi MM, et al. The electromyographic features of acute rhabdomyolysis. J Clin Neuromuscul Dis 2005;6:114–8.
46. Sugie K, Yamamoto A, Murayama K, et al. Clincopathological features of genetically confirmed Danon disease. Neurology 2002;58:1773–8.
47. Jaaskalainen S, Juel VC, Udd B, et al. Electrophysiological findings in X-linked myopathy with excessive autophagy. Ann Neurol 2002;51:648–52.
48. Petty RKH, Harding AE, Morgan-Hughes JA. The clinical features of mitochondrial myopathy. Brain 1986;109:915–38.
49. Dropcho EJ, Soong S. Steroid-induced weakness in patients with primary brain tumors. Neurology 1991;41:1235–9.

Electrodiagnostic Approach to Cranial Neuropathies

Kathleen D. Kennelly, MD, PhD

KEYWORDS

- Cranial nerves • Trigeminal nerve • Facial nerve
- Spinal accessory nerve • Blink reflex • Masseter reflex
- Electrodiagnosis

Many of the cranial nerves can be evaluated in clinical neurophysiology laboratories using well-studied, readily available techniques. These procedures can measure the functional integrity of the cranial nerves and can be helpful in initial diagnosis, prognosis, and long-term follow-up. This article is a general review of cranial nerve conduction studies, including techniques as well as interpretation of data. The needle examination of various cranial innervated muscles is also reviewed. The nerve conduction studies include the blink, masseter (jaw jerk), and masseter inhibitory reflexes, which evaluate the trigeminal (blink and jaw jerk) and facial nerves (blink), as well as trigeminal, facial, and spinal accessory motor stimulation. The needle examination techniques for certain voluntary muscles innervated by cranial nerves V, VII, X, XI, and XII are also described.

BLINK REFLEX: OVERVIEW AND TECHNIQUE

Overend[1,2] described the blink response after a tap on the forehead in 1896. Kugelberg[3] using electrical stimulus showed that it consisted of 2 responses: the early ipsilateral (R1) response and the late bilateral (R2) responses (**Fig. 1**). Rushworth[4] established that the afferent limb of the response travels in the first division of the trigeminal nerve with the afferent nerve cell body in the gasserian ganglion. R1 is mediated by the main sensory nucleus of the fifth nerve in the pons, connecting then to the facial nucleus. The R2 responses involve the spinal nucleus and tract of the fifth nerve through polysynaptic pathways in the pons and the medulla that connect to the nucleus of the facial nerve. The efferent limb is mediated by the motor axons of the facial nerve.[5–7]

The blink reflex study is usually performed with stimulation of the supraorbital nerve. The patient is supine and active electrodes are placed on the skin overlying each

Department of Neurology, Mayo Clinic Florida, 4500 San Pablo Road, Jacksonville, FL 32224, USA
E-mail address: kennelly.kathleen@mayo.edu

Neurol Clin 30 (2012) 661–684
doi:10.1016/j.ncl.2011.12.014
0733-8619/12/$ – see front matter © 2012 Elsevier Inc. All rights reserved.

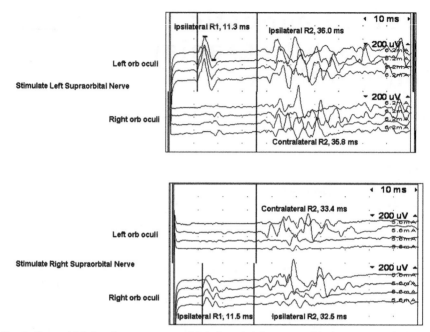

Fig. 1. Normal blink reflex responses with left and right supraorbital nerve stimulation.

orbicularis oculus muscle below the pupil, with reference electrodes placed laterally. Try to relax the patient because excessive background muscle activity can obscure the waveforms. The supraorbital nerve can be stimulated at the supraorbital notch either mechanically or electrically (**Fig. 2**). Recordings are made simultaneously from both sides (see **Fig. 1**). To prevent habitation, the stimuli are given irregularly at least 5 seconds apart. However, in approximately 5% to 10% of normal individuals a well-defined R1 response is not obtainable. Using paired stimuli with an interstimulus interval of 3 to 5 milliseconds may bring out the R1 response.[8]

Measurement of the blink responses include the absolute latencies as well as side-to-side comparisons between the R1 and R2 latencies.[7,9] Amplitude measurements are usually not significant because there can be as much as 40% variation in normal individuals.[10] If the stimulating electrode is too close to the midline a contralateral R1 response may be recorded (**Fig. 3**).[11] If paired stimuli are used it is important to observe the configuration of the R1 responses because the latencies may be erroneous. A double-peaked R1 response requires no change in the normal latency values. However, if a single peak is obtained then the R1 latency should be interpreted from the second shock artifact.[12] In young children the R1 latency may be prolonged with inconsistent R2 responses especially in children younger than 2 years of age.[13,14]

Besides the basic setup as noted earlier, the technique can be modified to stimulate either the infraorbital or mental nerve, which may be useful depending on the patient's symptoms.[9,15] Also in patients with aberrant reinnervation because of previous facial nerve injuries, synkinesis can be recorded with modification of the electrodes so that simultaneous recording is performed over the ipsilateral orbicularis oculus and the orbicularis oris or mentalis muscles.

In hemifacial spasm, a vascular loop or other structural lesions can compress the facial nerve causing focal demyelination and produce ephaptic transmission to other

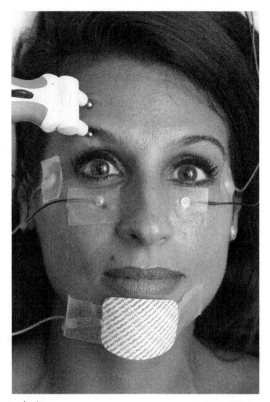

Fig. 2. Blink reflex technique.

axons near that site.[16–18] This abnormal communication has been termed "lateral spread" and can be identified by stimulating either the zygomatic branch of the facial nerve and recording over the mentalis muscle (**Fig. 4**) or stimulating the mandibular branch and recording over the orbicularis oculus.

INTERPRETATION OF THE BLINK REFLEX

The normal values recorded in milliseconds are as follows: R1 latency less than 13, ipsilateral R2 latency less than 41, contralateral R2 latency less than 44. The relative latency differences between sides should be no more than 1.2 milliseconds between each R1 and no more than 8 milliseconds between each R2. The blink reflex is most sensitive for lesions involving the first division of the trigeminal nerve. The clinical picture must also be considered to interpret the study correctly because abnormalities can be seen not only in peripheral nerve lesions but in central nervous system syndromes as well. The R1 response is less reliably obtained with infraorbital stimulation and rarely with stimulation of the mental nerve, and because R2 responses can be more variable, the results are more difficult to interpret.[15] Delayed or absent R1 responses indicate an abnormality in either or both the trigeminal and facial nerve on the stimulated side. If there are also abnormalities in the R2 responses, the examiner can usually localize the nerve involved.[9]

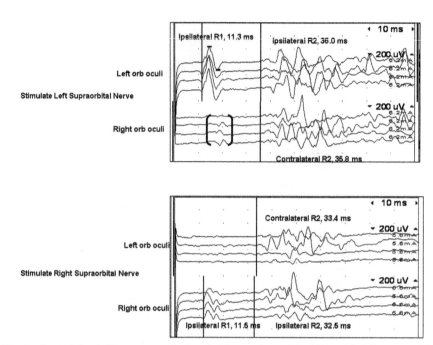

Fig. 3. Contralateral R1 response (*in brackets*) noted on right side with left supraorbital nerve stimulation (*left trigeminal neuralgia*).

Trigeminal Nerve Abnormalities

In trigeminal nerve lesions, the R1 latency can be delayed or absent on the affected side with prolongation of bilateral R2 latencies but both R1 and bilateral R2 latencies are normal with stimulation of the opposite, unaffected side.[19,20] If the trigeminal lesion is severe, with stimulation on the affected side, all responses may be absent, with normal responses obtained after stimulation on the opposite side.[19] These abnormalities can be seen with compressive lesions such as tumors in the region of the cerebellopontine angle,[21–23] collagen vascular diseases, and herpes, with the most common abnormality being a delay in the R1 response.[20] The blink reflex is usually normal in patients with idiopathic trigeminal neuralgia (see **Fig. 3**).[24,25] Although the blink reflex is not so sensitive in V2 and V3 abnormalities, a combination of both the blink and masseter reflexes may aid in localization of lesions in the midbrain and pons.

Facial Nerve Abnormalities

In facial nerve lesions, stimulation on the abnormal side can produce prolonged latencies or absent R1 and ipsilateral R2 responses with a normal contralateral R2 response. On the normal side, stimulation produces prolonged contralateral R2 latency or an absent response with normal R1 and ipsilateral R2 (**Fig. 5**). If both the blink reflex and direct facial nerve stimulation are used they can sometimes localize a demyelinating facial nerve injury as being either proximal or distal to the stylomastoid foramen. For example, in Bell palsy, early on the facial motor nerve response can be normal before degeneration distally occurs. However, because the blink reflex evaluates the entire facial nerve (including the interosseus portion), delayed or absent responses can be seen

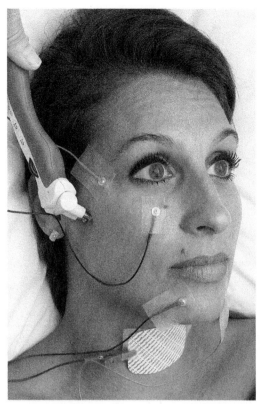

Fig. 4. Electrode placement to evaluate lateral spread in hemifacial spasm. G1 (*black*) active electrodes, G2 (*red*) reference electrodes. Stimulation shown here: zygomatic branch.

immediately. When the blink response is abnormal and facial nerve stimulation is normal, the lesion is located between the facial nucleus and the stylomastoid foramen. The blink response can also be useful in prognosis.[26–28] When the blink reflex is absent on the involved side, the prognosis is poor in most cases. When the reflex is normal or R1 is only delayed, the prognosis is excellent.[26,27] With serial studies, if the delayed or absent R1 and R2 responses return with continued normal facial motor stimulation, patients had a generally good recovery. If the blink responses did not return and the facial motor responses had smaller amplitudes then patients had poorer recovery.[26–28] Facial nerve abnormalities can be identified by the blink reflex in cerebellopontine angle tumors such acoustic neuromas or meningiomas **(Fig. 6)**[29,30] and traumatic facial nerve injuries.

In normal individuals, the stimulation of the supraorbital nerve produces contraction of only the orbicularis oculi muscles. If a patient has had a previous facial nerve injury that has led to aberrant reinnervation and subsequent synkinesis, responses may be seen in other facial muscles. This finding is also true for patients with hemifacial spasm. Although the blink reflexes are usually normal, sometimes the R1 amplitude may be very high, indicating hyperexcitability of the reflex. With adjustment of the stimulator and electrodes as previously described, the lateral spread response can also provide evidence of synkinesis.[8,17,18] In addition, needle examination of involved muscles may be helpful.

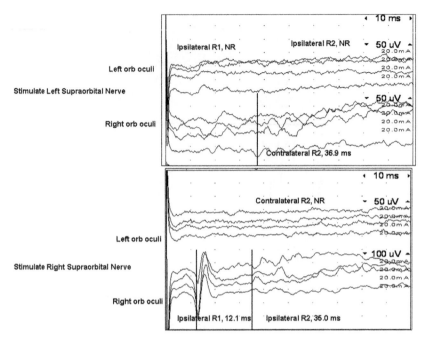

Fig. 5. Blink reflex findings in a patient with severe left Bell palsy. No response is recorded from the left orbicularis oculi with right or left supraorbital nerve stimulation.

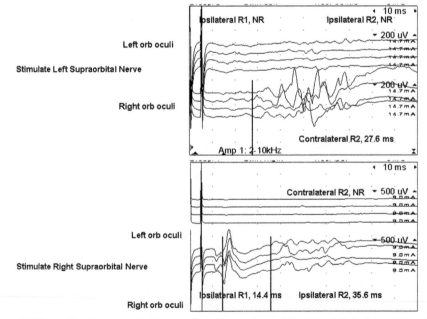

Fig. 6. Blink reflex (using paired stimulation) in a patient with severe left facial neuropathy secondary to a cerebellopontine angle tumor. No response is recorded from the left orbicularis oculi with right or left supraorbital nerve stimulation.

Peripheral Neuropathies

Latency prolongation may be found bilaterally in demyelinating neuropathies, including hereditary as well as acquired neuropathies such as acute and chronic inflammatory demyelinating polyradiculopathies.[31] In connective tissue disorders, prolonged latencies can also occur because of sensory neuropathies or neuronopathies.[31,32] The blink reflex is usually normal in axonal peripheral neuropathies.[8,9]

Central Nervous System Abnormalities

Abnormalities of the blink response have been noted in several central nervous system disorders such as multiple sclerosis, tumors, cerebrovascular disease, head trauma, and neurodegenerative disorders such as Parkinson disease and Huntington disease. The blink response can detect clinically silent lesions in multiple sclerosis with delay in R1 latencies.[33] In pontine gliomas, the R1 response is often delayed, frequently with a normal R2.[34] In patients with cerebral infarctions with hemiparesis, the R1 latency may be delayed or absent for 1 week and the R2 responses may be abnormal for several weeks after.[34,35] Thus acutely, the blink response cannot be used solely to determine if the facial weakness is caused by a central or peripheral disorder. Although not used routinely, the blink reflex may aid in prognosis of patients with coma related to head trauma, using serial studies; if there is progressive loss of R2 over time then the prognosis is poor.[36] Because general anesthesia abolishes the responses and sleep increases R2 latency and duration, the study is not useful in these situations.[8,9,36,37] In Parkinson disease and Huntington disease, habituation may be impaired with regularly applied electrical stimulus used in the blink response.[38,39]

Blink Reflex: Summary

The blink response is a useful technique to study pathways of the trigeminal and facial nerves. It can aid in localization of both peripheral and central nerve lesions. With simple modification of electrodes, information can be obtained in all divisions of the fifth nerve as well as unusual facial nerve disorders such as hemifacial spasm. In our laboratory the most frequent use is to obtain a sensory response in patients with diffuse conditions, such as demyelinating neuropathies. Often in severe peripheral neuropathies, the blink response may be the only sensory response recordable and can provide information about proximal nerve segments. When the blink response is used with other techniques including direct facial motor nerve stimulation, masseter reflex, masseter inhibitory reflex, and needle examination of cranial innervated muscles, lesions can be localized more accurately.

JAW JERK (MASSETER REFLEX): OVERVIEW AND TECHNIQUE

A monosynaptic muscle stretch reflex (masseter or jaw jerk) can be elicited by a tap on the jaw with a reflex hammer. This reflex is initiated by a stretch of the muscle spindles that sends afferent impulses through the motor root of the third division of the fifth cranial nerve intra-axially to the mesencephalic nucleus. Using a single synapse the motor nucleus of the fifth nerve is activated.[7,40] The efferent limb of the reflex arc causes the masseter to contract. The masseter reflex is potentiated by vibration.[41] The afferent nerve cell bodies are located centrally in the mesencephalic nucleus in the central nervous system rather than in the craniospinal ganglia as in the extremity deep tendon reflexes.[42,43]

The jaw jerk is performed as follows: the recording (G1) electrodes are taped symmetrically over each masseter muscle, two-thirds distance between the zygoma and the lower edge of the mandible. The reference (G2) electrodes are placed just below each zygomatic arch and anterior to the masseter. The sweep speed should be 2 ms/cm and gain between 100 and 500 mV/cm. A reflex hammer that is connected to the trigger initiates a sweep when it taps the examiner's finger over the individual's chin (**Fig. 7**).[8,9,44,45] If the patient's jaw is not relaxed, the background muscle activity may obscure the response, and because the tone of the muscle can change, 4 consecutive responses are obtained. The normal range of latencies is 6 to 10.5 milliseconds, with no more than 1 millisecond difference in side-to- side latency values. The amplitude is widely variable and measurement is not useful clinically (**Fig. 8**).[8,9,44,45]

INTERPRETATION OF THE MASSETER REFLEX

A unilateral latency delay or absent response suggests a lesion either in the trigeminal nerve or the brainstem (**Fig. 9**). However, the response can be difficult to obtain in some patients, and if the responses are absent bilaterally, no clinical interpretation can be made. Using the jaw reflex in conjunction with the blink response may help localize the lesion to the midbrain or pons. If the abnormality is limited to the masseter reflex, this suggests a midbrain lesion, but an abnormal R1 on blink testing indicates involvement of the rostral pons.[46] If there is denervation on needle examination of the masseter and other muscles of mastication, then a peripheral lesion is identified. Prolonged latencies can be seen in multiple sclerosis,[45,46] Chiari II malformations,[47] and vascular and neoplastic brainstem disorders.[45] The afferent nerve cell body is located in the mesencephalic nucleus, which lies intra-axially in the brainstem. The cell bodies that are involved in all other stretch reflexes are located

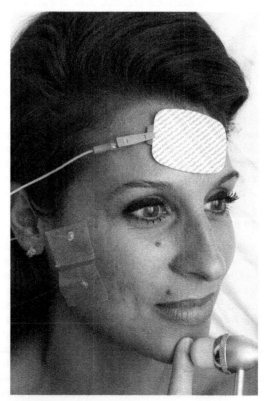

Fig. 7. Masseter reflex (jaw jerk) technique.

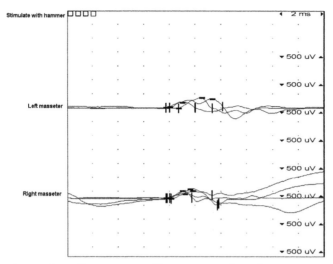

Fig. 8. Normal masseter reflex responses. The responses from 4 separate taps, recording from the left and right masseter, are superimposed.

extra-axially in the dorsal root ganglia. Therefore, patients with sensory symptoms caused by dorsal root ganglionopathies have normal masseter responses rather than a sensory neuropathy.[9,48] For this reason also, the response is normal in patients with Friedrich ataxia.[9,48]

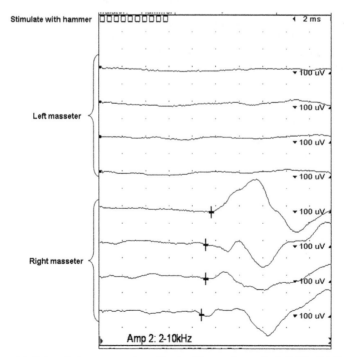

Fig. 9. Absent left jaw jerk response in patient with numbness in left V3 distribution and masseter weakness after face-lift (needle examination showed denervation in the masseter muscle).

The masseter (jaw jerk) reflex is useful in studying the reflex arc of the third division of the trigeminal nerve. In conjunction with other studies such as the blink reflex and needle examination of muscles of mastication, lesions can be more precisely localized both in the peripheral nervous system and the central nervous system.

MASSETER INHIBITORY REFLEX: OVERVIEW AND TECHNIQUE

If the masseter reflex is performed during jaw clenching, there is an electrically silent period in normal individuals. This silent period is caused by the suppression of masseter muscle activity by inhibitory interneurons in the brainstem. If mechanical stimulation is used 1 silent period (SP1) is recorded (**Fig. 10**), and if electrical stimulation is used, there are 2 silent periods (SP1 and SP2) (**Fig. 11**). The afferent impulses for SP1 are carried via the trigeminal sensory root, entering the ipsilateral trigeminal spinal tract and ascending to the trigeminal motor nuclei on both sides via interneurons. SP2 is caused by afferent fibers that also descend to the pontomedullary junction and lateral reticular formation.[9,43]

The masseter inhibitory reflex study uses the same setup as the jaw jerk. However, rather than having the patient relax the jaw muscles, the patient clenches his/her teeth and then using the triggering reflex hammer with a tap or using an electrical trigger the response is recorded. In normal individuals, SP1 starts between 11 and 15 milliseconds after the tap and lasts between 14 and 30 milliseconds. When using electrical stimulation, SP2 starts from 30 to 60 milliseconds after the stimulus. SP1 is the same response seen no matter whether mechanical or electrical stimulus is used.[8,9,44,47]

INTERPRETATION OF THE MASSETER INHIBITORY REFLEX

In patients with significant impairment of reflex mechanisms involved in chewing such as in sensory neuropathies or tetanus, the silent periods may be absent.[49-51] They can be unilaterally absent in patients with hemimasticatory spasm.[49] The latency of SP1 is often delayed in patients with demyelinating neuropathies.[51,52]

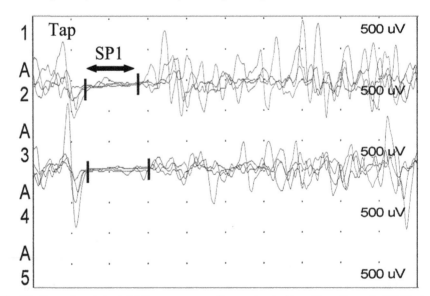

Fig. 10. Normal masseter inhibitory response after mechanical tap. (*From* Kennelly KD. Electrophysiological evaluation of cranial neuropathies. Neurologist 2006;12(4):195; with permission.)

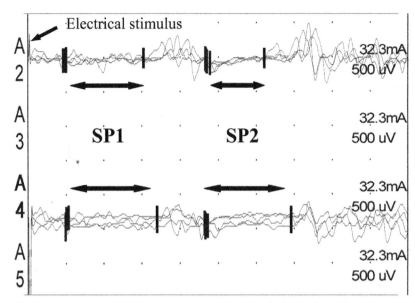

Fig. 11. Normal masseter inhibitory response after electrical stimulus. (*From* Kennelly KD. Electrophysiological evaluation of cranial neuropathies. Neurologist 2006;12(4):195; with permission.)

The masseter inhibitory reflex is a sometimes useful extension of the masseter (jaw jerk) reflex, because it can aid in identification of absent or delayed normal inhibitory responses that can occur in neuropathies as well as more unusual disorders such as tetanus.

TRIGEMINAL MOTOR NERVE STIMULATION: OVERVIEW AND TECHNIQUE

The trigeminal nerve repetitive stimulation technique was developed specifically to aid in the evaluation and diagnosis of myasthenia gravis.[53,54] With the patient supine, the active (G1) electrode is placed over the masseter muscle one-third between the angle of the mandible and the zygoma. The reference (G2) electrode is placed over the angle of the mandible. The ground electrode is on the neck. The masseter branch of the fifth cranial nerve is stimulated using a bare-tipped monopolar needle, which is inserted 0.5 to 1.0 cm into the mandibular notch between the coronoid process and the condyle of the mandible and below the zygomatic process. To protect the teeth, gauze pads are placed between the teeth. The stimulus is gradually increased to obtain a supramaximal response and then a train of 4 stimuli at 2 Hz is administered. The patient exercises the muscles by biting for 1 minute.[54] Technical errors can include movement of the stimulating needle away from the nerve, causing a false decrement, and direct muscle stimulation because of the proximity of the stimulating needle to the masseter muscle.[54]

INTERPRETATION OF REPETITIVE TRIGEMINAL MOTOR STUDIES

The yield of repetitive stimulation techniques in patients with myasthenia gravis depends on the distribution of muscle weakness. In general, more proximal muscles are more involved than distal muscles. Patients frequently have bulbar weakness before the development of more distal weakness.[55] With repetitive trigeminal nerve stimulation, results of 1 study showed abnormal decrement in 88% of patients with myasthenia gravis studied, including some patients with pure ocular symptoms.[53] In another study, the technique was less sensitive than using the facial or spinal accessory nerves.[54]

Repetitive stimulation of the trigeminal nerve may be a useful additive test in evaluating patients with myasthenia gravis.

FACIAL MOTOR NERVE CONDUCTION STUDIES: OVERVIEW AND TECHNIQUE

The facial nerve is primarily a motor nerve supplying the muscles of facial expression. However, in addition, sensation and parasympathetic fibers are carried as well in the nervus intermedius. The facial motor nucleus lies in the reticular portion of the caudal pons, and its nerve fibers along with the sensory and parasympathetic fibers leave the pons in the cerebellopontine angle entering the internal auditory meatus. At the end of the internal auditory meatus, it enters the facial canal, which is the narrowest region the nerve traverses and the common site for compression in Bell palsy. In the canal, efferent branches go to the glands and sensory fibers to the skin of the ear and mastoid, then as the nerve runs below the semicircular canal it gives off the nerve to the stapedius and the chorda tympani. The remaining nerve fibers exit the skull via the stylomastoid foramen and divide into the specific motor branches.[56,57] The motor axons of the facial nerve can be assessed using facial motor conduction studies.

This technique is usually performed with the active (G1) electrode placed over the nasalis muscles just lateral and 1 cm above the external nares and below the pupil. The reference (G2) electrode is placed in the same position on the opposite side. The stimulating electrodes contact the skin below and anterior to the lower tip of the mastoid beneath the earlobe. The anode is inferior to the cathode (**Fig. 12**). The distance from the cathode to the recording electrode must be identical on both sides.[9,58,59] Measurements include the latency from the shock artifact to the initial negative peak on the compound muscle action potential and the amplitude from the baseline to the negative peak (**Fig. 13**). Absolute values and comparisons from side to side are studied, so the distances must be equal between stimulating and recording electrodes on each side.[57] If the patient is not relaxed, excessive artifact can obscure the responses, and if too much stimulation is used, the masseter muscle may contract, causing an initial positivity. Other facial muscles can be tested as well, and again side-to-side comparison should be made with precise distance measurement.

Repetitive nerve stimulation is frequently performed on the facial innervated muscles for diagnosing defects of the neuromuscular junction, such as myasthenia gravis and Lambert-Eaton myasthenic syndrome. The technique starts with routine electrode placements, as noted earlier. In our laboratory, after supramaximal stimulation is achieved, 3 baseline trains of 4 repetitive stimuli at 2-Hz intervals are given. Then the patient exercises the muscle for 10 seconds (if the compound muscle action potential amplitude is low, such as seen in Lambert-Eaton myasthenic syndrome) or 60 seconds if the amplitude is normal. Exercise is followed by trains of stimuli. The first train is immediately after exercise and then the rest are performed at 30 seconds, 1, 2, 3, and then 4 minutes.[60,61] The most frequent error is excessive movement artifact as a result of patient discomfort, which can alter the recording electrodes or stimulator placement and cause false-positive results. Results should be reproducible.[60,61] In Lambert-Eaton myasthenic syndrome, if postexercise stimulation is not performed immediately, the incremental response may disappear because the amplitude of the compound muscle action potential can return to baseline after 60 seconds.[60]

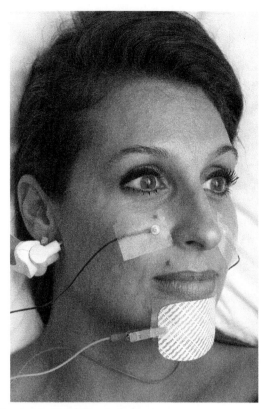

Fig. 12. Facial motor nerve stimulation technique.

INTERPRETATION OF FACIAL MOTOR CONDUCTION STUDIES

Normal values in our laboratory when the nasalis muscle is recorded are as follows: the amplitude greater than 1.8 mV and the latency less than 4.0 milliseconds.[58] Latency differences should be less than 0.6 milliseconds between sides.[56,57]

One of the most common uses for direct facial nerve stimulation is assessment of Bell palsy. The study can help both in localization of the peripheral seventh nerve lesion and may aid in prognosis. The latency and amplitude of the compound muscle action potential response and the minimal excitability of the facial nerve have all been previously studied in prognosis of Bell palsy.[9,57,58,62–64] In 1 study, performed at 5 to 7 days after onset, latency was evaluated. If the latency was normal then complete recovery was seen. If the latency was longer than 0.6 milliseconds than the normal side, good recovery could still occur, but there could be resultant facial synkinesis. If no response was obtained, there could be poorer recovery, including a higher incidence of facial synkinesis and the potential for permanent paralysis.[62] Another study used threshold excitability within 72 hours after insult. These investigators found that patients requiring more than 10 mA of stimulation to obtain a response have a poorer outcome.[64] Other studies compared the amplitude of the weak side with that of the normal side.[58,63] If within 5 to 7 days the amplitude is less than 10% of the normal side, recovery may take 3 times longer than if the amplitude is greater than 30% of the unaffected side (**Fig. 14**).[61] As noted in the section on blink reflex studies, the

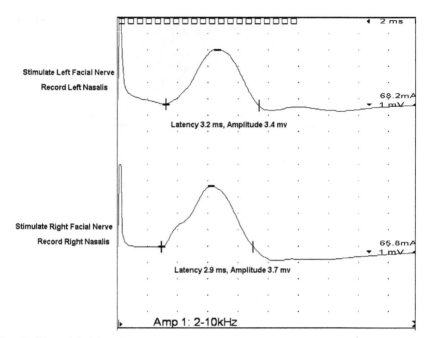

Fig. 13. Normal facial motor responses.

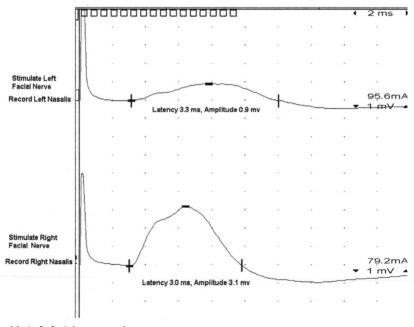

Fig. 14. Left facial neuropathy.

combination of direct facial nerve stimulation and the blink reflex study may help in localization of a facial nerve abnormality. Further evaluation with needle examination of facial innervated muscles can show active denervation and reinnervation.

Facial motor nerve stimulation may also be useful in inflammatory neuropathies because the facial nerve is the most frequent cranial nerve affected in Guillain-Barré syndrome. The facial weakness can occur early and especially when limb weakness is present. Nerve conduction abnormalities can include dispersion and conduction block. Depending on disease severity, axonal loss with small motor amplitudes may be noted later.[65]

When repetitive facial nerve stimulation is used in the diagnosis of a neuromuscular junction disorder, a decrement of at least 10% is considered abnormal. The decrement is greatest between the first and second response; this is the typical pattern for either presynaptic or postsynaptic neuromuscular junction disorders (**Fig. 15**). However, in a presynaptic neuromuscular junction disorder such as Lambert- Eaton myasthenic syndrome, the compound muscle action potentials have low amplitudes, which after brief exercise (10 seconds) facilitate immediately as much as 2 to 20 times the baseline amplitude.[60] In our laboratory an increase in amplitude of greater than 50% baseline amplitude is considered abnormal.

Facial motor nerve studies can help with localization of facial nerve lesions and may be useful in diagnosing more diffuse disorders such as seen in generalized neuropathies and neuromuscular junction disorders.

ACCESSORY MOTOR NERVE CONDUCTION STUDIES: OVERVIEW AND TECHNIQUE

The spinal root of the accessory nerve is derived from the motor neurons in the first 6 cervical spinal cord segments. These motor axons travel proximal through the foramen magnum, where they are joined by the nerve fibers arising from the nucleus ambiguus in the medulla. The spinal accessory nerve exits the skull via the jugular foramen and supplies first the sternocleidomastoid muscle. It then crosses the posterior triangle of the neck and supplies the trapezius muscle. Branches from C3 and C4 ventral rami join the accessory nerve under the trapezius muscle.[9,66]

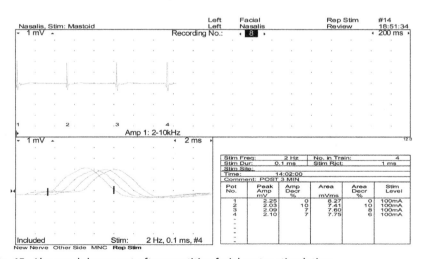

Fig. 15. Abnormal decrement after repetitive facial motor stimulation.

In nerve conduction studies of the accessory nerve, the patient is supine with head elevated and turned 45° to the opposite side. The active (G1) recording electrode is placed over the trapezius at one-half the distance between the C7 spinous process and the prominence of the acromioclavicular joint. The reference (G2) electrode is placed over the acromium. Stimulation is performed with the cathode behind the posterior border of the sternocleidomastoid muscle 10 cm from the active recording electrode. The anode is more proximal and placed along the course of the nerve (**Fig. 16**).[9,59] Distances from the cathode to the G1 electrode on each side need to be identical because side-to-side comparisons are performed. Result measurements include latency and amplitude, with the latency measured from shock artifact to initial negative peak and the amplitude of the compound muscle action potential from baseline to peak (**Fig. 17**).[9,59] This procedure evaluates primarily the innervation of the upper trapezius, and techniques have been described to evaluate latencies to both the middle and lower aspects of the muscle.[67]

Technical errors include poor relaxation of the patient or inadequate immobilization as well as inaccurate measurements. Because this study (like facial motor stimulation) is frequently used in repetitive stimulation, technical errors can lead to false-positive results.

INTERPRETATION OF ACCESSORY MOTOR NERVE CONDUCTION STUDIES

Damage to the nerve is usually caused by a peripheral process in the posterior triangle of the neck, with the most common cause being injury after lymph node biopsy or dissection.[68] Other causes include radical neck dissections as a result of cancer, postoperative radiation, rare complications of carotid endarterectomy, or cannulation of the internal jugular vein.[68–72] Blunt traumas to the posterior triangle of the neck can occur, as well as stretch injuries (eg, with rapid head turning).[68,73] Infections involving the cervical lymph nodes such as tuberculosis can involve the nerve.[68] Idiopathic causes such as brachial plexopathies can cause spinal accessory neuropathies and in 1 study were seen in 20% of brachial plexopathies.[74]

Intracranial damage is unusual but can occur as a result of tumors.[68,75,76] Vernet syndrome involves abnormalities of the spinal accessory, glossopharyngeal, and vagus nerves as they pass through the jugular foramen. This syndrome is most commonly secondary to metastatic disease but can occur with schwannomas.[68,77] Spinal accessory nerve conduction studies can help localize the site of the injury and aid in prognosis. These studies may show low-amplitude responses or

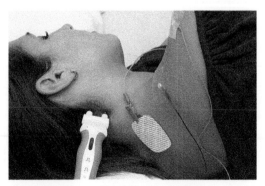

Fig. 16. Spinal accessory motor nerve stimulation technique.

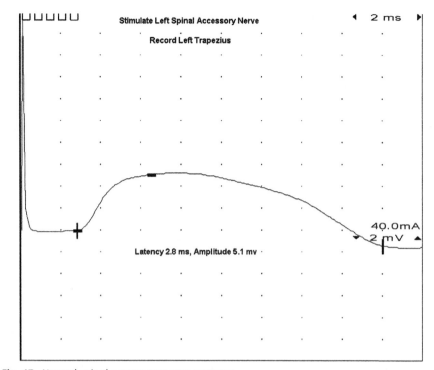

Fig. 17. Normal spinal accessory motor response.

conduction slowing or blocking. Decremental responses with repetitive stimulation can help with diagnosis of neuromuscular junction disorders (**Fig. 18**).

Spinal accessory motor studies can be useful in diagnosis and prognosis of spinal accessory nerve lesions but also in more diffuse processes such as brachial plexopathies, peripheral neuropathies, and disorders of the neuromuscular junction, as seen in myasthenia gravis.

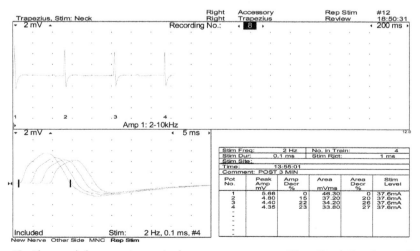

Fig. 18. Abnormal decrement on spinal accessory nerve repetitive stimulation in a patient with myasthenia gravis.

NEEDLE EXAMINATION OF CRANIAL INNERVATED MUSCLES OVERVIEW

The trigeminal, facial, spinal accessory, and hypoglossal innervated muscles are the most commonly evaluated cranial nerve-innervated muscles. The cranial innervated motor unit potentials in general smaller in amplitude and of shorter duration than motor unit potentials in limb muscles, being tested. Because of this, when there is poor relaxation, trying to study insertional activity and looking for fibrillation and fasciculation potentials can be challenging. There are several pictorial references describing the techniques for needle examination in these muscles.[78] The next sections review which muscles can easily be examined and some of the technical difficulties.

TRIGEMINAL NERVE (MUSCLES OF MASTICATION)

The muscles innervated by the third division of the fifth cranial nerve include the masseter, temporalis, and medial and lateral pterygoid muscles. The masseter and temporalis muscles are the easiest to examine. In needle examination of the masseter muscle, care should be used to avoid the parotid duct and gland. The parotid duct is localized close to the zygomatic arch. Part of the parotid gland is just posterior to the masseter muscle.[78] In needle examination of the temporalis muscle, avoid the temporal artery by locating the artery with palpation before needle insertion.[78]

FACIAL NERVE (MUSCLES OF FACIAL EXPRESSION)

The muscles innervated by the facial nerve are easy to examine as well. The most common muscles examined include the orbicularis oculus and oris, frontalis, and mentalis. In examination of the orbicularis oculus, the needle should be angled to avoid penetration of the orbit. The same principle applies to examination of the orbicularis oris. Insert the needle at an angle to the skin to avoid entering the oral cavity. Crossover innervation can be seen in the frontalis, orbicularis oris, and mentalis muscles, so insert the needle in the lateral aspect of these muscles.[9,78]

As described in the section on blink reflexes, hemifacial spasm and synkinesis can be identified with needle examination of the facial muscles (**Fig. 19**). Often in previous severe injuries reduced recruitment with large motor unit potentials is seen (**Fig. 20**). On clinical examination, hemifacial spasm consists of involuntary twitching of the eyelid, which can spread to involve other facial muscles. Electromyographic activity in hemifacial spasm consists of irregular repetitive motor unit discharges varying between 20 and 400 Hz, which can merge into a spasm lasting seconds. Vascular compression[79–81] of the facial nerve is the most common cause, including an unusual case of aneurysmal compression[82]; however, hemifacial spasm has also been seen in intramedullary tumors,[83] neurinomas in the cerebellopontine angle,[84] and basilar meningitis caused by tuberculosis.[85]

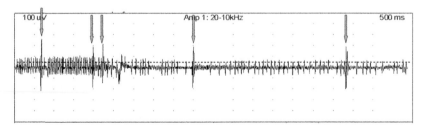

Fig. 19. Synkinesis in left facial nerve palsy in needle examination of orbicularis oris (*arrows* indicate blinking).

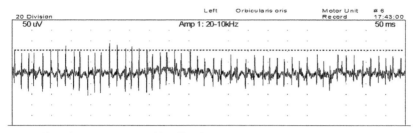

Fig. 20. Reduced recruitment in old Bell palsy.

VAGUS NERVE (LARYNGEAL MUSCLES)

The cricothyroid muscle innervated by the superior laryngeal nerve is the easiest laryngeal muscle to evaluate.[78] The thyroarytenoid muscle, innervated by the recurrent laryngeal nerve, is also accessible but is more difficult and more uncomfortable to examine.[78,86] Neither of these muscles is palpable, so the landmarks needed include the cricoid and thyroid cartilages and the cricothyroid membrane, which also can be difficult to identify in certain patients. Before needle examination of these muscles, a thorough otolaryngology examination should be performed to rule out structural abnormalities such as tumors. Technical difficulties include patient discomfort and penetration of the pharyngeal mucosal, which can cause coughing.

Most commonly, laryngeal needle examination is used to identify the thyroarytenoid muscle for injection of botulinum toxin for adductor laryngeal dystonia, which is the most common cause of spasmodic dysphonia.[86–88] Laryngeal needle examination can also detect neurogenic lesions affecting either the superior or recurrent laryngeal nerve, causing voice disorders. The extent of nerve damage can be assessed, and the serial studies may be helpful for prognosis after injury.[86–88]

SPINAL ACCESSORY NERVE (STERNOCLEIDOMASTOID AND TRAPEZIUS)

The spinal accessory nerve innervates the sternocleidomastoid and trapezius muscles. Both of these muscles are accessible to needle examination. In examining the sternocleidomastoid, palpable structures to avoid include the carotid artery and jugular vein. Also if the needle is inserted too deeply, the plexus could be pierced.[78] When examining the trapezius muscle, be careful again in inserting the needle too deeply to avoid the lung. Depending on the type of lesion, it can be useful to examine all 3 parts of the trapezius to quantify the extent of injury.[78] Needle electromyography of accessory innervated muscles can aid in confirming the extent of accessory nerve damage and help in prognosis.

HYPOGLOSSAL NERVE (TONGUE)

The hypoglossal nerve innervates the tongue, which consists of 3 paired muscles (genioglossus, hypoglossus, and styloglossus). Needle electromyography is most commonly performed in patients with suspected motor neuron disease, especially those with bulbar onset.[89] Needle electrode placement can be performed by 2 different methods, either inserting on the superior surface of the tongue or through the undersurface of the chin, which may be less painful.[78] The greatest challenge is obtaining relaxation, and therefore assessment of spontaneous activity can be difficult.

Although needle examination of cranial innervated muscles does involve special challenges not seen in limb musculature, examination of these muscles can be useful. Needle examination can aid in identifying the extent of a localized process, and with serial examinations recovery can often be measured.

SUMMARY

In clinical neurophysiology laboratories, many of the cranial nerves can be evaluated. The blink reflex is useful not only in localized lesions of the trigeminal and facial nerves but in diffuse disorders such as peripheral neuropathies. It should be normal in trigeminal neuralgia. Using the blink reflex in combination with the masseter reflex and facial motor nerve studies, more precise localizations can be made. Simple adjustments of the electrodes in blink studies and facial motor studies can also aid in localizing clinical lesions and identifying synkinesis and hemifacial spasm. The masseter and masseter inhibitory studies can be useful adjuncts to the more frequently used blink studies, especially in patients with muscles of mastication weakness and sensory symptoms in the V3 distribution. Not only are facial and spinal accessory nerve conduction studies useful for localized abnormalities but along with repetitive stimulation of the trigeminal nerve, repetitive stimulation of these nerves is frequently used in diagnosis of neuromuscular junction disorders. When the nerve conduction techniques are used with appropriate needle examination of cranial innervated muscles, the severity of the lesion can be determined.

ACKNOWLEDGMENTS

The author wishes to thank the technicians in our neurophysiology laboratory for their assistance (especially Lisa Thomas and Rebekah Lindsey) and our fellow, Dr Rachel DiTrapani.

REFERENCES

1. Overend W. Preliminary note on a new cranial reflex. Lancet 1896;1:619.
2. Fine EJ, Sentz L, Ssoria E. The history of the blink reflex. Neurology 1992;42: 450–4.
3. Kugelberg E. Facial reflexes. Brain 1952;75:385–96.
4. Rushworth G. Observations on blink reflexes. J Neurol Neurosurg Psychiatry 1962;25:93–108.
5. Tokunaga A, Oka M, Murao T, et al. An experimental study on facial reflex by evoked electromyography. Med J Osaka Univ 1958;9:397–411.
6. Shahani B. The human blink reflex. J Neurol Neurosurg Psychiatry 1970;33: 792–800.
7. Smith BE. Cranial reflexes and related techniques. In: Daube J, editor. Clinical neurophysiology. New York: Oxford University Press; 2009. p. 529–42.
8. Broggi G, Caraceni T, Negri S. An analysis of a trigemino-facial reflex in normal humans. Confin Neurol 1973;35:263–70.
9. Kennelly KD. Electrophysiological evaluation of cranial neuropathies. Neurologist 2006;12:199–203.
10. Stoehr M, Petruch F. The orbicularis oculus reflex: diagnostic significance of the reflex amplitude. Electromyogr Clin Neurophysiol 1978;18:217–24.
11. Soliven B, Meer J, Uncini A, et al. Physiologic and anatomic basis for contralateral R1 in blink reflex. Muscle Nerve 1988;11:848–51.

12. Rubin D, Dimberg E, Kennelly K. The effect of paired stimuli on blink reflex latencies in normal subjects. Muscle Nerve 2011;44(2):235–40.
13. Anday EK, Cohen ME, Hoffman HS. The blink reflex: maturation and modification in the neonate. Dev Med Child Neurol 1990;32:142–50.
14. Clay SA, Ramseyer JC. The orbicularis oculi reflex: pathologic studies in childhood. Neurology 1977;27:892–5.
15. Jaaskelainen SK. Blink reflex with stimulation of the mental nerve. Methodology, reference values, and some clinical vignettes. Acta Neurol Scand 1995;91:477–82.
16. Auger RG. Hemifacial spasm: clinical and electrophysiologic observations. Neurology 1979;29:1261–72.
17. Nielson VK. Pathophysiology of hemifacial spasm: I. Ephaptic transmission and ectopic excitation. Neurology 1984;34:418–26.
18. Nielsen VK. Pathophysiology of hemifacial spasm: II. Lateral spread of the supraobital nerve reflex. Neurology 1984;34:427–31.
19. Ongerboer de Visser BW, Goor C. Electromyographic and reflex study in idiopathic and symptomatic trigeminal neuralgias: latency of the jaw and blink reflexes. J Neurol Neurosurg Psychiatry 1974;37:1225–30.
20. Hagen NA, Stevens JC, Michet CJ. Trigeminal sensory neuropathy associated with connective tissue diseases. Neurology 1990;40:891–6.
21. Pulec JL, House WF. Facial nerve involvement and testing in acoustic neuromas. Arch Otolaryngol 1964;80:685–92.
22. Bender LF, Maynard FM, Hastings SV. The blink reflex as a diagnostic procedure. Arch Phys Med Rehabil 1969;50:27.
23. Eisen A, Danon J. The orbicularis oculi reflex in acoustic neuromas: a clinical and electrodiagnostic evaluation. Neurology 1974;24:306–11.
24. Goor C, Ongerboer de Visser BW. Jaw and blink reflexes in trigeminal nerve lesions. Neurology 1976;26:95–7.
25. Kimura J, Rodnitzky RL, Van Allen MW. Electrodiagnostic study of trigeminal nerve. Orbicularis oculi reflex and masseter reflex in trigeminal neuralgia, paratrigeminal syndrome, and other lesions of the trigeminal nerve. Neurology 1970;20:574–83.
26. Kimura J, Giron LT, Young SM. Electrophysiological study of Bell's palsy: electrically elicited blink reflex in assessment of prognosis. Arch Otolaryngol 1976;102:140–3.
27. Ghonim MR, Gavilan C. Blink reflex: prognostic value in acute peripheral facial palsy. ORL J Otorhinolaryngol Relat Spec 1990;52:75–9.
28. Heath JP, Cull RE, Smith IN, et al. The neurophysiological investigation of Bell's palsy and the predictive value of the blink reflex. Clin Otolaryngol 1988;3:85–92.
29. Nacimiento W, Podoll K, Graeber MB, et al. Contralateral early blink reflex in patients with facial nerve palsy: indication for synaptic reorganization in the facial nerve during regeneration. J Neurol Sci 1992;109:148–55.
30. Zileli M, Idiman F, Hicdonmez T, et al. A comparative study of brain-stem auditory evoked potentials and blink responses in posterior fossa tumor patients. J Neurosurg 1988;69:660–8.
31. Kimura J. An evaluation of the facial and trigeminal nerves in polyneuropathy: electrodiagnostic studies in Charcot-Marie-Tooth disease, Guillain-Barré syndrome and diabetic neuropathy. Neurology 1971;21:745–52.
32. Auger RG, Windebank AJ, Luchinetti CF, et al. Role of the blink reflex in the evaluation of sensory neuronopathy. Neurology 1999;53:407–8.
33. Kimura J. Electrically elicited blink reflex in diagnosis of multiple sclerosis. Brain 1975;98:413–26.

34. Kimura J. Electrodiagnostic study of brainstem strokes. Stroke 1971;2:576–86.
35. Berardelli A, Accornero N, Crucco G, et al. The orbicularis oculi response after hemispheral damage. J Neurol Neurosurg Psychiatry 1983;46:837–43.
36. Schmalohr D, Linke DB. The blink response in cerebral coma: correlations to clinical findings and outcome. Electromyogr Clin Neurophysiol 1988;28:233–44.
37. Kimura J, Harada O. Recovery curves of the blink reflex during wakefulness and sleep. J Neurol 1976;213:189–98.
38. Agostino R, Beradelli A, Cruccu G, et al. Correlation between facial involuntary movements and abnormalities of blink and corneal reflexes in Huntington's chorea. Mov Disord 1988;3(4):281–9.
39. Penders CA, Delwaide PJ. Blink reflex studies in patients with Parkinsonism before and during therapy. J Neurol Neurosurg Psychiatry 1971;34:674–8.
40. McIntyre AK, Robinson RG. Pathway for the jaw jerk in man. Brain 1959;82:468–74.
41. Godaux E, Demedt JE. Human masseter muscle: H- and tendon reflexes, their paradoxical potentiation by muscle vibration. Arch Neurol 1975;32:229–34.
42. Kimura J. H, T, masseter, and other reflexes. In: Kimura J, editor. Electrodiagnosis in diseases of nerve and muscle: principles and practice. 3rd edition. Philadelphia: FA Davis; 2001. p. 474–82.
43. Hopf HC. Topographic value of brainstem reflexes. Muscle Nerve 1994;17:475–84.
44. Hopf HC, Thomke F, Gutmann L. Midbrain vs. of masseter and blink reflexes. Muscle Nerve 1991;14:326–30.
45. Ongerboer De Visser BW, Cruccu G, Manfredi M, et al. Effects of brainstem lesions on the masseter inhibitory reflex: functional mechanisms of reflex pathways. Brain 1990;113:563–6.
46. Auger RG, McManis PG. Trigeminal sensory neuropathy associated with impaired oral sensation and absence of the masseter inhibitory reflex. Neurology 1990;40(5):759–63.
47. Koehler J, Scharz M, Urban PP, et al. Masseter reflex and blink reflex abnormalities in Chiari II malformation. Muscle Nerve 2001;24:425–7.
48. Auger RG. Preservation of the masseter reflex in Friedreich's ataxia. Neurology 1992;42:875–8.
49. Garcia- Mullen R, Daroff RB. Electrophysiological investigations of cephalic tetanus. J Neurol Neurosurg Psychiatry 1973;36:296–301.
50. Auger RG, Litchy WJ, Cascino TL, et al. Hemimasticatory spasm: clinical and electrophysiologic observations. Neurology 1992;42:875–8.
51. Auger RG. The latency of onset of the masseter inhibitory reflex in peripheral neuropathies. Muscle Nerve 1996;19:910–1.
52. Cruccu G, Agostino R, Inghilleri M, et al. Mandibular involvement in diabetic polyneuropathy and chronic inflammatory demyelinating polyneuropathy. Muscle Nerve 1998;21:1673–9.
53. Pavesi G, Cataaneo L, Tinchelli S, et al. Masseteric repetitive nerve stimulation in the diagnosis of myasthenia gravis. Clin Neurophysiol 2001;112:1064–9.
54. Rubin DI, Harper CM, Auger RG. Trigeminal nerve repetitive stimulation in myasthenia gravis. Muscle Nerve 2004;29:591–6.
55. Jablecki CK. Electrodiagnostic evaluation of patients with myasthenia gravis and related disorders. Neurol Clin 1985;3:557–72.
56. Brazis P. Localization of lesions affecting cranial nerve VII (the facial nerve). In: Brazis PW, Masdeu JC, Biller J, editors. Localization in clinical neurology. Boston: Little, Brown; 1990. p. 203–18.

57. Gilchrist JM. AAEM case report #26: seventh cranial neuropathy. Muscle Nerve 1993;16:447–52.
58. Dumitri D, Walsh NE, Porter LD. Electrophysiologic evaluation of the facial nerve in Bell's palsy. Am J Phys Med Rehabil 1988;67:137–44.
59. Watson J, Daube JR. Compound muscle action potentials. In: Daube JR, editor. Clinical neurophysiology. New York: Oxford University Press; 2009. p. 327–46.
60. Hermann RC. Repetitive stimulation studies. In: Daube JR, editor. Clinical neurophysiology. Philadelphia: FA Davis; 1996. p. 237–47.
61. Howard JF, Sanders DB, Massey JM. The electrodiagnosis of myasthenia gravis and the Lambert- Eaton myasthenic syndrome. Neurol Clin 1985;12:305–30.
62. Taverner D. Electrodiagnosis in facial palsy. Arch Otolaryngol 1965;81:470–7.
63. Olsen PZ. Prediction in recovery of Bell's palsy. Acta Neurol Scand 1975;(Suppl 61): 1–121.
64. Devi S, Challenor Y, Duarte N, et al. Prognostic value of minimal excitability of facial nerves in Bell's palsy. J Neurol Neurosurg Psychiatry 1978;41:649–52.
65. Forster F, Brown M, Merritt H. Polyneuritis with facial diplegia, a clinical study. N Engl J Med 1941;225:51–6.
66. Karuman PM, Soo KC. Motor innervation of the trapezius muscle: a histochemical study. Head Neck 1996;18(3):254–8.
67. Green RF, Brien M. Accessory nerve latency to the middle and lower trapezius. Arch Phys Med Rehabil 1985;66:23–4.
68. Stewart JD. Upper cervical spinal nerves, cervical plexus, and nerves of the neck. In: Stewart JD, editor. Focal peripheral neuropathies. 4th edition. West Vancouver BC (Canada): JBJ Publishing; 2010. p. 74–100.
69. Berry H, MacDonald E, Mrazak A. Accessory nerve palsy: a review of 23 cases. Can J Neurol Sci 1991;18:337–41.
70. Kim D, Cho Y, Tiel R, et al. Surgical outcomes of 111 spinal accessory nerve injuries. Neurosurgery 2003;53:1106–12.
71. Bostronm D, Dahlin L. Iatrogenic injury to the accessory nerve. Scand J Plast Reconstr Surg Hand Surg 2007;41:82–7.
72. Ewing M, Martin H. Disability following radical neck dissection; an assessment based on post operative evaluation of 100 patients. Cancer 1952;5:873–83.
73. Dellon A, Campbell J, Cornblath D. Stretch palsy of the spinal accessory nerve. Case report. J Neurosurg 1990;72:500–2.
74. Van Alfen N, Van Engelen B. The clinical spectrum of neuralgic amyotrophy in 246 cases. Brain 2006;129:438–50.
75. Christopherson L, Leech R, Grossman M. Intracranial neurilemoma of the spinal accessory nerve. Surg Neurol 1982;18:18–20.
76. Kaye A, Hahn J, Kinney S, et al. Jugular foramen schwannomas. J Neurosurg 1984;60:1045–53.
77. Greenberg H, Deck M, Vikran B, et al. Metastasis to the base of the skull: clinical findings in 43 patients. Neurology 1981;31:530–7.
78. Perotto AO. Muscles innervated by cranial nerves. In: Perotto AO, editor. Anatomical guide for the electromyographer. Springfield (IL): Charles C Thomas; 1994. p. 226–62.
79. Hjorth RJ, Willison RG. The electromyogram in facial myokymia and hemifacial spasm. J Neurol Sci 1973;20:117–26.
80. Auger R, Piepgras D, Laws E, et al. Microvascular decompression of the facial nerve for hemifacial spasm: clinical and electrophysiologic observations. Neurology 1981;31:346–50.
81. Harper CM Jr. AAEM case report #21: hemifacial spasm: preoperative diagnosis and intraoperative management. Muscle Nerve 1991;14:213–8.

82. Maroon JC, Lunsford LD, Deeb ZL. Hemifacial spasm due to aneurysmal compression of the facial nerve. Arch Neurol 1978;35:545–6.

83. O'Connor PJ, Wynn Parry CB, Davies K. Continuous muscle spasm in intramedullary tumors of the neuraxis. J Neurol Neurosurg Psychiatry 1966;29:310–4.

84. Revilla AG. Neurinomas of the cerebellopontine recess: a clinical study of one hundred and sixty cases including operative mortality and end results. Bull Johns Hopkins Hosp 1947;80:254–96.

85. Sandyk R. Hemifacial spasm in tuberculosis meningitis. Postgrad Med J 1983;59:570–1.

86. Walker FO. AAEM Course E: clinical diagnosis and electrodiagnosis of voice disorders. Rochester (MN): American Association of Electrodiagnostic Medicine; 1996.

87. Schaefer SD. Laryngeal electromyography. Otolaryngol Clin North Am 1991;24(5):1053–7.

88. Swenson MD. Electrodiagnostic Laryngeal Studies; An AAEM Workshop. Rochester (MN): American Association of Electrodiagnostic Medicine; 1997.

89. Rodriquez AA, Simpson DM. AAEM Course E: approach to the patient with bulbar symptoms. Rochester (MN): American association of Electrodiagnostic Medicine; 1996.

Technical Issues and Potential Complications of Nerve Conduction Studies and Needle Electromyography

Devon I. Rubin, MD

KEYWORDS

- Nerve conduction studies • Needle electromyography
- Complications • Pitfalls • Anomalous anatomy
- Anticoagulation • Pacemaker • Pain

Nerve conduction studies (NCS) and needle electromyography (EMG) provide important and complementary information as part of an electrodiagnostic study for evaluating patients with suspected neuromuscular disorders. The information obtained from these techniques helps to define the underlying pathologic changes that may involve nerves, neuromuscular junctions, or muscle fibers. Although the techniques are standardized and straightforward in experienced hands, potential technical problems that are encountered during the studies may interfere with accurate and reliable acquisition of information and interpretation of the data. Recognition, identification, and correction of various technical problems are critical to the reliable interpretation of any electrodiagnostic study.

Each of the techniques is safe and generally associated with only mild, transient discomfort when performed by experienced physicians. However, NCS involve the administration of electric current, thereby posing some potential risks in certain clinical circumstances. Similarly, because needle EMG involves inserting a needle percutaneously into muscle tissue, potential risks and complications may occur in rare instances. This article reviews technical aspects that should be considered to assist in accurate interpretation and safe performance of an electrodiagnostic study.

Department of Neurology, Mayo Clinic, 4500 San Pablo Road, Jacksonville, FL 32224, USA
E-mail address: rubin.devon@mayo.edu

Neurol Clin 30 (2012) 685–710
doi:10.1016/j.ncl.2011.12.008   neurologic.theclinics.com

TECHNICAL PROBLEMS DURING NCS

An NCS is performed by (1) placing an electrical stimulator on the skin directly over a nerve being tested, (2) placing recording electrodes at a distant site along the same nerve or over a muscle innervated by that nerve, and (3) applying an electrical stimulus sufficiently strong to depolarize all of the axons within the nerve. Technical problems may be encountered at each of these steps and, if not identified and corrected, may result in false-positive or false-negative interpretations of the study. When this occurs, the results may not truly reflect the integrity of the underlying neuromuscular anatomy being studied. Identifying technical problems requires a high degree of acumen and compulsiveness during the performance of the studies as well as close scrutiny of the waveforms, because the interpreting physician cannot identify these types of errors simply by reviewing the numerical data. Several types of technical, physiologic, and anatomic issues that may be encountered during an NCS are reviewed in this article.

Nerve Stimulation Problems

In order to adequately assess the integrity of a nerve during an NCS, all of the axons within the nerve being tested must be sufficiently depolarized. Insufficient or submaximal stimulation of the axons may occur when a nerve cannot be easily identified or when technical issues prevent the current administered on the surface of the skin from penetrating deeply enough through the subcutaneous tissues to depolarize the nerve in entirety. In contrast, administering excessive electrical current can produce abnormal responses as a result of current spread and depolarization of neighboring nerves. Both of these stimulation problems can alter the normal recorded response.

Imprecise nerve localization

During an NCS, the stimulator should be placed as close to the nerve as possible to ensure maximal stimulation with the lowest possible stimulus intensity and to minimize current spread to nearby nerves. In most of the common NCS performed, particularly at distal sites of stimulation such as the wrist or ankle, the nerves are superficial and readily identified. However, individual anatomic variation, soft tissue edema, limb deformities, postsurgical changes or scarring, and obesity can impair nerve identification. For example, in a patient with a subluxed ulnar nerve or who has had surgical transposition of the ulnar nerve, the nerve may lie anterior, rather than posterior, to the medial epicondyle, which may not be readily apparent when performing the study.

The optimal method to identify the location of a nerve is through the sliding technique, in which the stimulator is placed over the most likely site of the nerve being studied and the stimulus intensity is increased in small increments until a threshold, submaximal response is obtained. The stimulator is then moved a few millimeters in one direction parallel to the nerve without changing the stimulus intensity. A higher amplitude response indicates closer proximity to the nerve, whereas a lower amplitude response indicates that the stimulator has moved farther away from the nerve. The stimulator is moved several times in both directions until the site of the maximum amplitude waveform is identified. At that site, the stimulus intensity is then increased until a supramaximal response is obtained (**Fig. 1**).

Reversal of cathode-anode orientation

During routine NCS using a bipolar electrical stimulator, the cathode (the site of nerve depolarization) is placed directly over the nerve, pointed toward the recording electrodes, with the anode approximately 2 cm distant from the cathode. It is at these cathode stimulation sites that the conduction velocity (CV) distant measurements or

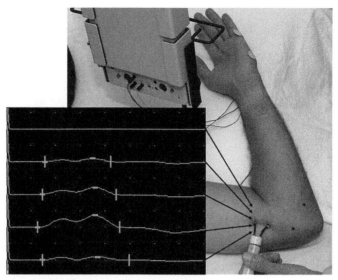

Fig. 1. Sliding technique on ulnar nerve conduction at the elbow. Note the different amplitudes with the same stimulation intensity at different sites at the elbow. The highest amplitude (at the fourth trace) indicates the site where the stimulator is closest to the nerve.

measurements for distal latency calculation are made. If the cathode and anode are inadvertently reversed, the nerve is depolarized approximately 2 cm farther away from the recording electrode, producing several technical abnormalities:

- Inaccurate CV. Because the site of nerve depolarization occurs approximately 2 cm farther than the suspected cathode site, reversal of the orientation at 1 of the 2 sites during assessment of CV along a nerve segment can produce an erroneously calculated CV (falsely slower or faster than normal, depending on whether the reversal occurred at the distal or proximal stimulation site).
- Falsely prolonged distal latency. When the cathode-anode reversal occurs at a distal stimulation site, the distance between the site of nerve depolarization and the recording electrode is 2 cm longer than expected; therefore, the distal latency may be prolonged by approximately 0.4milliseconds (**Fig. 2**).
- Anode block. A theoretic block of conduction of some of the fibers may occur as a result of hyperpolarization of axons at the anode. Anode block can lead to a higher stimulus intensity, which is necessary to depolarize the axons, and the excess current may spread to adjacent nerves, as described later.

Methods to eliminate inadvertent reversal of cathode and anode are listed in **Box 1**.

Submaximal nerve stimulation

The compound muscle action potential (CMAP) or sensory nerve action potential (SNAP) amplitude reflects the number and integrity of functioning axons. Appropriate interpretation and quantitation of an NCS requires stimulation of all axons within a nerve. If the nerve is not maximally stimulated, the number of conducting fibers is underestimated and the recorded amplitude may be falsely low, mimicking disease. Several physiologic factors, such as limb edema, fibrosis, obesity, or deep nerves at proximal sites may contribute to understimulation. In addition, high stimulator

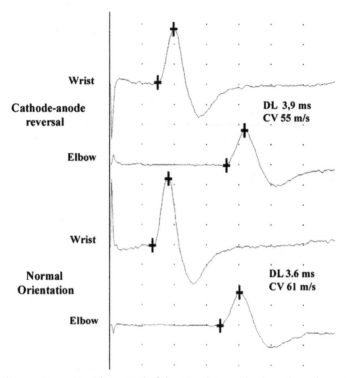

Fig. 2. Median sensory NCS with reversal of the stimulator cathode and anode causing a prolonged distal latency and inaccurate CV (*top*). Normal stimulus orientation (*bottom*). (Normal distal latency is <3.6 milliseconds.) DL, distal latency.

impedance also leads to submaximal stimulation. Submaximal stimulation may lead to the following findings (**Fig. 3**):

- Falsely low CMAP or SNAP amplitude. This finding may be misinterpreted as indicating a neuromuscular disorder. The occurrence at a proximal but not distal stimulation site may mimic a focal conduction block or anomalous innervation.
- Falsely prolonged distal latency or slowed CV. In a submaximally stimulated nerve, some of the large-diameter, faster conducting fibers are not depolarized. As a result, the maximal recorded CV is slower than normal and could mimic a focal mononeuropathy (eg, ulnar neuropathy at the elbow or median neuropathy at the wrist).

Box 2 lists methods that can be used to minimize or correct for submaximal stimulation.

Box 1
Methods to eliminate reversal of cathode and anode

- Ensure that the cathode is clearly noted on the stimulator (usually with a mark or – polarity sign)
- Observe the stimulator orientation before stimulation with every NCS

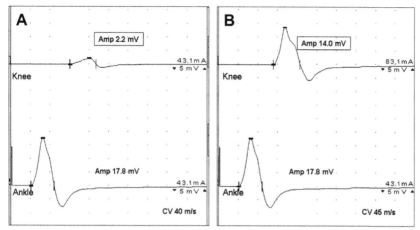

Fig. 3. Tibial motor (abductor hallucis recording) NCS. (*A*) Understimulation at the knee showing a low CMAP amplitude and slower CV. (*B*) Supramaximal stimulation at the knee.

Overstimulation of the nerve producing current spread to other nerves

An electrical stimulus applied to the skin overlying a nerve produces current flow through the extracellular tissue surrounding the nerve. Because these tissues have the ability to conduct electrical charge, increasing stimulus intensity increases the spread of the charge over a wider area (volume conduction). Excess stimulus intensity may result in spread of current to, and inadvertent depolarization of, neighboring nerves. Common sites of occurrence include areas where different nerves are in close proximity to each other and where a higher amount of current may be needed because of a deeper nerve location, such as the tibial nerve at the knee with spread to the peroneal nerve (and vice versa), median and ulnar nerves at the elbow, facial nerve stimulation (with spread to trigeminal), and at the Erb point during brachial plexus stimulation. Overstimulation and current spread leads to several potential problems (**Fig. 4**):

- Erroneously higher amplitudes. This problem is caused by the summation of responses from more than 1 nerve and muscles supplied by the additional nerve

---

Box 2
Methods to eliminate submaximal nerve stimulation

- The sliding technique to localize the nerve.
- Reduction of stimulator impedance with conducting paste.
- Closely observing the waveform following each stimulus for increasing amplitude with increasing stimulus intensity. If the amplitude increases without a significant change in waveform morphology, additional axons have been depolarized.
- Supramaximal stimulation is ensured when a 10% to 20% (usually 5–10 mA) increase in stimulus intensity produces no further increase in amplitude.
- Incrementally increasing the duration of the stimulus (eg, from 0.2 milliseconds to 1 millisecond) if a supramaximal response is not obtained with the maximal stimulus intensity (eg, 100 mA).
- Using a stimulator with a larger cathode and anode separation, a monopolar stimulator, or, in some cases, a monopolar needle stimulator for deeper nerves (eg, the tibial at the knee).

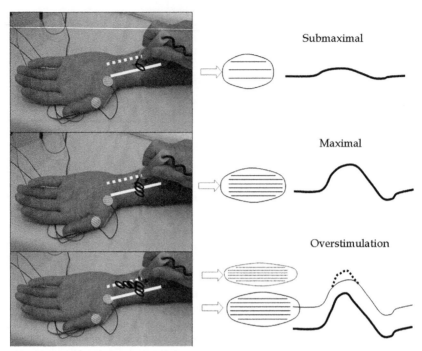

Fig. 4. The effect of overstimulation of the median nerve at the wrist during a median motor NCS. (*Top*) Submaximal nerve stimulation producing depolarization of less than 100% of muscle fibers from the abductor pollicis brevis (APB). (*Middle*) Maximal stimulation of the median nerve resulting in complete depolarization of 100% of APB muscle fibers. (*Bottom*) Overstimulation of the median nerve with spread to the ulnar nerve resulting in depolarization of 100% of median fibers and the addition of some ulnar-innervated muscle fibers in the region of the thenar eminence.

that is depolarized. The higher-than-normal amplitude may lead to a false-negative interpretation (interpreting the study as normal, when the actual response would be abnormally low). There is also typically a change in waveform morphology with overstimulation.

- Inaccurate onset latency and CV.
- False identification of anomalous anatomy. The findings may mimic anomalous innervation, such as a median-to-ulnar anastomosis (from overstimulation at the elbow) or accessory peroneal nerve (from overstimulation at the knee).
- False-negative repetitive stimulation. The current may spread directly to the muscle, bypassing the neuromuscular junction, and lead to a false-negative repetitive stimulation study in a patient with a neuromuscular junction disorder.

Clues to identify, and methods used to reduce, overstimulation are listed in **Box 3**.

Nerve Recording Problems

Appropriate application of the recording electrodes during an NCS is important to obtain an accurate and maximal response from the nerve or muscle. Problems related to the recording electrode size and placement can lead to abnormally recorded responses.

Box 3
Clues to identify, and methods to reduce, overstimulation

Clues

- Higher CMAP amplitude and area at proximal site of stimulation compared with distal site.
- Different waveform morphology between the proximal and distal sites of stimulation.
- Initial positive deflection (indicating volume conduction from a distant source).

Methods to reduce

- Reduce impedance with appropriate skin preparation (abrade the skin and use of electrode paste).
- Use the sliding technique to localize the nerve.
- Increase the stimulus intensity by small increments (ie, 5–10 mA) with each shock.
- Observe the waveform morphology following each stimulus increment. The point at which the morphology does not change with 1 or 2 small increases in intensity is the supramaximal point.
- Observe the muscle contraction to determine correct nerve stimulation (eg, dorsiflexion with peroneal nerve stimulation, plantar flexion with tibial nerve stimulation).

Electrode size

The recording electrodes should be large enough to record the action potential from all of the muscle fibers or nerves that are depolarized. Electrodes that are too small relative to the muscle may produce a lower response than normal because they record from a small portion of the muscle. For most NCS, electrodes 2 to 10 mm in diameter are sufficient. For large muscles or muscles such as the anterior tibialis or biceps, larger recording electrodes (2 cm or greater in diameter) should be used.

Electrode placement during motor NCS

Incorrect placement of either the active or reference electrode can alter the morphology of the waveforms and affect the recorded parameters (distal latency, amplitude, and CV). When recording over a muscle during a motor NCS, the active (G1) electrode should be placed directly over the muscle end-plate zone, whereas the reference (G2) electrode is placed at a variable but defined site, usually along the tendon of the muscle. The motor end-plate region is the site of origin of action potential generation along the muscle fibers following nerve stimulation. Once initiated, the action potentials travel along the fibers away from the end-plate zone. When G1 electrode placement is over the end-plate region, the initial waveform deflection is upward (negative). An initial downward (positive) deflection, or positive dip, indicates that the recorded muscle fiber action potentials have originated at a distance from the G1 electrode and are traveling toward, rather than away from, the electrode through the extracellular tissue (volume conduction). This positive initial deflection is present with all sites of stimulation (**Fig. 5**).

Although a positive dip is the most characteristic feature of G1 electrode placement off the end-plate region, a low CMAP amplitude, sometimes with an atypical waveform morphology, can also occur as a result of incorrect G1 placement. Therefore, a problem with G1 electrode placement should always be considered when an unexpectedly low CMAP amplitude is recorded (**Fig. 6**). Clues to identify, and methods to correct for, improper G1 electrode placement are listed in **Box 4**.

The placement of the G2 electrode also has an effect on the recorded CMAP.[1–3] Because the recording is performed using a differential amplifier, the difference in

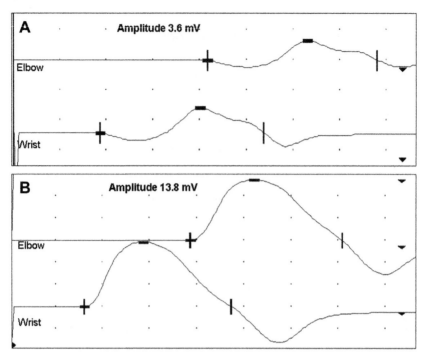

Fig. 5. Median motor NCS (abductor pollicis brevis recording) with incorrect G1 placement. (*A*) CMAP amplitude is reduced and a positive initial deflection is present at the wrist and elbow. (*B*) The normal response after the G1 electrode was moved.

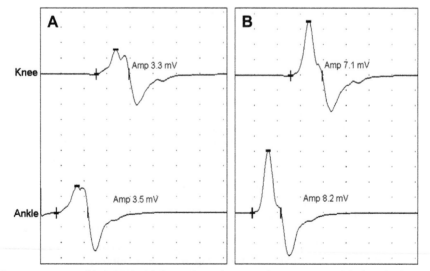

Fig. 6. A 40-year-old patient with leg pain and a normal examination. (*A*) The tibial CMAP amplitude is low (normal amplitude at knee >4.0 mV). (*B*) After moving the G1 electrode, the amplitude nearly doubles.

Box 4
Clues to identify, and methods to reduce, improper G1 electrode placement

Clues

- Initial positive deflection from baseline at all stimulation sites (proximal and distal)
- Unexpectedly low CMAP amplitudes
- Unusual CMAP waveform morphology

Methods to correct

- Know nerve conduction setup based on laboratory technique and reference values
- Carefully identify the muscle to be recorded before applying electrodes
- If initial positivity or unexpectedly low amplitude is observed, systematically move G1 until initial positivity disappears or amplitude becomes maximal
- Ensure that G1 and G2 inputs are correctly placed in the preamplifier

---

the electrical fields between the G1 and G2 electrodes is amplified. Although, in most standard motor NCS, the G2 electrode is placed over the muscle tendon, the G2 electrode is not electrically silent because it records a volume-conducted response traveling along the fibers toward the electrode. Therefore, the responses that are recorded and interpreted consist of the electrical fields recorded from each electrode. If the G1 and G2 electrodes are placed too close together, the responses obtained with each electrode will be similar, thereby reducing the recorded CMAP amplitude.

The normal effect of the G2 electrode on the CMAP morphology, even with placement over the muscle tendon, is greater with ulnar and tibial waveform morphologies than with other nerves. This difference results from the close proximity of ulnar or tibial innervated muscles in the hand or foot to the G2 electrode. As a result, the G2 recorded response contributes more to the final resulting CMAP than with other nerves where there are fewer muscles near the G2 electrode.[1–3] This contribution of the recorded potentials from intrinsic foot muscles recorded by the G2 electrode is the likely cause of the normal reduction in CMAP amplitude between the ankle and knee of up to 50% during the tibial motor NCS.[3] When interpreting the studies according to reference values that use standard recording montages, the effect of the G2 electrode placement is inherent in the normative data. Care must be taken to ensure that the same setup is used during each NCS that is used for the reference values.

Limb movement during the study
Once the electrodes have been applied over the muscle during motor NCS, any movement of the muscle or limb can shift the position of G1 and the relationship with the end-plate zone, thereby altering the morphology of the waveform. Careful attention to ensure that the limb position remains stable through each conduction study will reduce this problem.

Electrode placement during sensory NCS
Sensory NCS record a traveling volley of the summated sensory fiber action potentials traveling toward the recording electrodes along the nerve. During sensory NCS, the recording electrodes are placed as close as possible to the nerve to obtain the maximal response. The farther away the G1 recording electrode is from the action potential generator, the lower the amplitude of the response. This finding is particularly important in sensory studies, in which the amplitudes are much lower than motor

responses. The G1 and G2 electrodes should be placed 3.5 to 4 cm apart to maximize the summation of the potential as recorded with a differential amplifier. If the 2 electrodes are less than 3 cm apart, the SNAP amplitude decreases (**Fig. 7**).

Motor response interference with SNAP
Another source of error in sensory studies is mistaking a volume-conducted motor response for a sensory response. This error is most commonly seen in antidromic studies (particularly the ulnar) in which a mixed motor-sensory nerve is stimulated while recording over the sensory branches in a digit (**Fig. 8**). The volume-conducted motor response may interfere with or distort the sensory potential. When it is unclear whether a recorded waveform is a true sensory response or a volume-conducted motor response, moving the G1 recording electrode a short distance away from the stimulator will slightly prolong the latency of the sensory response, whereas the latency of the volume-conducted motor response will not change. Several methods can be used to correct for motor interference of the sensory response (**Box 5**).[4]

Distance Measurement Errors

During most NCS, the latency from the distal site of stimulation to the recording electrodes (distal latency) and the CV in a nerve segment are assessed. Both of these parameters rely on accurately measuring the length of the nerve between the stimulation and recording sites (**Fig. 9**). The measuring tape should always follow the course of the nerve with the limb remaining in the position tested. This rule applies especially in ulnar NCS when the study is performed with the arm in a flexed position. If the distance is measured with the arm extended after the stimulation is performed with the arm flexed, a falsely shorter distance than the actual length of the nerve will be measured, resulting in an apparently slower CV.

The result of a measurement error is proportional to the distance between the 2 stimulation sites, with a greater error the shorter the distance. For example, in a nerve with a CV of 50 m/s, a 5-mm error in distance measurement over a distance of 20 cm will produce a 2.4-m/s error in velocity. The same measurement error over a distance of 10 cm will produce a 4.8-m/s error in velocity. Methods to ensure correct distance measurements are listed in **Box 6**.

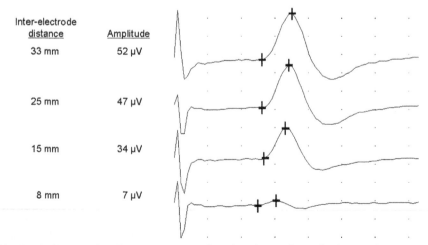

Inter-electrode distance	Amplitude
33 mm	52 µV
25 mm	47 µV
15 mm	34 µV
8 mm	7 µV

Fig. 7. Median antidromic sensory NCS with reduced interelectrode distance between G1 and G2 electrodes.

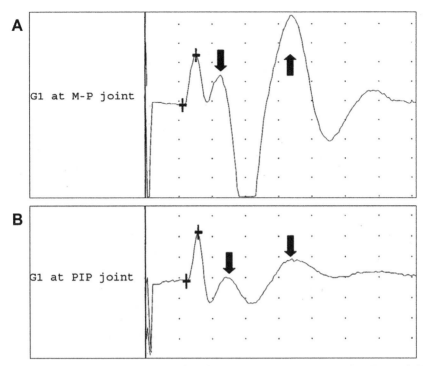

Fig. 8. (*A*) Ulnar sensory antidromic NCS showing prominent motor artifact (*arrows*) that mimics a sensory response. (*B*) Reduction in the motor artifact with movement of electrodes more distal on the digit. M-P, metacarpal-phalangeal; PIP, proximal interphalangeal joint.

Cool Limb Temperature

One of the more common pitfalls in the performance of NCS is not measuring limb temperature and performing a study on a cool limb. Cool limb temperatures can significant alter most NCS parameters and mimic focal or diffuse disease of the nerves. Lower temperatures affect the channel kinetics along the nerve by prolonging the duration of opening of the sodium and potassium channels and slowing electrotonic spread of the potential along the nerve.[5,6] These physiologic changes lead to (**Fig. 10**):

- Higher amplitude and prolonged durations of CMAP and SNAP responses
- Prolonged distal latencies (by approximately 0.2 milliseconds per °C decrease)
- Slowed CV (by 1.8–2.0 m/s per °C decrease)

Box 5
Methods to correct for motor interference of SNAP

- Use the smallest current necessary to produce a supramaximal response
- Move recording electrodes as far away as possible from the muscle groups generating the motor response (eg, place G1 near proximal interphalangeal joint rather than metacarpal-phalangeal joint on the ring finger during ulnar antidromic NCS)
- Shield the recording electrodes with gauze

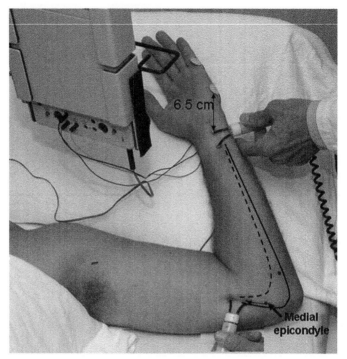

- - - - - - Measured Distance Wrist to Above Elbow: 305 mm
CV = 44 m/s

———— Actual Distance Wrist to Above Elbow: 325 mm
CV = 51 m/s

Fig. 9. Ulnar motor study showing differences in CV with different distance measurements between the wrist and elbow.

- Reduction in degree of conduction block (when present)
- Repair of neuromuscular transmission defect (lessens degree of decrement on repetitive nerve stimulation [RNS]).

The slowing of CVs or prolongation of the distal latencies that may occur with cool limb temperature can often lead to the erroneous interpretation of a study as indicating peripheral neuropathy, carpal tunnel syndrome, or ulnar neuropathy. Factors such as muscle atrophy, exposure to cold, and metabolic disorders such as hypothyroidism

---

Box 6
Methods to ensure correct distance measurement

- Mark site of stimulator cathode with a pen immediately after nerve stimulation (before the stimulator is removed from the skin)

- Hold the tape measure along the course of the nerve during measurement

- Use calipers for proximal nerve segments (eg, distance around shoulder or neck for brachial plexus or root stimulation)

- To ensure reliability, repeat measurement if an unexpected CV is obtained

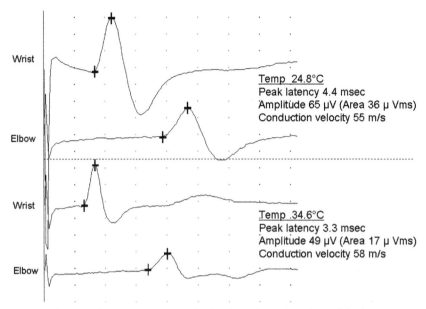

Fig. 10. Median antidromic sensory study. (*Top*) Performed with cool limb temperature causing a prolonged distal latency, mimicking carpal tunnel syndrome. (*Bottom*) After warming (normal distal latency <3.6 milliseconds).

may predispose a limb to cooling. In our laboratory, limb surface temperature should be greater than 32°C on the hand and greater than 30°C on the foot. Although the degree of slowing of CV per °C decrease in temperature is known, the relationship is not linear and therefore using a simple correction factor is not reliable, so maintaining warm limb temperature should be performed in all studies (**Box 7**).

Cool limb temperature can also affect repetitive stimulation studies, producing a false-negative study. Because cooler temperature prolongs the open time of the acetylcholine receptors and lowers the activity of acetylcholinesterase at the neuromuscular junction, thereby increasing the safety margin of neuromuscular transmission, the degree of decrement on repetitive NCS may be less in a cooler limb (comparable with the clinical ice-cube test).[7] Warming the limb has been shown to increase the yield of repetitive NCS.[8]

Technical Problems During RNS

The technical problems that occur during RNS include all of the issues related to routine NCS described earlier, but include another potential problem related to the need to ensure stability of the responses obtained following each of multiple, rapidly

---

Box 7
Methods to correct for a reduction in limb temperature

- Accurately measure limb temperature over the dorsum of the hand or foot during all studies.
- Warm a cool limb with a heat lamp, warm bath (10 minutes at 40°C), or heating pads. This procedure often improves the velocity and latencies and normalizes the study.

administered stimuli. With RNS technique, multiple sequential supramaximal stimuli are given at rates of 2 to 50 Hz. With each stimulus, the stimulator and recording electrodes must remain in a fixed position over the nerve and muscle, respectively. Movement of the stimulator off the nerve, change in the position of the recording electrodes over the muscle, or contraction of the limb all may alter the CMAP waveform between stimuli and produce false decrement. In most RNS studies, any decrement observed should first be considered the result of technical factors unless the typical physiologic features are shown. Characteristic features of true, physiologic decrement from a defect of neuromuscular transmission and patterns indicating false decrement caused by technical factors are listed in **Table 1** and shown in **Fig. 11**. Several methods can be helpful to minimize false decrement during RNS (**Box 8**).

Anatomic Nerve Variations with Anomalous Innervation

Variations in peripheral nerve anatomy are common and failure to recognize anomalous anatomy may lead to erroneous diagnoses when a study may be normal. The most commonly encountered anomalous variations in the arm and leg are the median-to-ulnar anastomoses (Martin-Gruber anastomosis [MGA], median-to-ulnar crossover) and accessory peroneal nerve, respectively. Although a detailed review of anomalous innervation is beyond the scope of this article, the main findings of MGA and accessory peroneal nerve are briefly reviewed.

MGA

The MGA is a common variation that is present in 15% to 31% of individuals and is bilateral in up to 68% of individuals.[9,10] This anatomic variation consists of a communication between the median and ulnar nerve fibers in the forearm, whereby fibers that are destined to supply ulnar-innervated muscles course through the median nerve in the upper arm and proximal forearm, and cross over to the ulnar nerve in the forearm before innervating the destined muscles. The fibers may branch off from the median nerve proper or the anterior interosseus branch.[11] Sensory fibers are not involved. In rare instances, the origin of the crossing over fibers may be more proximal and located above the elbow, thereby mimicking an ulnar neuropathy at the elbow on NCS.[12]

The muscles supplied by the crossing over fibers vary among individuals and include 1 or more of the following: (1) first dorsal interosseus (FDI), (2) abductor digiti

Table 1
Characteristic features of true and false decrement on RNS

Features of True Decrement	Features of False Decrement
Stable baseline without baseline noise	Fluctuating or unstable baseline
Tapering pattern of amplitude reduction	Higher amplitude with second or subsequent stimuli than with first stimulus or increasing amplitude from second to fourth stimuli
Largest decrease in amplitude/area between first and second stimuli	Largest decrease in amplitude/area between stimuli other than first and second
Repair of degree of decrement immediately following 10 s of exercise	Worsening of decrement immediately following 10 s of exercise
Reproducible degree of decrement with repeated trials	Markedly different degrees of decrement with repeated baseline trials at short intervals (eg, 20% decrement at trial 1, 3% decrement 60 s later)

A   **B**

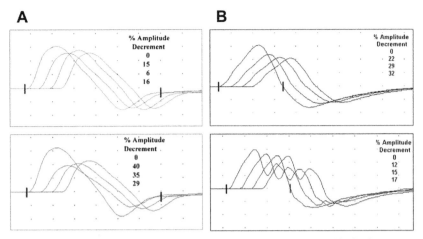

Fig. 11. (*A*) False decrement during repetitive stimulation at 2 Hz caused by limb movement. (*B*) True decrement in a patient with myasthenia gravis.

minimi (ADM), (3) adductor pollicis, or (4) flexor pollicis brevis. In approximately half of individuals with MGA, only 1 muscle is innervated by the crossing over fibers (FDI>adductor pollicis>ADM).[10,13–15] The patterns of findings seen on routine median and/or ulnar motor NCS in the presence of a MGA depend on which muscle(s) the crossing over fibers innervate.

Fibers supply the ADM

This type of MGA should be suspected during a routine ulnar motor NCS recording from the ADM, when the amplitude recorded with wrist stimulation is more than 20% higher than the response recorded with elbow stimulation. This CMAP amplitude reduction may simulate an ulnar neuropathy with a partial focal conduction block. Because the MGA fibers cross over to the ulnar nerve in the midforearm, stimulation of the ulnar nerve at the below-elbow site 5 cm distal to the medial epicondyle (proximal to the crossover fibers) yields an amplitude that is similar to the above-elbow stimulation site, in contrast with ulnar neuropathies at the elbow where the reduction occurs between the below-elbow and above-elbow stimulation sites. This type of MGA can be confirmed by stimulating the median nerve at the wrist and elbow while recording over the ADM (**Fig. 12, Table 2**).

Fibers supply FDI or flexor pollicis brevis

In this type of MGA, the crossing over fibers supply ulnar muscles that are located in the hand adjacent to the thenar region (FDI, adductor pollicis, or abductor pollicis brevis). This pattern of MGA is identified on a routine median motor NCS recording from

---

Box 8
Methods to minimize falsely abnormal decrement during RNS

- Perform 2 to 3 baseline studies at rest before exercise to ensure consistent results and technical reliability
- Stabilize the limb with wooden boards or Velcro straps to prevent movement of the limb during stimulation
- Ensure supramaximal nerve stimulation

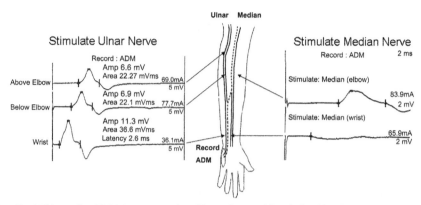

Fig. 12. MGA to the ADM (anastomosing fibers denoted by dashed line).

the thenar eminence. When the median nerve is stimulated at the elbow, in addition to recording from the usual median-innervated thenar muscles, the electrodes over the abductor pollicis brevis (APB) also record a volume-conducted response from the nearby ulnar-innervated muscles that are supplied through the crossing over fibers. This situation results in a higher-than-normal CMAP amplitude caused by the summation of the additional muscle fiber action potentials of the adductor pollicis, flexor pollicis brevis, and/or FDI. When the median nerve is stimulated at the wrist, distal to the crossover, the recorded response is a pure median response (**Fig. 13, Table 3**).

A distinctive pattern is seen in up to 20% of individuals with a type II MGA and a median neuropathy at the wrist (carpal tunnel syndrome).[16,17] With this combination, an initial positive deflection may be seen in the CMAP waveform with median nerve stimulation at the elbow, whereas, with wrist stimulation, no initial positivity is present (**Fig. 14**), resulting from focal slowing of the median fibers at the wrist, which delays the conduction of the true median fibers innervating the median muscles (eg, APB). As a result of this median fiber slowing, the crossing over fibers that supply the ulnar muscles in the thenar region conduct faster than the slowed median fibers and the response recorded from the crossing over fibers precedes the response from the true median fibers. The finding of a positive deflection with elbow stimulation has rarely been described in patients with carpal tunnel syndrome with otherwise normal

Table 2		
Findings of MGA to ADM		
Nerve Stimulated	**Recording Site**	**Findings**
Ulnar	ADM	CMAP with above-elbow stimulation >20% lower than wrist stimulation CMAP with below-elbow stimulation >20% lower than wrist stimulation (below-elbow and above-elbow responses are similar)
Median	APB	Normal results
Median	ADM	Performed to confirm MGA Initial negative CMAP obtained with elbow stimulation (normal individuals have no response) No response with wrist stimulation

Abbreviation: APB, abductor pollicis brevis.

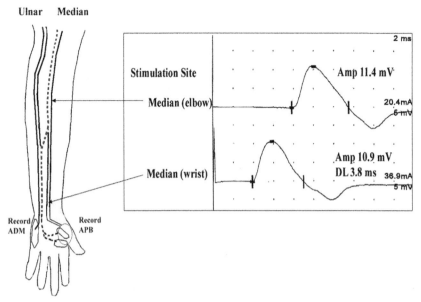

Fig. 13. MGA to the ulnar muscles in the thenar region (anastomosing fibers denoted by dashed line).

conduction studies.[17] In patients with more severe carpal tunnel syndrome and a higher degree of slowing in the median nerve, the response recorded from the crossing over fibers may be seen as a completely separate waveform from the true median waveform.[18]

Accessory peroneal nerve

In most individuals, the extensor digitorum brevis (EDB) is supplied by a branch of the deep peroneal nerve. In up to 28% of the population, the axons supplying the EDB travel within the superficial peroneal nerve and course around the lateral malleolus before innervating the EDB (termed the accessory peroneal nerve).[9,19] The accessory peroneal nerve innervates the fibers in the EDB muscle to a variable degree. In most cases, only a percentage of fibers (usually the lateral fibers) are supplied by the accessory branch, with the medial fibers supplied directly by the deep peroneal nerve, although in some cases the accessory peroneal nerve supplies the entire muscle.

Table 3
Findings of a MGA to the FDI/adductor pollicis/flexor pollicis brevis (thenar region muscles)

Nerve Stimulated	Recording Site	Findings
Median	APB	Higher CMAP amplitude with above-elbow than wrist stimulation Change in CMAP morphology between the above-elbow and wrist stimulation sites
Ulnar	ADM	Normal results. CMAP amplitude of above-elbow stimulation slightly lower than wrist stimulation
Ulnar	APB	CMAP recorded at wrist and elbow stimulation, with larger amplitude at wrist stimulation (this is also seen in individuals without MGA)

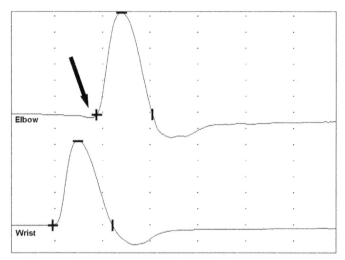

Fig. 14. MGA with superimposed carpal tunnel syndrome. The positive deflection with elbow stimulation reflects CMAP originating from the adductor pollicis and deep head of flexor pollicis brevis that are supplied through the crossing fibers.

An accessory peroneal nerve is identified by a higher CMAP amplitude (recorded from the EDB) with knee stimulation compared with ankle stimulation, and is confirmed by the presence of a recorded response from the EDB with stimulation behind the lateral malleolus (**Box 9, Fig. 15**). A higher CMAP amplitude at the knee than the ankle can also occur from overstimulation at the knee, and observation of the appropriate muscle twitch to ensure that current spread to the tibial nerve is not occurring is important.

In most situations, this finding is of no clinical significance. However, in lesions of the deep peroneal nerve, clinical and electrophysiologic sparing of the toe extensors could occur in the presence of an accessory peroneal nerve. Also, in laboratories where the peroneal nerve is stimulated at the ankle before the knee, caution should be used when a low CMAP amplitude is obtained, which could be misinterpreted as the result of underlying abnormality, and stimulation at the knee should always be performed.

Other anomalous anatomy

Other anatomic variations can produce confusing findings on NCS. One rare anomaly in the hand is the Riche-Cannieu anastomosis (all ulnar hand), in which all of the thenar muscles are supplied by the ulnar nerve.[20,21] This anomaly produces an absent

---

Box 9
NCS findings of an accessory peroneal nerve

- Higher CMAP amplitude with stimulation at the knee and fibular head than with stimulation at the ankle

- Stimulation behind the lateral malleolus produces an initially negative CMAP recorded from the EDB

- CMAP amplitude recorded from lateral malleolus stimulation typically equals the difference between the knee and ankle CMAP amplitudes

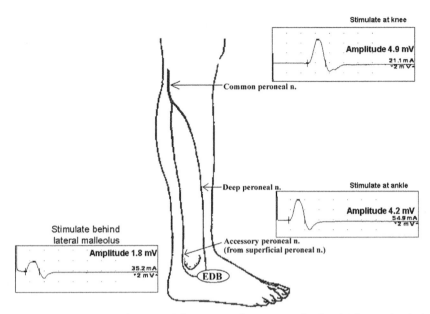

Fig. 15. Accessory peroneal nerve. Higher peroneal CMAP amplitude with knee stimulation compared with ankle stimulation. Stimulation behind the lateral malleolus produces a CMAP.

median motor response from the APB with median nerve stimulation at the elbow and wrist. This anastomosis should be suspected when a patient has an absent median motor CMAP response despite normal thenar muscle bulk and strength and normal findings on needle examination in the thenar muscles. The Riche-Cannieu anastomosis is confirmed by the presence of a normal CMAP response, with an initially negative deflection, following stimulation of the ulnar nerve and recording from the APB.

Another uncommon anomalous sensory innervation involving the hand is superficial radial sensory innervation to the dorsal, ulnar portion of the hand, which is normally supplied by the dorsal ulnar cutaneous (DUC) branch of the ulnar nerve. This anomaly has been identified in approximately 16% of normal individuals.[22] Consideration and testing for this anomaly is important in situations in which electrodiagnostic testing is performed to localize the site of an ulnar neuropathy and a low or absent DUC response is obtained. In this situation, checking for anomalous radial innervation can be performed by moving the stimulator to the radial nerve while recording over the dorsal ulnar hand.

RISKS OF NCS
Performance in Patients with Pacemakers or Cardiac Defibrillators

Because the performance of NCS requires the administration of a variable amount of electric current across the skin and into neighboring tissue, there is a theoretic risk when performing the studies in patients with pacemakers or cardiac defibrillators. In these patients, if the electric current administered reached the cardiac device, it could possibly be interpreted as a cardiac conduction signal and inhibit or trigger the device, leading to abnormal pacing or reprogramming of the device.[23–25] In some instances, repeated stimuli could potentially induce cardiac arrhythmias. Despite these theoretic concerns, studies of routine NCS in patients with implanted cardiac devices during continuous monitoring of the electrocardiogram and interrogation of the devices found that the electrical signals from NCS (with stimulation up to 100 mA and 0.5 milliseconds stimulus duration) of the leg, arm, and, in some patients, at the Erb point, were not sensed by, and never affected, the programming of the devices.[25] These studies suggested that NCS are safe in this patient population. The safety of NCS in patients with temporary transvenous cardiac pacemakers has not been studied and NCS should be avoided in patients with these types of pacemakers.

Performance in Patients with Peripheral Intravenous Lines

Similar to the risk to patients with cardiac devices, there is a theoretic risk of current flow to cardiac structures in patients with peripheral intravenous lines. With standard NCS using surface stimulation, the skin and subcutaneous tissues have a high resistance to current flow. However, patients with intravenous lines have a breach in the high-resistance tissue, possibly allowing current to flow through the intravascular fluid to cardiac tissue. In a study of NCS in 20 patients with peripheral intravenous lines and implanted cardiac devices that could monitor electrical activity in the heart, surface electrocardiograms never detected the peripherally administered current and there was no interference on the settings or function of the cardiac devices.[26] In this study, NCS were performed in the same limb as the intravenous lines, with stimulation performed at the wrist and elbow sites administering up to a 100-mA current with a duration of up to 0.5 milliseconds. Although only a small number of subjects were studied, these findings suggest that the performance of routine NCS on patients with peripheral intravenous lines is safe.

Studies have not been performed assessing the safety of NCS in patients with central venous lines or devices with external wires that are in close proximity to the heart. Although the risk of current flow through these structures may be low with routine NCS and stimulation in the leg or the distal arm, caution should be used and appropriate monitoring for cardiac conduction changes should be undertaken when NCS are performed in these patients. Similar cautions should be used if stimulation at proximal arm sites or Erb point is considered.

Needle Stimulation

In rare instances when supramaximal stimulation of a nerve located deep in a limb cannot be achieved with surface stimulation, near-nerve stimulation using a monopolar needle may be performed. When this technique is performed, the needle electrode is slowly advanced until it is in close proximity to the nerve to allow for nerve stimulation with as little current as possible. Although the risk of current administration through a needle is low, a theoretic risk of current spread to neighboring tissues is present. Because it is unlikely that needle stimulation would be performed on a nerve near the heart, there is little, if any, practical risk with this technique. However, a risk of hematoma formation or injury to structures within the pathway of the needle electrode is more common. For example, injury to the brachial plexus or the development of pneumothorax with puncture of the apex of the lung could occur with attempted needle stimulation of the brachial plexus at the Erb point, therefore needle stimulation at the Erb point should be avoided.

TECHNICAL PITFALLS OF NEEDLE EMG
Filter Settings

The typical frequency range of most of the EMG waveforms recorded during needle EMG is approximately 2 Hz to 30 kHz. To optimize the recorded signals with minimal distortion and to minimize nonphysiologic noise, the filters are usually set at 20 to 30 Hz low-frequency filter (LFF) or high-pass filter and 10 to 20 kHz high-frequency filter (HFF) or low-pass filter during most routine EMG studies. Alterations in the filter settings have an effect on the motor unit potential (MUP) morphology and can lead to an increase or decrease in the recorded duration of the MUP. Increasing the LFF reduces the amplitude and filters out more of the slower frequency tail components of the MUP, resulting in a reduction in the MUP duration. Higher LFF settings, typically of 500 to 2000 Hz, are used during single-fiber EMG. Although the LFF settings are not usually altered on the EMG equipment during routine studies, if unexpectedly short-duration MUPs are recorded in all muscles during a study, the examiner should always check to ensure that an inadvertent change in the filter settings has not occurred.

Needle Movement Problems

Reliable assessment of a muscle during needle EMG requires moving the needle through the muscle to different locations. Several problems can occur related to needle movement during needle EMG.

Too few sites examined

Neuromuscular diseases may involve axons or muscle fibers unequally. As a result, the electrical signals may be normal or minimally abnormal in one portion of a muscle but more severely abnormal in a different region. For example, dermatomyositis fibrillation potentials and short-duration MUP may be more prominent in superficial layers of the muscle, or peripheral nerve vasculitis may affect certain nerve fascicles more than others, thereby affecting motor units innervating different portions of a muscle unequally. Examination of only a single area of muscle may result in not identifying patchy abnormalities and an abnormal study may be interpreted as normal. This potential pitfall can be minimized by moving the needle through several different tracks during examination of each muscle.

Too rapid needle movements with minimal pauses

During an EMG study, a muscle is examined at rest to evaluate for abnormal spontaneous activity such as fibrillation potentials. Fibrillation potentials may fire at various frequencies with some firing as slow as 0.5 Hz, such as in some myopathies. Similarly, fasciculation potentials fire randomly and often infrequently. If needle movements are made quickly and without pausing for 0.5 to 1 second following each movement during examination of a resting muscle, slow-firing spontaneous discharges may be missed.

Too large needle movements

Adequately assessing multiple areas of the muscle with the needle electrode relies on patient tolerance and cooperation of the study. The technique and size of each needle movement can significantly affect study tolerance. The number of muscle fibers damaged by the needle electrode and the pain experienced during needle EMG correlate with the size of needle movements. Larger needle movements (>1 cm) have been shown to be more painful than small needle movements (<1 mm).[27] Electromyographers should perform each study using needle movements that are as small as possible to maximize patient tolerance.

Artifacts

Problems with interpretation of needle EMG findings may be encountered when electrical artifacts similar to pathologic waveforms are recorded. For example, a cardiac pacemaker artifact is recorded as a single spike, usually firing in a regular pattern at a rate of approximately 1 Hz. The regular firing pattern may be confused with, and interpreted as, a fibrillation potential. The pacemaker artifact is most often recorded in muscle closer to the pacemaker, such as the paraspinal muscles or proximal upper extremity muscles, but can be recorded from any muscle. It can often be distinguished from a fibrillation potential because it does not change or disappear with needle movement and the same spike firing at the same rate is found in more than 1 muscle. In addition, as a result of the square wave morphology of the pacemaker artifact, a pacemaker artifact has an artificial sound that is subtly different from a fibrillation potential.

Other artifacts can sometimes be confused with pathologic waveforms, such as 60-cycle or fluorescent light artifact, mimicking a complex repetitive discharge or an intermittently firing transcutaneous electrical nerve stimulator (TENS) or other electrical stimulator, mimicking a myokymic discharge. These electrical artifacts typically fire in a pattern that is more regular than even the regular patterns of physiologic waveforms, giving the waveforms artificial sounds.

POTENTIAL RISKS DURING NEEDLE EMG

Needle EMG is generally a safe procedure when performed by experienced physicians. However, because the technique involves insertion of a needle through the skin and up to several centimeters into a muscle, potential complications may rarely occur.[28] Risks related to the performance of needle EMG include examining patients on antiplatelet or anticoagulant medications, examining patients with a variety of cutaneous issues, and examining muscles that are in close proximity to other organs or structures. In addition, the discomfort associated with needle EMG can affect the ability to optimally record the electrical activity throughout a muscle. Awareness of these potential complications, and adjustment in the technique to reduce the risks, are critical for a safe study and optimizing patient care.

EMG in Patients on Anticoagulation or with Bleeding Disorders

Needle examination can generally be performed without complications in patients on anticoagulants, antiplatelet agents, or with bleeding complications, although adjustments in technique and limitations may apply. The risk of performance of the needle examination in these patients is excessive bleeding and hematoma formation. If this were to occur in a closed compartment, such as the anterior compartment of the leg, there is the potential for development of compartment syndrome and tissue necrosis.[29] The magnitude of the risk is low and there have been only a few reports of paraspinal hematoma, calf hematoma, and calf artery pseudoaneurysm development following needle examination in patients on anticoagulation.[30–32] In a survey of 47 EMG laboratories in the United States, 9% of laboratories reported experiencing at least 1 episode of bleeding complication requiring medical or surgical intervention caused by needle EMG.[32]

Despite these concerns, in a recent study using ultrasound to assess for hematoma formation in the anterior tibialis muscle following needle EMG in patients on warfarin (with international normalized ratio [INR] >1.5 and <4.2) and antiplatelet agents (aspirin or clopidogrel), only 2 of 101 patients on warfarin and 1 of 57 patients on antiplatelet agents developed small (2–3 mm wide by 2–3 cm long), subclinical hematomas.[33] At this time, there is no standard of practice or consensus in electrodiagnostic medicine regarding the highest level of anticoagulation at which a needle examination can safely be performed without additional risk. Therefore, each case must be considered individually and the necessity and benefits of the study must be weighed against the potential risks. In the ideal situation, anticoagulants should be discontinued before the study, although this increases the risk of potential thrombotic complications. Most electromyographers prefer to know the level of anticoagulation (INR) before the study to determine the level of risk, and the decision of whether to perform an entire or partial study is individual. If the needle examination is performed on patients on anticoagulation, some adjustment in the technique of the study may help to minimize potential bleeding complications (**Box 10**).

Similar precautions should be taken in patients with thrombocytopenia. If the platelet count is more than 30,000/mm^2, the study can usually be performed safely. For patients with hemophilia and uncommon bleeding disorders, the patient's hematologist should be consulted before performance of the needle examination.

EMG in Patients with Skin Problems

Several dermatologic conditions should lead to avoidance or limitation of the needle examination. The needle electrode should not be inserted through infected skin (eg, cellulitis) or into an area of prominent vasculature (eg, varicose veins or arteriovenous dialysis shunt). In addition, patients with thin skin, such as those on corticosteroids, may be more prone to bleeding or tearing of the skin and extra caution should be taken during the examination.

EMG in Lymphedema

Examining a limb with lymphedema poses the risk of persistent leaking of serous fluid, potentially increasing the risk of the development of cellulitis. Despite the absence of studies assessing this risk, a position statement by the American Association of Neuromuscular and Electrodiagnostic Medicine (AANEM) suggested that "reasonable caution should be exercised in performing needle examinations in lymphedematous regions."[34]

Examining Peripleural Muscles

Examination of muscles adjacent to or near the lung poses a risk of puncturing the pleura and inducing pneumothorax. This problem may occur with examination of the diaphragm, rhomboids, serratus anterior, trapezius, supraspinatus, and cervical and thoracic paraspinals. Experience in examining these muscles, and precise knowledge of the location and anatomy of these muscles and their relationship to the pleura, are critical to preventing this complication. Techniques used to reduce the risk of pneumothorax when examining these muscles have been reviewed.[28] In all cases, when any of these muscles are examined, the needle electrode should be advanced slowly and smoothly, listening for the sharp, clicky sound of the MUPs (indicating close proximity). When the sound of the potentials becomes more dulled with slow needle advancement, the needle is likely nearing the distant portion of the muscle

---

Box 10
Technique adjustments during needle examination in patients on anticoagulation or with bleeding disorders

- Examine the least number of muscles necessary to make the diagnosis
- Avoid deep muscles (eg, paraspinals, diaphragm)
- Avoid muscles in tight fascial spaces (eg, tibialis anterior)
- Avoid muscles in close proximity to arteries (eg, iliopsoas, flexor pollicis longus)
- Place pressure on the puncture site for 1 to 2 minutes following the examination

and should be withdrawn. Listening for a respiratory pattern of MUP firing, indicating the approach to the peripleural muscles, should prompt caution with continued forward advancement of the needle. The increasing use of ultrasonography during EMG studies to identify and observe needle insertion into the peripleural muscles may further help to reduce this complication.

Performance of Needle EMG in Patients with Pacemaker or Defibrillator

There is no contraindication to performing the needle examination in patients with a pacemaker or other automated defibrillator. Recognition of pacemaker artifact is important to avoid misinterpretation of the artifact as a fibrillation potential.

Performance of Needle EMG in Patients with Prosthetic Cardiac Valves

The risk of needle EMG in patients with rheumatic or other types of valvular heart disease or with prosthetic valves is similar to that of repeated venipuncture, and prophylactic antibiotics are not necessary.

Reducing Pain Associated with Needle EMG

Most patients are able to tolerate the discomfort of the needle examination without difficulty, but a few need a special approach. Pain minimization requires attention to interactions with the patient, and particularly the technique of the needle examination. Techniques such as distraction, continued reassurance, and an empathetic approach to the patient during the study may improve the patient's tolerance of the study. The technique of needle movement has a significant impact in pain reduction. Studies have shown that needle movements of less than 1 mm when using concentric needle electrodes are significantly less painful than needle movements of approximately 1 cm.[27,35]

SUMMARY

NCS and needle EMG can be safely performed in most patients with appropriate technique and precautions in certain circumstances. Attention to detail of technique, awareness of technical factors that can affect reliable interpretation of the study, and appropriate troubleshooting are imperative for quality performance and accurate interpretation of the study.

REFERENCES

1. Kincaid JC, Brashear A, Markand ON. The influence of the reference electrode on CMAP configuration. Muscle Nerve 1993;16:392–6.
2. Brashear A, Kincaid JC. The influence of the reference electrode on CMAP configuration: leg nerve observations and an alternative reference site. Muscle Nerve 1996;19:63–7.
3. Barkhaus PE, Kincaid JC, Nandedkar SD. Tibial motor nerve conduction studies: an investigation into the mechanism for amplitude drop of the proximal evoked response. Muscle Nerve 2011;44:776–82.
4. Rutkove SB. Reduction of motor artifact in antidromic ulnar sensory studies. Muscle Nerve 1999;22:520–2.
5. Rutkove SB, Kothari MJ, Shefner JM. Nerve, muscle, and neuromuscular junction electrophysiology at high temperature. Muscle Nerve 1997;20:431–6.
6. Franssen H, Wieneke GH, Wokke JH. The influence of temperature on conduction block. Muscle Nerve 1999;22:166–73.

7. Hubbard JI, Jones SF, Landau EM. The effect of temperature change upon transmitter release, facilitation, and post-tetanic potentiation. J Physiol 1971;216: 591–609.

8. Rutkove SB, Shefner JM, Wang AK, et al. High temperature repetitive nerve stimulation in myasthenia gravis. Muscle Nerve 1998;21:1414–8.

9. Guttman L. AAEM minimonograph #2: important anomalous innervations of the extremities. Muscle Nerve 1993;16:339–47.

10. Wilbourn AJ, Lambert EH. The forearm median-to-ulnar nerve communication: electrodiagnostic aspects. Neurology 1976;26:368.

11. Srinivasan R, Rhodes J. The median-ulnar anastomosis (Martin-Gruber) in normal and congenitally abnormal fetuses. Arch Neurol 1981;38:418–9.

12. Whitaker CH, Felice KJ. Apparent conduction block in patients with ulnar neuropathy at the elbow and proximal Martin-Gruber anastomosis. Muscle Nerve 2004; 30:808–11.

13. Sun SF, Streib EW. Martin-Gruber anastomosis: electromyographic studies: part II. Electromyogr Clin Neurophysiol 1983;23:271–85.

14. Kimura I, Ayyar DR. The hand neural communication between the ulnar and median nerves: electrophysiological detection. Electromyogr Clin Neurophysiol 1984;24:409–14.

15. Kimura J, Murphy MJ, Varda DJ. Electrophysiological study of anomalous innervation of intrinsic hand muscles. Arch Neurol 1976;33:842–4.

16. Gutmann L. Median-ulnar nerve communications and carpal tunnel syndrome. J Neurol Neurosurg Psychiatry 1977;40:982–6.

17. Gutmann L, Gutierrez A, Riggs JE. The contribution of median to ulnar communication in diagnosis of mild carpal tunnel syndrome. Muscle Nerve 1986;9:319–21.

18. Rubin DI, Dimberg EL. Martin-Gruber anastomosis and carpal tunnel syndrome: morphologic clues to identification. Muscle Nerve 2010;42:457–8.

19. Lambert EH. The accessory deep peroneal nerve: a common variation in innervation of extensor digitorum brevis. Neurology 1969;19:1169–76.

20. Sachs GM, Raynor EM, Shefner JM. The all ulnar hand without forearm anastomosis. Muscle Nerve 1995;18:309–13.

21. Dimitru D, Walsh NE, Weber CF. Electrophysiologic study of the Riche-Cannieu anomaly. Electromyogr Clin Neurophysiol 1988;28:27–31.

22. Leis AA, Wells KJ. Radial nerve cutaneous innervation to the dorsum of the hand. Clin Neurophysiol 2008;119:662–6.

23. Nora LM. American Association of Electrodiagnostic Medicine guidelines in electrodiagnostic medicine: implanted cardioverters and defibrillators. Muscle Nerve 1996;19:1359–60.

24. LaBan MM, Petty D, Hauser AM, et al. Peripheral nerve conduction stimulation: its effect on cardiac pacemakers. Arch Phys Med Rehabil 1988;69:358–62.

25. Schoeck AP, Mellion ML, Gilchrist JM, et al. Safety of nerve conduction studies in patients with implanted cardiac devices. Muscle Nerve 2007;35:521–4.

26. Mellion ML, Buxton AE, Iyer V, et al. Safety of nerve conduction studies in patients with peripheral intravenous lines. Muscle Nerve 2010;42:189–91.

27. Strommen JA, Daube JR. Determinants of pain in needle electromyography. Clin Neurophysiol 2001;112:1414–8.

28. Al-Shekhlee A, Shapiro BE, Preston DC. Iatrogenic complications and risks of nerve conduction studies and needle electromyography. Muscle Nerve 2003; 27:517–26.

29. Farrell CM, Rubin DI, Haidukewych GJ. Acute compartment syndrome of the leg following diagnostic electromyography. Muscle Nerve 2003;27:374–7.

30. Rosioreanu A, Dickson A, Lypen S, et al. Pseudoaneurysm of the calf after electromyography: sonographic and CT angiographic diagnosis. Am J Roentgenol 2005;185:282–3.
31. Butler ML, Dewan RW. Subcutaneous hemorrhage in a patient receiving anticoagulant therapy: an unusual EMG complication. Arch Phys Med Rehabil 1984; 65:733–4.
32. Gruis KL, Little AA, Zebarah VA, et al. Survey of electrodiagnostic laboratories regarding hemorrhagic complications from needle electromyography. Muscle Nerve 2006;34:356–8.
33. Lynch SL, Boon AJ, Smith J, et al. Complications of needle electromyography: hematoma risk and correlation with anticoagulation and antiplatelet therapy. Muscle Nerve 2008;38:1225–30.
34. AANEM Position Statement. Needle EMG in certain uncommon clinical contexts. Muscle Nerve 2005;31:398–9.
35. Walker WC, Keyser-Marcus LA, Johns JS, et al. Relation of electromyography-induced pain to type of recording electrodes. Muscle Nerve 2001;24:417–20.

Coding and Reimbursement of Electrodiagnostic Studies

Neil Busis, MD[a,b,*]

KEYWORDS

- Coding • Billing • Reimbursement
- Electrodiagnostic medicine • Practice management

This article reviews the *Current Procedural Terminology* (*CPT*) codes for electrodiagnostic procedures for 2012. The most frequently asked questions (FAQs) about these codes are included along with the correct answers. *CPT* code modifiers and the global period for some procedures are presented. The final sections discuss the creation and revision of neurologic *CPT* codes, their ties to reimbursement, and regulations regarding the physician supervision of diagnostic tests. Relevant print and Internet resources are listed.

The current *CPT* codes and their definitions are derived from *Current Procedural Terminology: CPT 2012* published by the American Medical Association (AMA). All definitions of *CPT* codes and modifiers in this article are taken directly from *Current Procedural Terminology: CPT 2012* (*CPT only © 2011 American Medical Association. All Rights Reserved*). The author developed the comments on the codes and FAQs along with American Academy of Neurology (AAN) staff and members of the AAN Medical Economics and Management Committee.

For 2012, there are important changes in electromyographic (EMG) procedure codes to be used when the patient also receives nerve conduction studies. New and revised codes for 2012 are marked as <new> and <rev>, respectively.

There will most likely be major changes in coding for electrodiagnostic procedures for 2013. The 2013 codes will be released to the public in late 2012.

The *CPT* codes for neurologic procedures are not defined to include consultation or other evaluation and management (E/M) services. When appropriate, therefore, codes for these services and skills may be submitted in addition to the codes for any neurologic procedures performed on a given patient on a given date.

[a] Section of Neurology, Division of Medicine, UPMC Shadyside Hospital, Pittsburgh, PA, USA
[b] Neurodiagnostic Laboratory, UPMC Shadyside Hospital, 5230 Centre Avenue, Pittsburgh, PA 15232, USA
* 532 South Aiken Avenue, Suite 507, Pittsburgh, PA 15232.
E-mail address: nab@neuroguide.com

Neurol Clin 30 (2012) 711–730
doi:10.1016/j.ncl.2012.01.001
0733-8619/12/$ – see front matter © 2012 Elsevier Inc. All rights reserved.
neurologic.theclinics.com

CPT RESEQUENCING INITIATIVE

In an effort to meet the growing demands for available numbers in *CPT* code sets while adhering to the principles of health information technology, the AMA introduced a resequencing system to integrate new code concepts into existing code families regardless of the availability of sequential numbers. The numbers assigned to some *CPT* codes will not necessarily fit into the numerical order of some code families. Codes introduced under the resequencing initiative are marked by "#".

RESULTS, TESTING, INTERPRETATION, AND REPORT

The "Introduction" at the beginning of the *CPT 2012* manual defines the meaning of "report." Results are the technical components of a service. Testing leads to results; results lead to interpretation. Reports are the work product of the interpretation of test results.

Certain procedures or services described in the *CPT* codebook involve a technical component (eg, tests), which produces results (eg, data, images, slides). For clinical use, some of these results require interpretation. Some *CPT* descriptors specifically require interpretation and reporting to report that code.

INTRODUCTION TO THE SECTION ON NEUROLOGY AND NEUROMUSCULAR PROCEDURES

From the *CPT 2012* manual: "Neurologic services are typically consultative, and any of the levels of consultation (99241–99255) may be appropriate. In addition, services and skills outlined under Evaluation and Management levels of service appropriate to neurologic illnesses should be reported similarly.

The EEG, autonomic function, evoked potential, reflex tests, EMG, NCV, and MEG services (95812–95829 and 95860–95967) include recording, interpretation by a physician, and report. For interpretation only, use modifier 26. For EMG guidance, see 95873, 95874."

ADD-ON CODES

Some of the listed procedures are commonly performed in addition to the primary procedure performed. These additional or supplemental procedures are designated as add-on codes. Add-on codes in *CPT* can be readily identified by specific descriptor nomenclature, which includes phrases such as "each additional" or "list separately in addition to primary procedure." All add-on codes found in *CPT* are exempt from the multiple procedure concept. They are exempt from the use of modifier 51 because these procedures are not reported as stand-alone codes.

NERVE CONDUCTION STUDIES, REFLEX AND LATE RESPONSE TESTING

Codes 95900 to 95904 apply to nerve conduction tests. These codes describe nerve conduction tests when performed with individually placed stimulating, recording, and ground electrodes. The placement of stimulating, recording, and ground electrodes and the test design must be individualized to the patient's unique anatomy. Nerves tested must be limited to the specific nerves and conduction studies needed for the particular clinical question being investigated. The stimulating electrode must be placed directly over the nerve to be tested and stimulation parameters properly adjusted to avoid stimulating other nerves or nerve branches. In most motor nerve conduction studies, and in some sensory nerve conduction studies, both proximal and distal stimulation are used. Recordings of motor nerve conduction studies must be made from electrodes placed directly over the motor point of the specific muscle to be tested. Recordings of sensory nerve conduction studies must be made from electrodes placed directly over the specific nerve to be tested. Waveforms must be reviewed on-site in real time, and the technique (stimulus site, recording site, ground site, filter settings) must be adjusted, as appropriate, as the test proceeds to minimize artifact and the chances of unintended stimulation of adjacent nerves and unintended recording from adjacent muscles or nerves. Reports must be prepared on-site by the examiner and must consist of the work product of the interpretation of numerous test results, using well-established techniques to assess the amplitude, latency, and configuration of waveforms elicited by stimulation at each site of each nerve tested. This includes the calculation of nerve conduction velocities, sometimes including specialized F-wave indices, along with comparison with normal values, summarization of clinical and electrodiagnostic data, and physician or other qualified health care professional interpretation.

Code 95905 describes nerve conduction tests when performed with preconfigured electrodes customized to a specific anatomic site.

95900: Nerve conduction, amplitude and latency/velocity study, each nerve; motor, without F-wave study
95903: motor, with F-wave study
95904: sensory

> Report 95900, 95903, and/or 95904 only once when multiple sites on the same nerve are stimulated or recorded.
> <new>Use 95885–95887 in conjunction with 95900–95904 when performing EMG with nerve conduction studies.<new>

95905: Motor and/or sensory nerve conduction, using preconfigured electrode arrays, amplitude and latency/velocity study, each limb, includes F-wave study when performed, with interpretation and report

> Report 95905 only once per limb studied.
> <rev>Do not report 95905 in conjunction with 95885, 95886, 95900–95904, and 95934–95936.<rev>

95933: Orbiculars oculi (blink) reflex, by electrodiagnostic testing
95934: H-reflex, amplitude, and latency study; record gastrocnemius/soleus muscle
95936: record muscles other than gastrocnemius/soleus muscle (to report a bilateral study, use modifier 50)
51792: Stimulus-evoked response (eg, measurement of bulbocavernosus reflex latency time)

Changes to Reflect the New EMG Codes Reported When Nerve Conduction Studies are Done on the Same Date

In support of the establishment of the 3 add-on codes, 95885 to 95887, for needle EMG performed in conjunction with nerve conduction studies, a parenthetic note has been added after code 95904, instructing the appropriate use with the new codes. An exclusionary parenthetic note has also been added after code 95905, precluding its use with codes 95885, 95886, 95900 to 95904, and 95934 to 95936.

Rationale for Code 95905

Code 95905 was established to report the performance of motor and sensory nerve conduction using preconfigured arrays. Introductory language assists in differentiating nerve conduction studies performed with individually placed stimulating electrodes from those performed with preconfigured electrodes.

- Testing should be limited to those nerves necessary to address the clinical question being investigated.
- Standardized screening tests are not the same as carefully designed nerve conduction studies and do not entail the same physician work.
- Waveforms must be reviewed on-site.
- Reports must be prepared on-site.

The Proper Use of Codes 95900 to 95904

There have been 2 major ambiguities in the nerve conduction study code definitions:

- How to code for studies of 2 or more branches of a given motor or sensory nerve
- How to code for a mixed nerve conduction study

Numbers of Motor and Sensory Nerve Studies

With the approval of the AMA CPT Editorial Panel, the American Association of Neuromuscular and Electrodiagnostic Medicine (AANEM, formerly American Association of Electrodiagnostic Medicine) developed a list of all motor and sensory nerve conduction studies that can be coded as separate procedures. If a procedure was on this list, it could be coded as a separate unit of 95900, 95903, or 95904.

The list of nerves became the official *CPT* policy in 2006. The latest version is included in "Appendix J" of *CPT 2012* (**Box 1**) and is specifically referenced in the section on nerve conduction studies (for listing of nerves considered for separate study, see Appendix J). There is no need to refer to any versions of the list that appeared in the earlier publications.

The statement "Report 95900, 95903, and/or 95904 only once when multiple sites on the same nerve are stimulated or recorded" has remained in *CPT 2012*, however. It now serves solely as a reminder that a nerve conduction study assessing different segments of a single nerve cannot be coded as separate units. For example, a study of the 4 segments of the right ulnar motor nerve (without F waves), (1) axilla-above elbow, (2) above-below elbow, (3) below elbow-wrist, and (4) wrist-abductor digiti minimi muscle, can only be coded as 1 unit of 95900.

Mixed Nerve Conduction Studies

Mixed nerve conduction studies are coded using *CPT* code 95904. Mixed nerves contain sensory and motor fibers. To perform a mixed nerve conduction study, the examiner stimulates a mixed nerve and records from another site over that nerve. A mixed nerve conduction study is a totally separate study from sensory or motor nerve conduction studies of a given nerve. For example, a thorough assessment of the median nerve across the carpal tunnel can consist of all 3 studies:

- Median motor (stimulate at wrist, record over abductor pollicis brevis muscle)
- Median sensory (stimulate at wrist, record sensory fibers supplying digit III)
- Median mixed nerve conduction (stimulate median mixed nerve in the palm, containing sensory fibers and motor fibers to lumbrical muscles; record at wrist)

Box 1
Electrodiagnostic medicine listing of sensory, motor, and mixed nerves

This summary assigns each sensory, motor, and mixed nerve with its appropriate nerve conduction study code to enhance accurate reporting of 95900, 95903, and 95904. Each nerve constitutes one unit of service. This list is published as "Appendix J" of *Current Procedural Terminology: CPT 2012.*

Codes 95900 and 95903 involve the following motor nerves:

I. Upper extremity/cervical plexus/brachial plexus motor nerves

   A. Axillary motor nerve to the deltoid

   B. Long thoracic motor nerve to the serratus anterior

   C. Median nerve

      1. Median motor nerve to the abductor pollicis brevis

      2. Median motor nerve, anterior interosseous branch, to the flexor pollicis longus

      3. Median motor nerve, anterior interosseous branch, to the pronator quadratus

      4. Median motor nerve to the first lumbrical

      5. Median motor nerve to the second lumbrical

   D. Musculocutaneous motor nerve to the biceps brachii

   E. Radial nerve

      1. Radial motor nerve to the extensor carpi ulnaris

      2. Radial motor nerve to the extensor digitorum communis

      3. Radial motor nerve to the extensor indicis proprius

      4. Radial motor nerve to the brachioradialis

   F. Suprascapular nerve

      1. Suprascapular motor nerve to the supraspinatus

      2. Suprascapular motor nerve to the infraspinatus

   G. Thoracodorsal motor nerve to the latissimus dorsi

   H. Ulnar nerve

      1. Ulnar motor nerve to the abductor digiti minimi

      2. Ulnar motor nerve to the palmar interosseous

      3. Ulnar motor nerve to the first dorsal interosseous

      4. Ulnar motor nerve to the flexor carpi ulnaris

   I. Other

II. Lower extremity motor nerves

   A. Femoral motor nerve to the quadriceps

      1. Femoral motor nerve to vastus medialis

      2. Femoral motor nerve to vastus lateralis

      3. Femoral motor nerve to vastus intermedialis

      4. Femoral motor nerve to rectus femoris

   B. Ilioinguinal motor nerve

   C. Peroneal (fibular) nerve

      1. Peroneal motor nerve to the extensor digitorum brevis

      2. Peroneal motor nerve to the peroneus brevis

      3. Peroneal motor nerve to the peroneus longus

      4. Peroneal motor nerve to the tibialis anterior

  D. Plantar motor nerve

  E. Sciatic nerve

  F. Tibial nerve

      1. Tibial motor nerve, inferior calcaneal branch, to the abductor digiti minimi

      2. Tibial motor nerve, medial plantar branch, to the abductor hallucis

      3. Tibial motor nerve, lateral plantar branch, to the flexor digiti minimi brevis

  G. Other

III. Cranial nerves and trunk

  A. Cranial nerve VII (facial motor nerve)

      1. Facial nerve to the frontalis

      2. Facial nerve to the nasalis

      3. Facial nerve to the orbicularis oculi

      4. Facial nerve to the orbicularis oris

  B. Cranial nerve XI (spinal accessory motor nerve)

  C. Cranial nerve XII (hypoglossal motor nerve)

  D. Intercostal motor nerve

  E. Phrenic motor nerve to the diaphragm

  F. Recurrent laryngeal nerve

  G. Other

IV. Nerve roots

  A. Cervical nerve root stimulation

      1. Cervical level 5 (C5)

      2. Cervical level 6 (C6)

      3. Cervical level 7 (C7)

      4. Cervical level 8 (C8)

  B. Thoracic nerve root stimulation

      1. Thoracic level 1 (T1)

      2. Thoracic level 2 (T2)

      3. Thoracic level 3 (T3)

      4. Thoracic level 4 (T4)

      5. Thoracic level 5 (T5)

      6. Thoracic level 6 (T6)

      7. Thoracic level 7 (T7)

      8. Thoracic level 8 (T8)

      9. Thoracic level 9 (T9)

     10. Thoracic level 10 (T10)

     11. Thoracic level 11 (T11)

    12. Thoracic level 12 (T12)

  C. Lumbar nerve root stimulation

    1. Lumbar level 1 (L1)

    2. Lumbar level 2 (L2)

    3. Lumbar level 3 (L3)

    4. Lumbar level 4 (L4)

    5. Lumbar level 5 (L5)

  D. Sacral nerve root stimulation

    1. Sacral level 1 (S1)

    2. Sacral level 2 (S2)

    3. Sacral level 3 (S3)

    4. Sacral level 4 (S4)

Code 95904 involves the following sensory and mixed nerves:

I. Upper extremity sensory and mixed nerves

  A. Lateral antebrachial cutaneous sensory nerve

  B. Medial antebrachial cutaneous sensory nerve

  C. Medial brachial cutaneous sensory nerve

  D. Median nerve

    1. Median sensory nerve to the first digit

    2. Median sensory nerve to the second digit

    3. Median sensory nerve to the third digit

    4. Median sensory nerve to the fourth digit

    5. Median palmar cutaneous sensory nerve

    6. Median palmar mixed nerve

  E. Posterior antebrachial cutaneous sensory nerve

  F. Radial sensory nerve

    1. Radial sensory nerve to the base of the thumb

    2. Radial sensory nerve to digit 1

  G. Ulnar nerve

    1. Ulnar dorsal cutaneous sensory nerve

    2. Ulnar sensory nerve to the fourth digit

    3. Ulnar sensory nerve to the fifth digit

    4. Ulnar palmar mixed nerve

  H. Intercostal sensory nerve

  I. Other

II. Lower extremity sensory and mixed nerves

  A. Lateral femoral cutaneous sensory nerve

  B. Medial calcaneal sensory nerve

  C. Medial femoral cutaneous sensory nerve

  D. Peroneal nerve

1. Deep peroneal sensory nerve

2. Superficial peroneal sensory nerve, medial dorsal cutaneous branch

3. Superficial peroneal sensory nerve, intermediate dorsal cutaneous branch

E. Posterior femoral cutaneous sensory nerve

F. Saphenous nerve

1. Saphenous sensory nerve (distal technique)

2. Saphenous sensory nerve (proximal technique)

G. Sural nerve

1. Sural sensory nerve, lateral dorsal cutaneous branch

2. Sural sensory nerve

H. Tibial sensory nerve (digital nerve to toe 1)

I. Tibial sensory nerve (medial plantar nerve)

J. Tibial sensory nerve (lateral plantar nerve)

K. Other

III. Head and trunk sensory nerves

A. Dorsal nerve of the penis

B. Greater auricular nerve

C. Ophthalmic branch of the trigeminal nerve

D. Pudendal sensory nerve

E. Suprascapular sensory nerves

F. Other

From Current Procedural Terminology 2012. CPT copyright 2011 American Medical Association. All rights reserved.

Conventional motor and sensory nerve conduction studies should not be bundled together into a single mixed nerve conduction study. They can and should be coded separately. If a carrier still attempts to bundle motor and sensory nerve conduction study codes together, modifier 59 should be used with motor nerve conduction study codes to make sure that the codes remain unbundled.

Numbers of Studies that Should be Performed

Many physicians indicate that they are not being paid for nerve conduction studies (sensory or motor). Reasons for rejections include statements that the number of nerves tested is not necessary or the *International Classification of Diseases, Ninth Revision, (ICD-9)* codes that have been used are not appropriate. The April, 2002, *CPT Assistant* article on electrodiagnostic medicine essentially reprinted the key points in the AANEM "Recommended Policy for Electrodiagnostic Medicine" that address these questions and many others. For example, this article included a table outlining the recommended numbers of motor and sensory nerve conduction studies that can be used to diagnose 90% of patients with certain common conditions and symptoms. Like the list of nerves, this table is included in "Appendix J" of *CPT 2012* (**Table 1**). The table, as carriers adopt it, should alleviate many, if not all, of the major coding problems associated with these electrodiagnostic procedures.

Table 1
Type of study/maximum number of electrodiagnostic tests necessary in 90% of cases

Indication	Needle EMG (95860–95864, 95867–95870)	Nerve Conduction Studies (95900, 95903, 95904)			Other EMG Studies (95934, 95936, 95937)	
		Motor Nerve CS With and/ or Without F wave	Sensory Nerve Conduction Studies	H Reflex	Neuromuscular Junction Testing (Repetitive Stimulation)	
Carpal tunnel (unilateral)	1	3	4	—	—
Carpal tunnel (bilateral)	2	4	6	—	—
Radiculopathy	2	3	2	2	—
Mononeuropathy	1	3	3	2	—
Polyneuropathy/ mononeuropathy multiplex	3	4	4	2	—
Myopathy	2	2	2	—	2
Motor neuronopathy (eg, amyotrophic lateral sclerosis)	4	4	2	—	2
Plexopathy	2	4	6	2	—
Neuromuscular junction	2	2	2	—	3
Tarsal tunnel syndrome (unilateral)	1	4	4	—	—
Tarsal tunnel syndrome (bilateral)	2	5	6	—	—
Weakness, fatigue, cramps, or twitching (focal)	2	3	4	—	2
Weakness, fatigue, cramps, or twitching (general)	4	4	4	—	2
Pain, numbness, or tingling (unilateral)	1	3	4	2	—
Pain, numbness, or tingling (bilateral)	2	4	6	2	—

The following table provides a reasonable maximum number of studies performed per diagnostic category necessary for a physician to arrive at a diagnosis in 90% of patients with that final diagnosis. The numbers in each column represent the number of studies recommended. The appropriate number of studies to be performed is based upon the physician's discretion. This table is published in the AMA's *CPT 2012* as *Appendix J*.

From Current Procedural Terminology 2012. CPT copyright 2011 American Medical Association. All rights reserved.

CPT Changes 2006: an Insider's View explained the rationale behind this table as follows:

"The maximum number of studies table summarizes the recommended maximum number of studies per diagnostic category necessary for a physician to arrive at a diagnosis in 90% of patients with that final diagnosis, when performing needle EMG tests (95860–95864 and 95867–95870); nerve conduction studies (95900, 95903, and 95904); and other EMG studies (95934, 95936, and 95937). The numbers in the table are to be used as a tool to detect outliers to assist in appropriate reporting. Each number in the table represents one study or unit. The maximum numbers are designed to apply to a diverse range of practice styles as well as practice types, including those at referral centers where more complex testing is frequently necessary. In simple, straightforward cases, fewer tests will be necessary. This is particularly true when results of the most critical tests are normal. In complex tests, the maximum numbers in the table will be insufficient for the physician to arrive at a complete diagnosis. In cases where there are borderline findings, additional tests may be required to determine if the findings are significant.

The appropriate number of studies to be performed should be left to the judgment of the physician performing the electrodiagnostic (EDX) evaluation; however, in the small number of cases that require testing in excess of the numbers listed in the table, the physician should be able to provide supplementary documentation to justify the additional testing. Such documentation should explain what other differential diagnostic problems needed to be ruled out in that particular situation. In some patients, multiple diagnoses will be established by EDX testing, and the recommendations listed in the table for a single diagnostic category will not apply. It should be noted that in some situations it is necessary to test an asymptomatic contralateral limb to establish normative values for an individual patient. Normal values based on the general population alone are less sensitive than this approach; therefore, restrictions on contralateral asymptomatic limb testing will reduce the sensitivity of electrodiagnostic tests."

Other FAQs: Nerve Conduction, F-wave, and H-Reflex Studies (95900–95904, 95934–95936)

Some payers reject code 95900 and/or code 95903 on a consistent basis whenever they are reported together for the same patient, indicating 95900 is a component code of 95903. This is true, of course, if reported for the same nerve, but not true if reported for different nerves. The AAN has suggested submitting a paper claim with the report indicating the number of nerves tested. This works in some cases but not others. The Centers for Medicare & Medicaid Services (CMS) has suggested that modifier 59 be used with each code to indicate that it is a distinct procedural service being performed on a different area of the body (different nerve). This may work for reimbursement but is incorrect coding. These codes are designed to be billed per nerve (no modifier needed), yet payers do not recognize this and reject them on a regular basis. It is probably simpler to perform all motor nerve conduction studies on a given patient on a given date either with or without F waves, if possible.

EMG

<rev>Needle EMG procedures include the interpretation of electrical waveforms measured by equipment that produces both visible and audible components of electrical signals recorded from the muscles studied by the needle electrode.

The code 95870 or 95885 must be used when 4 or fewer muscles are tested in an extremity. The codes 95860 to 95864 or the code 95866 must be used when 5 or more muscles are tested in an extremity.

EMG codes (95860–95864 and 95867–95870) must be used when no nerve conduction studies (95900–95904) are performed on that day. Codes 95885, 95886, and 95877 must be used for EMG services when nerve conduction studies (95900–95904) are performed in conjunction with EMG on the same day.

Either 95885 or 95886 must be reported once per extremity. Codes 95885 and 95886 can be reported together up to a combined total of 4 units of service per patient when all 4 extremities are tested<rev>.

95860:   Needle EMG; 1 extremity with or without related paraspinal areas
95861:   two extremities with or without related paraspinal areas (for dynamic EMG performed during motion analysis studies, see 96002–96003)
95863:   three extremities with or without related paraspinal areas
95864:   four extremities with or without related paraspinal areas
95865:   larynx

Do not report modifier 50 in conjunction with 95865.
For unilateral procedure, report modifier 52 in conjunction with 95865.

95866:   hemidiaphragm
95867:   cranial nerve–supplied muscles, unilateral
95868:   cranial nerve–supplied muscles, bilateral
95869:   thoracic paraspinal muscles (excluding T1 or T12)
95870:   limited study of muscles in 1 extremity or nonlimb (axial) muscles (unilateral or bilateral) other than thoracic paraspinal muscles, cranial nerve–supplied muscles, or sphincters

To report a complete study of the extremities, see 95860 to 95864.
For anal or urethral sphincter, detrusor, urethra, and perineum musculature, see 51785 to 51792.
For eye muscles, use 92265.

95872:   Needle EMG using single fiber electrode, with quantitative measurement of jitter, blocking, and/or fiber density; any/all sites of each muscle studied
<new>#+95885:   Needle EMG, each extremity, with related paraspinal areas; when performed, done with nerve conduction, amplitude, and latency/velocity study; limited (list separately in addition to code for primary procedure)
<new>#+95886:   complete, 5 or more muscles studied, innervated by 3 or more nerves or 4 or more spinal levels (list separately in addition to code for primary procedure)

<new>Use 95885 and 95886 in conjunction with 95900 to 95904.
<new>Do not report 95885 and 95886 in conjunction with 95860 to 95864, 95870, and 95905.
<new>#+95887: Needle EMG, nonextremity (cranial nerve supplied or axial) muscles done with nerve conduction, amplitude, and latency/velocity study (list separately in addition to code for primary procedure).

<new>Use 95887 in conjunction with 95900 to 95904.

<new>Do not report 95887 in conjunction with 95867to 95870 and 95905.

95875:	Ischemic limb exercise test with serial specimen acquisition for muscle metabolites
51784:	EMG studies of anal or urethral sphincter; other than needle, any technique
51785:	Needle EMG studies of anal or urethral sphincter, any technique
92265:	Needle oculoelectromyography, 1 or more extraocular muscles, 1 or both eyes, with interpretation and report

About the EMG Section Descriptor

The paragraph at the beginning of the *Electromyography* section defines what constitutes a needle EMG study. Not all techniques that purport to assess electrophysiologic aspects of muscle function in health and disease are covered by the *CPT* codes in this section. For example, this family of codes does not cover surface EMG.

New Codes for EMG Studies Done with Nerve Conduction Studies

To address the concerns of the AMA/Specialty Society Relative Value Scale Update Committee (RUC) related to the screening of codes that are performed together more than 75% of the time, 3 add-on codes and an introductory language for needle EMG performed in conjunction with nerve conduction studies have been established. Code 95885 has been established for reporting a limited needle EMG study per extremity when performed with a nerve conduction study. Code 95886 is for reporting a complete study, per extremity, performed with a nerve conduction study. Codes 95885 and 95886 can be reported together up to a combined total of 4 units of service per patient when all 4 extremities are tested.

Code 95887 has been established reporting needle EMG procedures performed on a nonextremity muscle (cranial nerve supplied or axial) performed in conjunction with a nerve conduction study. The AAN's position is that code 95887 was written and valued to be used per site tested. Sites recognized are unilateral face and cervical and lumbar paraspinal muscles without needle EMG examination of corresponding limb muscles, thoracic paraspinal muscles, larynx, hemidiaphragm, thoracic muscles, and abdominal muscles. For example, if EMG of bilateral face muscles is performed, the physician should report 2 units of service of 95887. At the time this was written, this point is being clarified by the AMA.

Codes 95885, 95886, and 95887 appear with a number symbol (#) to indicate that these codes appear out of numerical sequence. Reference notes have been added (where these codes would have been found numerically) to direct users to the appropriate code range 95860 to 95887. These new needle EMG add-on codes are reported in addition to the nerve conduction codes 95900 to 95904 when nerve conduction studies are performed in conjunction with EMG on the same day.

As indicated in the instructional parenthetic note, codes 95885, 95886, and 95887 are excluded from use in conjunction with new EMG codes 95860 to 95864, 95867 to 95870, and 95905.

FAQs: EMG (95860–95875)

There are many questions regarding problems in getting paid for these procedures in various states (not quite as much a problem as nerve conduction studies but nevertheless substantial). The primary issues seem to be the limited number of *ICD-9* codes considered appropriate by the payer to justify EMGs and the number of limbs that can be studied in a given patient. The AANEM-recommended national policy addresses these issues. The readers are referenced to the article on electrodiagnostic medicine in the *CPT Assistant*, April 2002 issue (Volume 12, Issue 4), parts of which are included in "Appendix J" of *CPT 2012* (see **Table 1**).

A common question concerns how many muscles should/need to be studied per limb to use the limb EMG codes. The proper procedure for Medicare patients has been outlined in the Federal Register (issue of October 31, 1997, vol. 62, No. 211, page 59090).

Another frequent question is whether one can bill codes for limited study of specific muscles (*CPT* codes 95869 and 95870) multiple times for each muscle and so forth. CMS clearly sets forth the procedures to be followed (see later).

Proper Use of Needle EMG CPT Codes 95860 to 95870

Starting in 2012, these codes can only be reported for patients who do not have nerve conduction studies done on the same date. The CMS has previously established the following policies regarding the numbers of muscles that must be tested for proper use of these codes:

CPT codes 95860, 95861, 95863, and 95864 (needle EMG of 1, 2, 3, or 4 limbs with or without related paraspinal areas)
To bill these codes, extremity muscles innervated by 3 nerves (for example, radial, ulnar, median, tibial, peroneal, or femoral nerves and not subbranches) or 4 spinal levels must be evaluated, with a minimum of 5 muscles studied per limb. One cannot bill paraspinal muscles separately with these codes, unless studying paraspinal muscles between T3 and T11, in which case code 95869 is to be used.
CPT code 95869 (needle EMG, thoracic paraspinal muscles)
This *CPT* code should be used when exclusively studying thoracic paraspinal muscles, excluding T1 or T12. One unit can be billed, despite the number of levels studied or whether unilateral or bilateral. This code cannot be billed with *CPT* codes 95860, 95861, 95863, or 95864 if only T1 and/or T2 are studied when an upper extremity was also studied.
CPT code 95870 (needle EMG, other than paraspinal [eg, abdomen, thorax])
This *CPT* code can be billed at 1 unit per extremity. The code can also be used for muscles on the thorax or abdomen (unilateral or bilateral). One unit may be billed for studying cervical or lumbar paraspinal muscles (unilateral or bilateral), regardless of the number of levels tested. This code should not be billed when the paraspinal muscles corresponding to an extremity are tested and when the extremity codes 95860, 95861, 95863, or 95864 are also billed.
Principles of CPT Coding, Sixth Edition, states, "That code may be used more than once. For example, if three muscles are tested in each upper extremity, use code 95870 with two units of service, rather than code 95861" (page 453).

About Codes 95865 and 95866

Starting in 2012, these codes can only be reported for patients who do not have nerve conduction studies done on the same date. *CPT* codes 95865 (EMG of larynx) and 95866 (EMG of hemidiaphragm) were created because it was thought that the existing needle EMG codes did not properly cover certain difficult EMG studies. Code 95865 is defined as a bilateral code. Unilateral studies of the larynx should be coded with modifier 52 (reduced services), and modifier 50 (bilateral procedure) should never be used with this code. Code 95866 is defined as a unilateral code because it is described as an EMG of the hemidiaphragm, not the diaphragm. Presumably, a bilateral study (if one was ever done) would be coded as 95866-50 or 2 units of 95866 based on payer preference.

Needle EMG of the larynx is typically performed to diagnose laryngeal nerve and muscle disorders, for intraoperative monitoring during procedures performed on the larynx, and during administering botulinum toxin (Botox) injections to the laryngeal muscles. Needle EMG of the larynx is typically performed on both sides. Needle EMG of the diaphragm is performed to diagnose respiratory muscle disorders and, less frequently, for intraoperative monitoring.

Incidentally, some coding ambiguity was introduced by the inclusion of code 95865: the larynx is innervated by a cranial nerve, and existing codes 95867 and 95868 are for needle EMG of cranial nerve–supplied muscles. This ambiguity should not pose a problem in practice.

NEUROMUSCULAR JUNCTION TESTING

95857:   Cholinesterase inhibitor challenge test for myasthenia gravis
95937:   Neuromuscular junction testing (repetitive stimulation, paired stimuli), each nerve, any 1 method

Changes in Code 95857 for 2011

Code 95857 was revised by deleting the term *Tensilon* and replacing it with the term *cholinesterase inhibitor challenge*. Tensilon is a drug that is no longer available.

BOTULINUM TOXIN INJECTIONS

64612:   Chemodenervation of muscles, muscles innervated by facial nerve (eg, for blepharospasm, hemifacial spasm)
64613:   neck muscles (eg, for spasmodic torticollis, spasmodic dysphonia)
64614:   extremities and/or trunk muscles (eg, for dystonia, cerebral palsy, multiple sclerosis)

For chemodenervation guided by needle EMG or muscle electrical stimulation, see 95873 and 95874.
For chemodenervation for strabismus involving the extraocular muscles, use 67345.
For chemodenervation of internal anal sphincter, use 46505.

67345:   Chemodenervation of extraocular muscle
For chemodenervation for blepharospasm and other neurologic disorders, see 64612 and 64613.
46505:   Chemodenervation of internal anal sphincter

For chemodenervation of other muscles, see 64612, 64614, and 64640.
Report the specific service in conjunction with the specific substances or drugs provided.

64611:   Chemodenervation of parotid and submandibular salivary glands, bilateral.

Report 64611 with modifier 52 if fewer than 4 salivary glands are injected.

64650: Chemodenervation of eccrine glands, both axillae
64653: other areas (eg, scalp, face, neck) per day

Report the specific service in conjunction with codes for the specific substances or drugs provided.
For chemodenervation of extremities (eg, hands or feet), use 64999.

64999: unlisted procedure, nervous system

Neurophysiologic Guidance of Botulinum Toxin Injections

+95873: Electrical stimulation for guidance in conjunction with chemodenervation (list separately in addition to code for primary procedure)
+95874: Needle EMG for guidance in conjunction with chemodenervation (list separately in addition to code for primary procedure)

Use 95873 and 95874 in conjunction with 64612 to 64614.
Do not report 95874 in conjunction with 95873.
Do not report 95873 and 95874 in conjunction with 95860 to 95870.

Proper Use of the Botulinum Toxin Injection Codes

Before *CPT 2001*, codes 64612 and 64613 described chemodenervation (including the use of botulinum toxin) of muscles of the face and neck only. There was no specific code for injections of botulinum toxin administered to the muscles of the limbs, even though this was becoming a common procedure in clinical practice. Code 64614, introduced in 2001, describes this procedure for use in the limbs and trunk muscles to treat dystonia, spasticity, and muscle spasms.

Codes 64612 and 64613 were revised in 2001 to omit the phrase *destruction by neurolytic agent*. The term *destruction* does not apply to these procedures because the nerve is not technically destroyed but chemodenervated, meaning the effect of the injected drug is largely or completely reversible over time.

Can CPT Codes 64612 to 64614 be Billed More Than Once on a Date of Service

Codes 64612 to 64614 involve chemodenervation of muscles in the face, neck, extremities, and/or trunk. These services may involve injections of single muscle groups or multiple muscle groups.

The 2001 coding guidance published in the AMA *CPT Assistant* newsletter indicates that "codes 64612–64614 should be reported only one time per procedure even if multiple injections are performed in sites along a single muscle or if several muscles are injected" (CPT Assistant. April 2001;11[4]). Therefore, it is important to ascertain each individual payer's billing guidelines when billing for these services. It is incorrect to assume that if the bill was paid, the service was billed correctly. To reduce the risk of denials, recoupment actions, or other challenges about proper billing, each individual payer must be checked with. Getting it right allows providers to receive appropriate reimbursement for these services.

Can the Codes be Billed Bilaterally

Chemodenervation code 64612 is identified in the Medicare Physician Fee Schedule (MPFS) database as a code for which the allowance for procedures performed bilaterally will be 150% of allowance for the unilateral service. Bilateral procedures may be reported on a single line using modifier -50 and reporting 1 unit of service. Under the MPFS, Medicare payment is set as the lesser of the fee schedule allowance or the actual charge. Alternatively, for non-Medicare payers, bilateral procedures may be reported on 2 lines using the RT and LT (right side and left side, respectively) modifiers and reporting 1 unit of service for each.

Chemodenervation codes 64613 and 64614 are currently valued in the MPFS database as bilateral services. Both codes are assigned a bilateral indicator of 2, meaning the bilateral surgery payment rules do not apply (MLN Matters: MM7319). The modifier -50 should not be used with these codes. Some, but not all, Medicare carriers allow billing 1 unit of service per body area. Body areas are defined by CMS as

- One eye (including all muscles surrounding the eye and both upper and lower lids)
- One side of the neck
- One side of the face
- All muscles of 1 limb and the associated girdle muscles

It is important to familiarize oneself with what constitutes a body area under the CMS definition.

The administration of botulinum toxin injection to both sides of the neck in a patient would be reported to Medicare contractors who allow billing of 1 unit of service per body area as 64613 and 64613-59. The -59 modifier denotes the separate body area.

Anecdotally, there are differing policies among payers. Therefore, individual providers will need to check with their local contractor and/or payers to determine the proper billing procedure for these codes in their locality for the specific payer to whom a claim is submitted.

To review local coverage decisions for their respective CMS contractor, providers must consult with their Medicare Administrative Contractor's Part B policy related to botulinum toxin. It must be noted that coverage even for a single carrier may vary by region.

Can CPT Codes 64612 to 64614 be Billed Together

Different chemodenervation procedures performed for the same patient on the same date of service can be reported together using different codes on different lines using modifier -51 for the procedures with lower fee schedule amounts. Modifier -51 is used when 2 different procedures (reported by 2 different CPT codes) are performed for the same patient on the same date of service.

Although these procedures are gaining acceptance by payers for many diagnoses, coverage policies vary. CPT policy explicitly excludes the use of these codes to report injections for facial wrinkles or hyperhidrosis, but coverage for other diagnoses is determined at the carrier level. To ensure efficient processing and limit rejections, it is best to check with individual carriers and understand their coverage policies before submitting claims.

These codes do not include guidance by EMG or electrical stimulation, if done at the time of the injection, or the drug itself.

The Global Period for Chemodenervation Procedures

There is a 10-day global period for chemodenervation procedures. This means that payment for these procedures includes any related services performed 1 day preoperatively, on the day of the procedure, and 10 days postoperatively. Any E/M service related to the chemodenervation procedure that is performed within the first 10 days postoperatively would not be paid separately. If E/M services rendered in the postoperative period are unrelated to the reason for chemodenervation, then modifier 24 needs to be appended to the E/M code for it to be paid, and a different diagnosis code must be used on that claim. A separately identifiable E/M service on the date of injection should be billed with modifier 25 or, if it was a decision for surgery, modifier 57.

Payment Adjustment Rule for Multiple Chemodenervation Procedures

In the Medicare fee schedule, standard payment adjustment rules for multiple procedures apply to chemodenervation codes. If the procedure is reported on the same day as another procedure with an indicator of 1, 2, or 3, the procedures must be ranked by fee schedule amount and the appropriate reduction to this code (100%, 50%, 50%, 50%, 50%, and by report) must be applied. The payment must be based on the lower of (1) the actual charge or (2) the fee schedule amount reduced by the appropriate percentage.

About the Codes for Neurophysiologic Guidance of Botulinum Toxin Injections

Before the chemodenervation procedure, it is sometimes necessary to more precisely localize needle placement before the chemical is injected. Therefore, the physician may perform electrical stimulation or needle EMG to achieve this localization.

Providers must be aware of the correct *CPT* codes to use for EMG-guided botulinum toxin injections. Starting in 2006, there are 2 new add-on *CPT* codes to describe these 2 neurophysiologic guidance techniques (electrical stimulation and needle EMG) used during chemodenervation procedures. The 2 codes should be used only in conjunction with codes 64612 to 64614. They cannot be used together. Other needle EMG codes cannot be used in conjunction with these new codes. Of botulinum toxin injection guidance codes 95873 and 95874, one can be billed per botulinum toxin injection code these represent separate and distinct services.

CPT CODE MODIFIERS

A modifier provides a means by which a practitioner can indicate that a service or procedure was altered by specific circumstances but not changed in its definition or code. Modifiers can be reported by appending the 2-digit modifier number to the service or procedure number that is usually reported.

The following *CPT* code modifiers can be used with many of the *CPT* codes discussed in this article, under the proper circumstances:

- 24: Unrelated E/M service by the same physician during a postoperative period
  This modifier may be used with the chemodenervation codes under the circumstances described in that section.
- 25: Significant, separately identifiable E/M service by the same physician on the same day of the procedure or other service
  A classic example of the use of modifier 25 is performance of a lumbar puncture and E/M service on the same date. Modifier 25 is appended to the E/M code to indicate that both a significant E/M service and a procedure were performed on a given date. Some carriers may require that modifier 25 be appended to E/M services that are provided on the same date as neurodiagnostic procedures.
- 26: Professional component
  For interpretation and reporting only (for example, when a hospital owns the EMG equipment and pays the technician's salary), modifier 26 is added to the code for the neurodiagnostic procedure. Physicians cannot directly bill for the technical component of a procedure even when they use their own equipment in the hospital. The diagnosis-related group system, by law,

covers the technical component of Medicare services for inpatients. Thus, for Medicare, physicians must bill the institution by a separate agreement if they are to receive reimbursement for the technical component for these studies. This rule does not apply to other payers unless they track the Medicare policy.

50: Bilateral procedure

51: Multiple procedures

   Modifier 51 should not be appended to report an E/M service and a procedure performed on the same patient on the same date (modifier 25 appended to the E/M code serves this purpose).

   Modifier 51 should not be used with any of the nerve conduction codes. These codes are already defined on a "per nerve basis." *CPT 2012* specifically flags these codes as exempt from modifier 51.

52: reduced services

53: Discontinued procedure

   This modifier is not to be confused with modifier 52, which is used to describe a procedure that was partially reduced at the physician's discretion.

57: Decision for surgery

   This modifier may be used with the chemodenervation codes under the circumstances described in that section.

59: Distinct procedural service

   Modifier 59 should not be appended to an E/M service. To report a separate and distinct E/M service with a non-E/M service performed on the same date, see modifier 25.

99: Multiple modifiers

Healthcare Common Procedure Coding System Level II Modifiers

The Healthcare Common Procedure Coding System (HCPCS) level II modifiers can be used in addition to the modifiers discussed earlier in certain circumstances. There are HCPCS modifiers for procedures performed on the left or right sides of the body:

- LT: left side (used to identify procedures performed on the left side of the body)
- RT: right side (used to identify procedures performed on the right side of the body)

These modifiers cannot probably be used with neurodiagnostic procedures. To differentiate between separate and distinct EMG and nerve conduction studies, modifier 59 (distinct procedural service) is the correct choice. RT and LT are not appropriate for any of the evoked potential codes because these are all inherently bilateral.

PHYSICIAN SUPERVISION OF DIAGNOSTIC TESTING

The CMS (Health Care Financing Administration at that time) has stated that some degree of physician supervision is required for every diagnostic test payable under the physician fee schedule with few exceptions. These rules were published in a Program Memorandum to Carriers on April 19, 2001, and became effective on July 1, 2001. The memorandum can be accessed via the Web at http://www.cms.hhs.gov/Transmittals/downloads/B0128.pdf.

   These regulations apply to outpatient testing only.

ADDITIONAL INFORMATION ON *CPT* CODES FOR NEUROLOGIC PROCEDURES

Post-*CPT* code modifications alter how payers process claims.

1. Reimbursement and coding issues are separate
2. Bundling of codes (National Correct Coding Initiatives Edits)
3. Limits on diagnoses used with codes
4. Quotas on numbers of codes/diagnosis
5. Limits on rate of repetition of codes
6. Carriers can use/define codes differently
7. Proprietary carrier-specific codes or interpretation of code definitions

It is worth emphasizing: reimbursement and coding issues are separate! No fee schedules, basic unit values, relative value guides, conversion factors or scales, or components thereof are included in *CPT*.

REVISING *CPT* CODES AND RELATIVE VALUE UNITS FOR NEUROLOGIC PROCEDURES

There is a yearly cycle that determines the next year's *CPT* codes and their reimbursement values.

1. Specialty societies refine old *CPT* code definitions and develop new codes.
2. New codes or code revisions are presented to the *CPT* editorial panel, which accepts, modifies, or rejects the submissions
3. New or substantially revised *CPT* codes go to the Relative Value Scale Update Committee to be assigned physician work Relative Value Units (RVUs).
4. Established RVUs are regularly reviewed.
5. Practice expense RVUs are assigned by the Practice Expense Review Committee (PERC).
6. The RUC and the PERC transmit their recommendations to the CMS.
7. Final RVUs and annual conversion factor updates are decided by the CMS and the Congress, respectively

REFERENCES/RESOURCES
Print Resources

The *CPT* bible is the *Current Procedural Terminology: CPT 2012*. The AMA publishes several editions. Consider acquiring the *CPT* Professional edition. In addition to the features of the standard *CPT* manual, this edition includes color keys, illustrations, cross-references to the *CPT Assistant* newsletter (see later), and preinstalled thumb-notch tabs. Electronic packages are also available.

The *CPT Changes 2012: An Insider's View*, written by the *CPT* coding staff, provides the official AMA interpretations and explanations for each *CPT* code and guideline change in *CPT 2012*.

The *CPT Assistant*, a monthly newsletter published by the AMA, is an excellent source of information on *CPT* issues.

Internet Resources

AAN, http://www.aan.com/
American Academy of Physical Medicine & Rehabilitation, http://www.aapmr.org/
AANEM, http://www.aanem.org/
AMA, http://www.ama-assn.org/
CMS, http://www.cms.gov/
HCPCS, http://www.cms.hhs.gov/MedHCPCSGenInfo/

ACKNOWLEDGMENTS

I thank Mary McDermott, William Henderson, Bryan Soronson, and David Evans, my neurologist colleagues and AAN staff, for very helpful reviews of earlier versions of this coding information.

A Day in the EMG Laboratory: Case Studies of 10 Patients with Different Clinical Problems

Rachel DiTrapani, MD, Devon I. Rubin, MD*

KEYWORDS

- Electromyography • Nerve conduction studies • Algorithm
- Neuromuscular disorders

Other articles in this issue have reviewed basic concepts of nerve conduction studies (NCSs) and needle electromyography (EMG), and have detailed the electrodiagnostic features and approaches that are used to evaluate different types of neuromuscular disorders. This article discusses 10 representative case vignettes that may be encountered during a day in the EMG laboratory, which demonstrate the approaches used in our EMG laboratory to evaluate patients presenting with specific symptoms and a variety of suspected neuromuscular conditions. Each case presents a brief description of the patient's symptoms and clinical findings, suggests the suspected localization or diagnosis that was considered based on the clinical features before the performance of the electrodiagnostic study, and then presents the NCS and needle EMG data that were actually gathered from that patient. Comments and instructive electrodiagnostic considerations as they relate to each case are discussed at the end of the case. Although it would be uncommon to encounter all of these patients in a single day in the EMG laboratory, it would surely be an interesting and educational workday.

CASE 1. A HOSPITAL VOLUNTEER WITH HAND NUMBNESS
Clinical History

A 79-year-old woman, who worked as a volunteer at the information desk of our hospital, complained of numbness and paresthesias in her right thumb and index finger. Her symptoms were constant, but worse when she would drive to work in the morning and during the night when she was trying to sleep. She noted that rubbing

Department of Neurology, Mayo Clinic, 4500 San Pablo Road, Jacksonville, FL 32224, USA
* Corresponding author.
E-mail address: rubin.devon@mayo.edu

Neurol Clin 30 (2012) 731–755
doi:10.1016/j.ncl.2011.12.010
0733-8619/12/$ – see front matter © 2012 Elsevier Inc. All rights reserved.

or shaking her hand improved the symptoms slightly. She denied weakness; however, she reported dropping objects that she was holding in her hand on occasion. She also reported some achiness of her shoulder and entire arm, and occasional mild neck stiffness. She did not experience any similar symptoms in her left hand.

Physical Examination

The pertinent neurologic examination findings were decreased sensation to pinprick on the flexor surface of the thumb, index, and middle fingers. There was no weakness or atrophy noted in the right thenar or other arm muscles. Reflexes were normal and symmetric in her upper extremities.

Differential Diagnosis

The clinical features were most suspicious for a right median neuropathy at the wrist (carpal tunnel syndrome [CTS]). However, other localizations that may present with similar features and should be considered include a C6-C7 radiculopathy (especially given some neck and arm discomfort), a proximal median neuropathy, or, less likely, a brachial plexopathy.

Electrodiagnostic Summary and Interpretation

The electrodiagnostic studies (NCSs and needle examination) are shown in **Tables 1** and **2**. The NCSs demonstrated prolonged right median motor and sensory distal latencies and a low median sensory amplitude with a mildly slowed conduction velocity. Needle EMG was normal. The findings indicate a moderately severe right median neuropathy at the wrist (CTS).

Case Comment

This case demonstrates typical features of a median neuropathy at the wrist, such as occurs in CTS, with conduction slowing identified in motor and sensory fibers in the distal median nerve across the wrist. In this case, motor NCSs were performed first and because the median motor fibers demonstrated a prolonged distal latency, the antidromic sensory techniques were selected for the sensory studies. Had the median motor NCSs been completely normal, the orthodromic (palmar) sensory studies or other comparison studies (median–radial to thumb or median–ulnar to ring finger) would have been performed to increase the sensitivity of identifying a very mild distal median neuropathy. The needle examination consisted of evaluation of muscles supplied by the median nerve as well as those innervated by the C5 through T1 roots to exclude a superimposed cervical radiculopathy (although a cervical radiculopathy at any level would not affect the median sensory NCSs). Given the normal median

Table 1
Case 1: nerve conduction studies

Stimulate (Record)	Amplitude (mV or μV)			Velocity (m/s)			Distal Latency (ms)			F-Wave Latency (ms)		
	R	L	NL	R	L	NL	R	L	NL	R	L	Est
Ulnar, m (hypothenar)	12.7		>6	55		>51	3.0		<3.6	27		24.8
Ulnar, s anti (fifth)	33		>10	60		>54	3.0		<3.1			
Median, m (thenar)	7.7	8	>4	51	58	>48	5.1	3.4	<4.5	27.3	28.0	28.6
Median, s anti (index)	10	20	>15	51	66	>56	4.6	3.0	<3.6			

Abbreviations: Est, estimate; NL, normal values.

| Table 2 | | | |
| Case 1: needle examination of the right upper extremity | | | |
Muscle	Insertional Activity	Fibrillation Potentials	MUP
Deltoid	NL	0	NL
Biceps	NL	0	NL
Triceps	NL	0	NL
Pronator teres	NL	0	NL
Abductor pollicis brevis	NL	0	NL
Flexor pollicis longus	NL	0	NL
First dorsal interosseous	NL	0	NL

Abbreviations: MUP, motor unit potential; NL, normal.

compound muscle action potential (CMAP) amplitude, the yield of identifying significant abnormalities in the abductor pollicis brevis was relatively low; however, because the median motor NCS was not entirely normal, the muscle was examined in this case.[1]

The study was interpreted as showing a moderately severe median neuropathy. Different grading scales are used to grade the severity of median neuropathies at the wrist: mild cases typically demonstrate only sensory NCS abnormalities, whereas moderately severe cases are those in which there is slowing of conduction in median motor fibers across the wrist without a loss of amplitude, and severe cases have reduction in the motor amplitude. Documenting an electrophysiologic grade of the degree of the median neuropathy at the wrist is useful in the EMG report, because it may guide the referring physician's decision on treatment. However, the degree of electrodiagnostic abnormalities and the clinical symptoms may not always correlate well. Although this patient did not have any symptoms in her left hand, sensory NCSs were performed to assess for subclinical involvement of her left hand because CTS is frequently bilateral. This patient did not have a median neuropathy on the left.

CASE 2. A COMPUTER PROGRAMMER WITH A NUMB PINKY AND WEAK HAND
Clinical History

A 31-year-old man who works as a computer programmer presented with numbness of his left fifth (pinky) digit. He noted that he frequently would rest his elbow on a pad at his desk in an effort to keep his wrists in line while typing, to avoid developing CTS. By the end of his workday, he noticed a tingling radiating down the medial aspect of his forearm into his left ring and pinky finger. This progressed to persistent numbness involving his left fifth digit specifically. He also complained of occasional elbow discomfort. He denied any weakness in his hand or arm.

Physical Examination

The pertinent findings included decreased sensation to pinprick over the medial aspect of the fourth and fifth digits of the left hand. There was equivocal weakness but no atrophy in his hypothenar and interosseous muscles. Reflexes were normal and symmetric.

Differential Diagnosis

The clinical history suggests a left ulnar neuropathy, probably localized at the elbow given his history of resting his elbow on a pad while at work. Additional considerations include a distal ulnar neuropathy at the wrist, a C8 or T1 radiculopathy, or a brachial plexus lesion involving the lower trunk or medial cord.

Electrodiagnostic Summary and Interpretation

The electrodiagnostic studies (NCSs and needle examination) are shown in **Tables 3** and **4**. NCSs demonstrated low left ulnar sensory (antidromic) nerve amplitude. With elbow stimulation, no reliable response was recorded and, therefore, conduction velocity could not be determined. Short segmental incremental stimulation (inching) along the left ulnar nerve showed a partial motor conduction block of 28% in amplitude and 30% in the area localized adjacent to the medial epicondyle (**Fig. 1**). Needle examination demonstrated only reduced recruitment in the first dorsal interosseous and abductor digiti minimi. No fibrillation potentials or other motor unit potential (MUP) morphologic changes were seen. There is electrodiagnostic evidence of a mild left ulnar neuropathy in the region of the elbow that is localized to the medial epicondyle, characterized primarily by focal demyelination.

Case Comment

This case demonstrates typical features of an ulnar neuropathy at the elbow. In this patient the sensory NCSs demonstrated low ulnar sensory amplitudes, which supports axonal degeneration of the ulnar sensory fibers. However, in isolation this finding could be seen with an ulnar neuropathy localized proximal to the wrist, but could also be seen with a lower trunk or medial cord plexopathy. In this case, palmar studies were also performed to assess for slowing across the wrist, as may be seen in a distal ulnar neuropathy at the Guyon canal. If there was a high index of suspicion for a lesion at the wrist, the dorsal ulnar cutaneous sensory study would have been useful because it would be normal in an ulnar nerve lesion at the wrist and abnormal (low amplitude) in a lesion at the elbow.

The standard ulnar motor NCS, with stimulation at the wrist and above the elbow, was normal, including the conduction velocity across the elbow, making it difficult to precisely localize the process to the ulnar nerve at the elbow. However, this case demonstrates the value of inching along the ulnar nerve in 2-cm segments across the elbow to assist in more precise localization of a mild ulnar neuropathy characterized by very focal demyelination. The inching study demonstrated a segment

Table 3				
Case 2: nerve conduction studies of the left upper extremity				
Stimulate (Record)	Amplitude (mV or μV) (Normal)	Velocity (m/s) (Normal)	Distal Latency (ms) (Normal)	F-Wave Latency (ms) (Estimate)
Ulnar, m (hypothenar)	8.8 (>6)	53 (>51)	2.5 (<3.6)	30 (30)
Ulnar, s anti (fifth)	7 (>10)	NR (>54)	2.7 (<3.1)	
Ulnar, s palmar (fifth)	13 (>15)	NR (>54)	1.9 (<2.3)	
Median, m (thenar)	7.7 (>4)	58 (>48)	3.4 (<4.5)	28 (28.6)
Median, s palmar (wrist)	197 (50)	66 (>55)	1.9 (<2.3)	

Abbreviation: NR, no response obtained.

Table 4
Case 2: needle examination of the left upper extremity

Muscle	Insertional Activity	Fibrillation Potentials	MUP	Recruitment (Reduced)
Deltoid	NL	0	NL	
Biceps	NL	0	NL	
Triceps	NL	0	NL	
Pronator teres	NL	0	NL	
Extensor indicis	NL	0	NL	
Flexor digitorum profundus III and IV	NL	0	NL	
First dorsal interosseous	NL	0	NL Duration	1+
Flexor carpi ulnaris	NL	0	NL Duration	
Abductor digiti minimi	NL	0	NL Duration	1+

Abbreviation: NL, normal findings.

where a definite conduction block (>10% over a 2-cm segment) and a focal shift in latency (1.4 milliseconds in this case) were identified between two sites of stimulation (see **Fig. 1**). This finding, when present, provides localizing value in identifying the precise site of compression or injury to the ulnar nerve.

In this case, the needle examination only demonstrated subtle abnormalities (reduced recruitment) in ulnar innervated hand muscles. As the only finding, the reduced recruitment would be compatible with underlying pathophysiology of

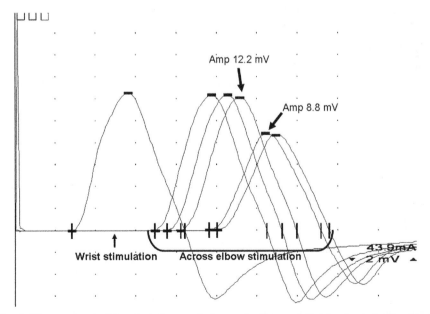

Fig. 1. Ulnar motor inching study in case 2, demonstrating a partial focal conduction block at the medial epicondyle. The responses at each stimulation site are superimposed. The first response on the left is stimulation at the wrist. The remaining responses occur from stimulation around the elbow in 2-cm increments.

focal demyelination and partial conduction block without evidence of axonal loss (in which fibrillation potentials or long-duration MUPs would be expected). Other, nonulnar C8-T1 muscles, such as the abductor pollicis brevis and extensor indicis proprius, were normal and helped to exclude those localizations. In this case, and in some ulnar neuropathies at the elbow, the proximal ulnar muscles (flexor carpi ulnaris and flexor digitorum profundus) were normal. These muscles may have been spared because the branches to those muscles often exit the ulnar nerve proximal to the elbow (and thus proximal to the lesion) or because the nerve fascicles to those muscles may have been preferentially spared. In cases such as this where the pathologic changes suggest focal demyelination, the prognosis is generally favorable if the offending cause of the ulnar neuropathy is eliminated.

CASE 3. A CANCER PATIENT WITH TINGLING TOES
Clinical History

An 18-year-old woman with a history of cancer presented with decreased sensation in her feet. Her symptoms began shortly after the completion of a course of chemotherapy, which included vincristine and cyclophosphamide. She reported decreased sensation in both feet and described a feeling of "walking on staples." She felt generally weaker in her arms and legs. She denied any pain in her extremities.

Physical Examination

The pertinent neurologic examination abnormalities included decreased sensation to pinprick, temperature, vibration, and joint position in both feet up to the level of the ankles bilaterally. Reflexes were diminished in her upper limbs and absent in her quadriceps and ankles bilaterally. Strength testing revealed bilateral weakness of foot dorsiflexion, eversion, inversion, and plantar flexion (Medical Research Council [MRC] grade 4/5). Her Romberg sign was present and her gait examination was notable for a sensory ataxia.

Differential Diagnosis

Given the temporal relationship between the patient's chemotherapy and development of symptoms, the most likely diagnosis is a chemotherapy-associated, length-dependent, peripheral neuropathy involving sensory and motor fibers. Another possibility is a polyradiculoneuropathy or sensory ganglionopathy (which would be less likely with true weakness). In addition, other unlikely considerations are bilateral lumbosacral radiculopathies or lumbosacral plexopathies.

Electrodiagnostic Summary and Interpretation

The electrodiagnostic studies (NCSs and needle examination) are shown in **Tables 5** and **6**. NCSs demonstrated absent sensory responses diffusely, an absent peroneal motor response, low tibial motor amplitude with a slowed conduction velocity, and a slowed median motor conduction velocity with a prolonged distal latency. Needle examination demonstrated mild long-duration MUPs in the anterior tibialis. The findings are those of a severe, length-dependent, large-fiber, peripheral neuropathy involving mainly sensory fibers, with milder involvement of motor fibers.

Case Comment

In this case a peripheral neuropathy was suspected, based on the clinical history of having received chemotherapeutic agents known to be associated with a peripheral neuropathy, and the typical clinical examination findings of distal sensory loss, hyporeflexia, mild distal weakness, and sensory ataxia. NCSs and EMG were performed to

Table 5
Case 3: nerve conduction studies

Stimulate (Record)	Amplitude (mV or μV) (Normal)	Velocity (m/s) (Normal)	Distal Latency (ms) (Normal)	F-Wave Latency (ms) (Estimate)
Ulnar, m (hypothenar)	7.2 (>6)	53 (>51)	2.8 (<3.6)	31.4 (23.8)
Ulnar, s anti (fifth)	NR	NR	NR	
Radial, s (wrist)	NR		NR	
Median, m (thenar)	8.7 (>4)	48 (>48)	5.2 (<4.5)	28 (28.6)
Median, s anti (index)	NR	NR	NR	
Peroneal, m (extensor digitorum brevis)	NR	NR	NR	
Sup. Peroneal, s (ankle)	NR		NR	
Tibial, m (abductor hallucis)	3.1 (>4)	32 (>40)	4.7 (<6.1)	66.8 (73.2)
Plantar, medial, s (ankle)	NR		NR	

Abbreviation: NR, no response.

characterize the distribution of involvement, differentiate between sensory and motor components, differentiate between axonal degeneration or demyelination as the primary pathologic changes, exclude multiple radiculopathies or a plexopathy, and assess severity.

The most prominent finding on NCSs was the diffusely absent sensory responses. This finding can be seen in a diffuse severe sensory neuropathy or sensory ganglionopathy, which is difficult to distinguish on an electrophysiologic basis. The performance of blink reflexes may help, although absent blink reflex responses can be seen in either process. Some have advocated using the masseter (jaw-jerk) response in situations in which all sensory responses, including blink reflexes, are absent (see the article on Cranial Neuropathies by Lacomis elsewhere in this issue). Because the jaw-jerk reflex is a monosynaptic reflex with the mesencephalic ganglion located within the brainstem rather than extramedullary, the response should be preserved in ganglionopathies but be abnormal in sensory neuropathies. However, this reflex is technically difficult to elicit in some normal people, so interpretation should be made with caution.

Table 6
Case 3: needle examination

Muscle	Insertional Activity	Fibrillation Potentials	MUP	Duration (Long)	Amplitude (High)
First dorsal interosseous	NL	0	NL		
Tensor fascia lata	NL	0	NL		
Vastus medialis	NL	0		±	±
Gluteus maximus	NL	0	NL		
Tibialis anterior	NL	0		±	±
Medial gastrocnemius	NL	0	NL		

Abbreviation: NL, normal.

In this case the motor conduction studies were mildly abnormal, indicating that the neuropathy involved motor fibers to some degree in addition to the more severely affected sensory fibers. The tibial and median motor conduction velocities were mildly slowed but not in the range of definite demyelination. To be confident that the neuropathy is primarily due to demyelination in the case of a low tibial motor amplitude, the conduction velocity should be less than 50% of the lower limit of normal, which in this case was not. In addition, the median motor distal latency was prolonged with a normal amplitude, suggesting that there may be a possible superimposed median neuropathy at the wrist.

The NCS findings could also be seen in a diffuse, patchy polyradiculoneuropathy. The needle examination demonstrated only mild abnormalities in the distal leg muscles, and the proximal leg muscles were normal. Examination of proximal muscles is important to exclude a polyradiculopathy, in which distal and proximal muscles supplied by the same roots would be expected to be abnormal. In this case, the discrepancy between the moderately severe lower extremity motor NCS abnormalities and the very mild needle examination abnormalities in the distal leg muscles may reflect the possibility that only the very distal motor fibers to the distal foot muscles were predominantly affected. Needle examination was not performed in foot muscles, such as the abductor hallucis or first dorsal interosseous pedis in this case; had those muscles been examined, they may have shown more significant abnormalities than the leg muscles. The features of this case are typical for chemotherapy-induced peripheral neuropathy.

CASE 4. A WOMAN WITH PAINLESS, PROXIMAL WEAKNESS
Clinical History

A 48-year-old woman presented with a 1-year history of progressive, painless, proximal muscle weakness. She described difficulty walking around her block, which she had done regularly for years. She noted weakness with climbing stairs, and difficulty raising her arms over her head while blow-drying her hair. She reported no speech or swallowing impairment and did not experience double vision or drooping of her eyelids. She denied muscle tenderness or pain and had no systemic symptoms, such as skin abnormalities or pulmonary complaints. Bowel and bladder function was also normal.

Physical Examination

The findings were notable for symmetric, moderately severe weakness of proximal shoulder muscles, hip flexors and abductors, and foot dorsiflexors bilaterally. Sensory examination was normal. Reflexes were normal diffusely.

Differential Diagnosis

The clinical possibilities in this case include a myopathy, a disorder of neuromuscular junction transmission, such as myasthenia gravis or Lambert-Eaton myasthenic syndrome (LEMS), or polyradiculopathy (such as chronic inflammatory demyelinating polyradiculopathy).

Electrodiagnostic Summary and Interpretation

The electrodiagnostic studies (NCSs and needle examination) are shown in **Tables 7** and **8**. NCSs of the left upper and lower extremities were normal. Needle examination demonstrated fibrillation potentials and short-duration MUPs with rapid recruitment in several proximal muscles. There was decreased insertional activity and markedly

Table 7				
Case 4: nerve conduction studies of the left side				
Stimulate (Record)	Amplitude (mV or μV) (Normal)	Velocity (m/s) (Normal)	Distal Latency (ms) (Normal)	F-Wave Latency (ms) (Estimate)
Ulnar, m (hypothenar)[a]	8 (>6)	77 (>51)	2.6 (<3.6)	26.2 (20.2)
Median, s anti (index)	16 (>15)	63 (>56)	3 (<3.6)	
Peroneal, m (extensor digitorum brevis)	3.6 (>2)	46 (>41)	4 (<6.6)	51.6 (49.6)
Tibial, m (abductor hallucis)	5.2 (>4)	51 (>40)	4.3 (<6.1)	55.6 (45.4)
Sural, s (malleolus)	4 (>0)	47 (>40)	3.9 (<4.5)	

[a] Repetitive stimulation at 2 Hz (no decrement).

reduced recruitment of short-duration MUPs in the anterior tibialis. The findings were consistent with a patchy myopathy, mainly involving lower extremity muscles.

Case Comment

The electrodiagnostic approach to this patient began with standard motor and sensory conduction studies in the legs, which were most clinically affected, as well as screening conduction studies in an arm. The normal findings on the NCSs would make a polyradiculopathy less likely, but could be seen in myopathies and neuromuscular junction disorders. Repetitive stimulation studies were performed on the ulnar nerve, using 2-Hz stimulation at rest, to screen for a neuromuscular junction disorder. Had the index of suspicion for a neuromuscular junction disorder been high or had the routine needle examination demonstrated marked MUP variation, repetitive stimulation of additional proximal nerves, such as the spinal accessory nerve, would have been performed.

Her needle examination consisted of examination of moderately weak muscles and demonstrated changes typical for myopathy, including short-duration, low-amplitude, polyphasic MUPs with rapid recruitment in proximal muscles. The findings of reduced recruitment (along with short-duration MUPs) in the anterior tibialis were consistent with end-stage myopathic changes. The presence of fibrillation potentials suggests underlying pathologic changes of muscle fiber necrosis or splitting, or vacuolar

Table 8							
Case 4: needle examination of the left side							
Muscle	Insertional Activity	Fibrillation Potentials	MUP	Recruitment	Duration	Amplitude	Phases
Deltoid	Increased	1+		NL	1+ short	1+ low	25%
Biceps	NL	0	NL	±			
First dorsal interosseous	NL	0	NL				
Vastus medialis	Increased	2+		Rapid 1+	2+ short	2+ low	25%
Tensor fascia lata	Increased	1+		Rapid 1+	1+ short	1+ low	50%
Tibialis anterior	Decreased	0	NL	Reduced 2+	3+ short	3+ low	
T10 paraspinal	Increased	1+	0	Rapid 1+	1+ short	1+ low	

Abbreviation: NL, normal.

damage to muscle fibers. These findings would raise the possibility of an inflammatory myopathy, such as polymyositis, although many other types of myopathies can produce similar findings on EMG (see the article on Myopathies elsewhere in this issue). Although neuromuscular junction disorders can occasionally be associated with fibrillation potentials and mild short-duration MUPs in some muscles, the findings in this patient are much more pronounced than what would be expected in myasthenia gravis or LEMS, and the rapid recruitment is more compatible with a myopathy.

This patient underwent a muscle biopsy of her deltoid, the findings of which were consistent with polymyositis.

CASE 5. A GOLFER WITH NECK PAIN
Clinical History

A 74-year-old man presented with a 6-week history of neck pain and intermittent sharp pain that radiated down his left arm into the middle finger. His symptoms began approximately 6 weeks previously, after playing in a golf tournament. He had a previous history of occasional neck pain that would last for several weeks at a time but never radiated down his arm. He reported a vague sense of heaviness in his arm and described some numbness in his hand.

Physical Examination

The pertinent findings included mild weakness of elbow and wrist extension, and a depressed left triceps muscle deep tendon reflex. Neck movement to the left caused pain to radiate from the neck, down the arm, and into the middle finger (positive Spurling sign). Placing the left arm over the head relieved his symptoms temporarily. Sensory examination was normal.

Differential Diagnosis

In this case the distribution of the patient's subjective symptoms and findings on his neurologic examination, as well as the reproducibility of his symptoms with neck movement, suggested that the most likely diagnosis was a left C7 radiculopathy. Other less likely possibilities included a posterior cord or middle trunk brachial plexus lesion or a radial neuropathy.

Electrodiagnostic Summary and Interpretation

The electrodiagnostic studies (NCSs and needle examination) are shown in **Tables 9** and **10**. The NCSs of the left upper extremity were normal. Needle examination demonstrated a mild degree of increased insertional activity and fibrillations in left C7 innervated muscles. There was increased polyphasia and mild long-duration,

| Table 9 | | | | |
| Case 5: nerve conduction studies | | | | |
Stimulate (Record)	Amplitude (mV or μV) (Normal)	Velocity (m/s) (Normal)	Distal Latency (ms) (Normal)	F-Wave Latency (ms) (Estimate)
Ulnar, m (hypothenar)	7.6 (>6)	55 (>51)	3.2 (<3.6)	31.9 (27.7)
Ulnar, s anti (fifth)	13 (>10)	56 (>54)	2.8 (<3.1)	
Median, m (thenar)	10.0 (>4)	50 (>48)	3.6 (<4.5)	28.1 (30.2)
Median, s anti (index)	33 (>15)	60 (>56)	3 (<3.6)	

Table 10
Case 5: needle examination

Muscle	Insertional Activity	Fibrillation Potentials	MUP	Recruitment (Reduced)	Duration (Long)	Amplitude (High)	Phases
Deltoid	NL	0	NL				
Biceps	NL	0	NL				
Triceps	Increased	1+		1+	±	±	75%
Extensor indicis proprius	NL	0	NL				
Pronator teres	Increased	±		1+	±	±	50%
Extensor carpi radialis	Increased	±		1+	±	±	50%
First dorsal interosseous	NL	0	NL				
C7 paraspinal	Increased	1+		1+			75%

Abbreviation: NL, normal.

high-amplitude MUPs in the C7 distribution. The findings were consistent with a subacute, active, left C7 radiculopathy.

Case Comment

In this case, the clinical features were very typical of a cervical radiculopathy. Because the most frequently affected root in a cervical radiculopathy is the C7 root and also because the clinical findings fit within this root distribution, it might be argued that the performance of electrodiagnostic testing provides little additional information and that an EMG could be bypassed in place of imaging studies. Although in certain cases this approach would not be incorrect, EMG does have utility and may provide complementary information to imaging studies regarding the problem. The goal of electrodiagnostic studies in the evaluation of a suspected cervical radiculopathy is not only to confirm that the process is at the root level and to localize which root(s) is (are) involved, but also to assess severity and activity (ie, whether there is denervation of the muscles innervated by the root).

In this case routine motor NCSs (median and ulnar) were performed and were normal, which would be expected in all cervical radiculopathies outside of the C8 or T1 distribution. In patients with suspected C7 (or C6) radiculopathies, other more proximal motor NCSs, such as the radial (extensor digitorum communis recording) in C7 radiculopathies or musculocutaneous (biceps recording) in C6 radiculopathies, could be performed. However, the more proximal NCSs are more technically challenging and would typically still be normal unless there was significant axonal loss. Therefore, these conduction studies are not routinely performed and the C5 to C7 roots are mostly assessed by needle EMG. The F-wave latencies may occasionally be prolonged in root disorders (or plexus lesions), although the median and ulnar F waves again only assess conduction through the C8 and T1 roots.

The sensory NCSs may perhaps be more useful than motor NCSs when evaluating patients with suspected cervical radiculopathies. The sensory responses should always be normal in cervical radiculopathies, because the roots are typically injured proximal to the dorsal root ganglia, thereby sparing the distal axons in the arm. In this case, the median sensory (antidromic) study assessed the sensory pathway through the median nerve, lateral cord and upper/middle trunk of the plexus, and through the C6/7 root, whereas the ulnar antidromic sensory study assessed the pathway through the ulnar nerve, lower trunk, medial cord, and C8 root. Had either of these been abnormal, a lesion involving the distal nerve or brachial plexus would have been considered. In this case, no radial NCSs were performed. Although radial neuropathy was in the differential diagnosis given the distribution of weakness, it was not strongly suspected because the patient had significant neck pain. Had the index of suspicion for a radial neuropathy been high, radial motor and sensory NCSs would have been performed.

Needle EMG is typically the most sensitive and useful component of the evaluation in cervical radiculopathies. In this case the focus was on the muscles supplied by the C7 root (triceps, pronator teres, extensor carpi radialis, and C7 cervical paraspinals), but muscles innervated by other roots were also examined to help define the localization. The C7 innervated muscles demonstrated fibrillation potentials, which indicated denervated muscle fibers, and often implies an active radiculopathy (in which there is either denervation from an ongoing process or a process that is resolving but in which reinnervation has not yet occurred). The MUP abnormalities were mainly an increased percentage of polyphasic MUPs with only minimally increased duration. This pattern of MUP changes occurs early in reinnervation, usually after about a month, and is helpful in defining the temporal profile of the process, which was subacute in this case. Although the findings in the limb muscles could also have been seen with a middle-trunk brachial plexopathy, the presence of abnormalities in the cervical paraspinals and the absence of an abnormal median sensory NCS confirm the process at the root level.

CASE 6. A TRAVELING BUSINESSMAN WITH LEG PAIN
Clinical History

A 48-year-old business executive who traveled overseas each month presented with a 4-month history of lower back and leg pain. He did not recall any precipitating single event but would experience more pain the week after his trips. The pain was described as a deep ache in his low lumbar region with a deep, achy pain that radiated into his right hip and occasionally down his buttock and posterior thigh to the knee. He denied experiencing any weakness but had noted that he nearly tripped a few times while walking quickly through the airport. The symptoms would improve but did not resolve completely after a week of minimal activity.

Physical Examination

His neurologic examination demonstrated mild weakness of the right foot dorsiflexion and foot eversion, and equivocal weakness of right hip abduction. Sensory testing reveals decreased pinprick sensation of the right lateral leg and dorsum of the foot. Reflexes were normal and symmetric in his lower extremities.

Differential Diagnosis

The clinical history and physical examination findings were most concerning for a right lumbosacral radiculopathy, localized to the L5 or S1 nerve roots. However, a lumbosacral plexopathy, sciatic neuropathy, or peroneal neuropathy was also a consideration.

Electrodiagnostic Summary and Interpretation

The electrodiagnostic studies (NCSs and needle examination) are shown in **Tables 11** and **12**. The NCSs demonstrated a low right peroneal CMAP amplitude with a mildly slowed conduction velocity. The peroneal F wave was absent. The superficial peroneal sensory response was present but the amplitude was approximately 50% of

Table 11
Case 6: nerve conduction studies

Stimulate (Record)	Amplitude (mV or μV)			Velocity (m/s)			Distal Latency (ms)			F-Wave Latency (ms)		
	R	L	NL	R	L	NL	R	L	NL	R	L	Est
Peroneal, m (extensor digitorum brevis)	1.7	4.2	>2	39	42	>41	5.5	5.3	<6.6	NR		
Superficial peroneal, s (ankle)	5	13	>0				3.8	3.7	<4.1			
Tibial, m (abductor hallucis)	5.9		>4	43		>40	4.5		<6.1			
Sural, s (malleolus)	11		>6	45		>40	3.9		<4.5			

Abbreviations: Est, F-wave estimate; NL, normal values.

the amplitude on the left. Needle EMG demonstrated fibrillation potentials and long-duration MUPs in right L5 innervated muscles. These findings were interpreted as consistent with a subacute to chronic, active right L5 radiculopathy.

Case Comment

This case brings up several important points related to the electrodiagnostic features of a lumbosacral (particularly L5) radiculopathy. The lower extremity motor NCSs demonstrated a low peroneal CMAP amplitude, which was consistent with, but not specific for, an L5 radiculopathy. A low peroneal CMAP can also be seen in a sacral plexus, sciatic nerve, or a peroneal nerve lesion. Given this finding and because the patient had sensory loss on the dorsum of his foot, the superficial peroneal sensory nerve was performed in addition to the sural sensory NCSs. In this case, the superficial sensory response was present but the amplitude was possibly low (slightly less than 50% of the unaffected side). Although a low sensory nerve action potential (SNAP) amplitude typically indicates a postganglionic process, such as a lumbosacral plexopathy, sciatic neuropathy, or peroneal neuropathy, in some individuals the dorsal root ganglion at the L5 level is situated more proximal in the spinal canal, and a lateral disk may directly compress the ganglion rather than the proximal rootlet.[2] Therefore, a low superficial peroneal SNAP can occur with an L5 radiculopathy, complicating the interpretation and localization of the process based on NCSs alone in this case. The fact that the tibial motor and sural responses were normal (although were not

Table 12
Case 6: needle examination

Muscle	Insertional Activity	Fibrillation Potentials	MUP	Recruitment (Reduced)	Duration (Long)	Amplitude (High)
Vastus medialis	NL	0	NL			
Tensor fascia lata	Increased	1+			1+	1+
Medial gastrocnemius	NL	0	NL			
Tibialis anterior	Increased	±			±	±
Tibialis posterior	Increased	2+		1+	2+	2+
Peroneus longus	Increased	2+		1+	2+	2+
Gluteus maximus	Increased	0	NL			
L5 paraspinal	Increased	1+			± Long	

Abbreviation: NL, normal.

compared with the other side, so could potentially be of low amplitude) would make a sciatic neuropathy or sacral plexopathy less likely. In this patient, the peroneal F waves were absent. Absent peroneal F waves may occur in normal individuals and therefore do not necessarily indicate a proximal nerve or root lesion.

The needle examination included assessment of muscles in the L5, as well as the L4 and S1, distribution. Because the NCS findings raised the possibility of a peroneal neuropathy versus an L5 root, the needle EMG incorporated L5 muscles that were not supplied through the peroneal nerve (such as the posterior tibialis and tensor fascia lata). The needle examination demonstrated fibrillation potentials and long-duration, polyphasic MUPs in L5 innervated muscles. However, each muscle with L5 innervation was not affected to a similar degree. In particular, the anterior tibialis, which is a very commonly examined muscle when screening for an L5 or lumbosacral radiculopathy, was much less abnormal than the posterior tibialis or peroneus longus because the latter muscles often have more L5 innervation than the anterior tibialis, which usually has more L4 innervation. Therefore, in patients in whom there is a strong suspicion of an L5 radiculopathy, distal and proximal muscles that are predominantly supplied by the L5 root (posterior tibialis or peroneus longus and tensor fascia lata or gluteus medius) should be examined.

The pattern of findings on the needle examination, with long-duration MUPs and fibrillation potentials, indicated a relatively long-standing process, which has likely been present for or recurrent for months (because there is evidence of substantial rein-nervation). The presence of fibrillation potentials in distal and proximal L5 muscles suggests an active process with ongoing denervation. Had fibrillation potentials only been present in the distal L5 muscles, without proximal fibrillations, it would have suggested that the process may be old or resolving, with adequate reinnervation proximally.

CASE 7. A WOMAN WITH WRIST DROP
Clinical History

A 54-year-old woman underwent an uneventful minor surgical procedure on her right wrist. About a week after the surgery, she awoke one morning and noted that she was unable to extend her fingers or wrist on the right. She had some possibly mild numbness in her hand, but denied experiencing any pain in her arm or neck. She had no symptoms in the left hand.

Physical Examination

The abnormal findings included severe weakness in the finger extensors, wrist extensors, and supinator on the right. The remaining muscles, including elbow extensors, were normal. She was able to feel pinprick throughout her right hand but thought that the sensation was slightly diminished on the dorsum of her hand compared with the left. Reflexes were normal.

Differential Diagnosis

The clinical history and examination findings suggested a radial neuropathy as the cause of the patient's symptoms. The distribution of deficits fits mostly into the radial nerve distribution, although the triceps seemed to be spared. However, other less likely possibilities included a posterior cord brachial plexopathy or C7 to C8 radiculopathy.

Electrodiagnostic Summary and Interpretation

The electrodiagnostic studies (NCSs and needle examination) are shown in **Tables 13** and **14**. The electrodiagnostic study was performed about 3 weeks after the onset of

Table 13
Case 7: nerve conduction studies

Stimulate (Record)	Amplitude (mV or µV)			Velocity (m/s)			Distal Latency (ms)			F-Wave Latency (ms)		
	R	L	NL	R	L	NL	R	L	NL	R	L	Est
Median, m (APB)	8.4		>4	51		>48	4.2		<4.5	26.7		27.7
Ulnar, m (ADM)	14.1		>6	53		>51	3.1		<3.6	26.1		23.2
Median, s (index)	34		>15	58		>56	3.4		<3.6			
Ulnar, s (5th)	21		>10	57		>54	2.8		<3.1			
Radial, m (EDC)	1.2	6.2			55		2.0	2.1				
Superficial radial, s	26	28	>20				1.7	2.0	<2.9			

Abbreviations: ADM, abductor digiti minimi; APB, abductor pollicis brevis; EDC, extensor digitorum communis; NL, normal values.

the patient's symptoms. NCSs demonstrated normal median and ulnar motor and sensory responses. The right radial motor amplitude was low compared with the left. Inching along the radial nerve around the spiral groove demonstrated an 80% drop in amplitude over a 2-cm segment at the proximal spiral groove (**Fig. 2**). The radial sensory amplitude was normal and similar to that of the left. Needle examination demonstrated fibrillation potentials and no voluntary MUP activation in radial inner-vated muscles, apart from the triceps and anconeus. The findings were consistent with a right radial neuropathy located at the proximal spiral groove, characterized by focal demyelination with some degree of axonal loss.

Case Comment

This case demonstrated findings of an uncommon upper extremity mononeuropathy: a radial neuropathy at the spiral groove. The goal of the electrodiagnostic study in this patient was to confirm localization to the radial nerve and exclude other possibilities, such as a posterior cord plexopathy or a C7 to C8 radiculopathy. In addition, the elec-trodiagnostic studies were helpful in determining the precise site of the nerve lesion. In

Table 14
Case 7: needle examination

Muscle	Insertional Activity	Fibrillation Potentials	MUP	Recruitment
First dorsal interosseous	NL	0	NL	
Pronator teres	NL	0	NL	
Triceps	NL	0	NL	
Anconeus	NL	0	NL	
Brachioradialis	Increased	2+		No activation
Supinator	Increased	2+		No activation
Extensor digitorum communis	Increased	2+		No activation
Extensor indicis proprius	Increased	2+		No activation
Biceps	NL	0	NL	
Deltoid	NL	0	NL	

Abbreviation: NL, normal findings.

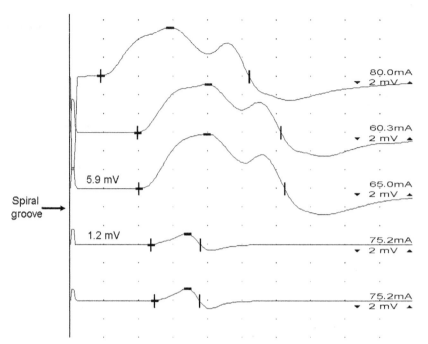

Fig. 2. Radial motor (inching) nerve conduction study in case 7, demonstrating a focal conduction block at the spiral groove.

this case standard, nonradial motor and sensory conduction studies were performed to ensure that there was no evidence of a more diffuse process or localization outside of the radial nerve distribution. The radial motor NCSs demonstrated a normal amplitude at the distal stimulation site (at the elbow), and even demonstrated a normal response when stimulation was performed at the distal portion of the spiral groove. Had stimulation not been performed at the proximal spiral groove, as occurred during the inching study, the severe focal conduction block would not have been identified on NCSs. This finding demonstrates the instructive point that if a patient has significant weakness believed to be caused by a peripheral nerve process and the motor conduction study to the weak muscle is normal, stimulation more proximally along the nerve (or even at the plexus or root) to assess for proximal conduction block should be considered.

The needle examination demonstrated abnormalities in the radial muscles distal to the anconeus. The triceps and the anconeus are the only two radial innervated muscles whose nerve branches emanate from the radial nerve proximal to the spiral groove. The presence of fibrillation potentials indicates some degree of axonal loss (in addition to the focal demyelination noted by the conduction block). This temporal progression from conduction block to axonal loss is common with many nerve compression lesions.

It is also notable that the radial sensory amplitude was spared, likely because the major pathophysiologic change was conduction block and because the typical radial sensory study is performed with stimulation distal to the site of block (at the wrist). Identifying proximal conduction block in sensory fibers is very difficult because of the normal dispersion of the SNAPs over long distances. This patient was thought to have a "Saturday night palsy."

CASE 8. A MAN WITH ARM PAIN AND WEAKNESS AFTER YARD WORK
Clinical History

A 54-year-old man presented with right upper extremity weakness and pain. The morning after a day of yard work, he experienced severe pain in his right shoulder that worsened with movement of his arm. The pain continued over the next week, during which he noted weakness of his right arm. Over the next 2 weeks his pain reduced and was present only intermittently; however, he continued to note weakness of his arm. He described weakness in raising his right arm and some weakness on gripping objects. He had some mild numbness in his right shoulder. He did not complain of any symptoms in his left arm.

Physical Examination

The only abnormal findings were seen in the patient's right arm. Muscle strength testing in the right arm was as follows (graded on the MRC scale): deltoid 4, biceps 4, infraspinatus 2, supraspinatus 2, triceps 5, pronation 4, supination 4, wrist extension 5, wrist flexion 5, flexor digitorum profundus (index and middle digits) 2, flexor digitorum profundus (fourth and fifth digits) 5, flexor pollicis longus 2, extensor digitorum communis 5, interossei 5, and abductor pollicis brevis 5. There was prominent atrophy of his right supraspinatus and infraspinatus. Reflexes were normal. There was mild decreased pinprick sensation over his right shoulder.

Differential Diagnosis

In this patient, the onset of pain in the arm after a day of yard work would first raise the concern for a cervical radiculopathy. The pattern of weakness on his neurologic examination is complicated and difficult to localize into a specific root distribution. One possibility was that of a C5 to C6 root lesion, although the weakness in some of his more distal arm muscles would suggest a possible C8 to T1 lesion. Other possibilities would include multiple mononeuropathies (axillary, musculocutaneous, and partial median), a brachial plexopathy, or a central cord lesion (although he did not have features of a myelopathy).

Electrodiagnostic Summary and Interpretation

The electrodiagnostic studies (NCSs and needle examination) are shown in **Tables 15** and **16**. NCSs demonstrated a reduced right suprascapular CMAP amplitude relative to the left (**Fig. 3**). The right lateral antebrachial and radial sensory amplitudes were

Table 15
Case 8: nerve conduction studies

Stimulate (Record)	Amplitude (mV or µV)			Velocity (m/s)			Distal Latency (ms)			F-Wave Latency (ms)		
	R	L	NL	R	L	NL	R	L	NL	R	L	Est
Median, m (APB)	6.8		>4	52		>48	4.4		<4.5	29		30
Ulnar, m (ADM)	12.2		>6	60		>51	3.5		<3.6	29		25
Median, s (index)	44		>15	58		>56	3.3		<3.6			
Ulnar, s (5th)	39		>10	61		>54	3.2		<3.1			
Lateral antebrachial, s	19	39					2.0	2.0				
Suprascapular, m	5.9	9.8					2.0	2.2				
Superficial radial, s	20	42	>20				2.4	2.2	<2.9			

Table 16
Case 8: needle examination

Muscle	Insertional Activity	Fibrillation Potentials	MUP	Recruitment (Reduced)	Duration (Long)	Amplitude (High)	Phases
Rhomboid major	NL	0	NL				
Infraspinatus	Inc	2+		2+	2+	1+	100%
Deltoid	Inc	1+			1+		
Biceps brachii	Inc	1+			±		
Supraspinatus	Inc	±		2+	2+	2+	100%
Triceps brachii	NL	0	NL				
Extensor digitorum communis	NL	0	NL				
Pronator teres	NL	0	NL				
Flexor pollicis longus	Inc	2+		2+	1+	1+	
Pronator quadratus	Inc	2+		2+	1+		
Abductor pollicis brevis	NL	0	NL				
First dorsal interosseous	NL	0	NL				
C6 paraspinal	NL	0	NL				

Abbreviations: Inc, increased; NL, normal.

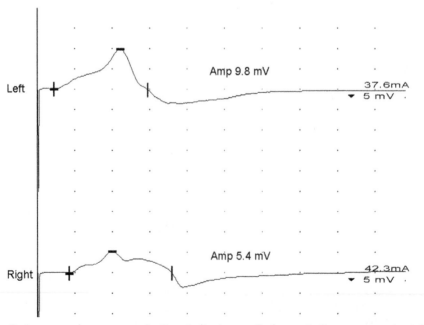

Fig. 3. Suprascapular nerve conduction studies in case 8, demonstrating an approximately 50% amplitude reduction in the affected (right) side compared with the unaffected side.

mildly low relative to the left. Concentric needle EMG demonstrated fibrillation poten-tials and long-duration, polyphasic MUPs with markedly reduced recruitment in the right supraspinatus, infraspinatus, flexor pollicis, and pronator quadratus, and similar, but much milder, findings in the deltoid and biceps. The remaining muscles were normal. The study was interpreted as a complex study with evidence of a patchy process, most likely involving the upper trunk of the brachial plexus (and mainly the fibers to the suprascapular nerve) and the anterior interosseous branch of the median nerve. The pattern of findings, primarily involving 2 individual nerves, would be compatible with a patchy inflammatory process involving the nerve, such as seen in neuralgic amyotrophy.

Case Comments

This is a complicated case, in which the pattern of abnormalities is difficult to precisely localize into a single site within the peripheral nervous system. The initial concern based on the history and clinical examination was for multiple cervical radiculopathies, a brachial plexopathy, or multiple mononeuropathies. The study began with standard motor and sensory NCSs (median and ulnar). Despite the patient's weakness in some median-innervated muscles, the normal responses obtained on median motor (abductor pollicis brevis) and sensory (recorded from the index finger) argued against a process involving the proximal median nerve. However, routine median NCSs do not reliably assess the anterior interosseous branch of the median nerve (AION) (in which less commonly performed NCSs, such as recording from the pronator quadratus, would need to be performed). In addition, because most of his weakness outside of the AION was in the shoulder girdle muscles (especially the spinati), the routine NCSs do not thoroughly assess for a C5 to C6 root lesion or an upper trunk plexop-athy. Because these localizations were strongly considered, additional sensory NCSs of fibers that course through the upper trunk (lateral antebrachial cutaneous and superficial radial) were performed. The reduction in amplitudes in both of these indicated a lesion that was distal to the dorsal root ganglion and supported a brachial plexopathy (or multiple mononeuropathies). The suprascapular motor NCS was also performed to provide an objective measure of the degree of nerve dysfunction, although assessment of this nerve could have also been made solely on the needle examination of the supraspinatus and infraspinatus.

The needle examination demonstrated findings of a neurogenic process that again was difficult to precisely localize into a single lesion. The most severe abnormalities were present in muscles supplied by the suprascapular and AION, but there were also mild abnormalities in other muscles supplied by the upper trunk of the brachial plexus.

The pattern of electrodiagnostic findings, in the context of the patient's history, was typical of neuralgic amyotrophy (Parsonage-Turner syndrome). This entity is catego-rized as an inflammatory or immune-mediated brachial plexopathy; however, prefer-ential involvement of a single or multiple individual nerves in addition to other portions of the brachial plexus is very common.[3] This entity may have a predilection to certain nerves, such as the long thoracic, suprascapular, and AION. As a result of the patchy nature of involvement, neuralgic amyotrophy may be one of the most diffi-cult entities to study from an electrodiagnostic standpoint. Maintaining a high index of suspicion, performing a very thorough clinical neuromuscular examination before per-forming any electrodiagnostic studies, and liberalizing the number of NCSs (often with side-to-side comparisons) and muscles examined with needle EMG are important steps in an appropriate assessment of these patients.

CASE 9. A MAN WITH POSTOPERATIVE DIPLOPIA, DYSARTHRIA, AND FATIGUE
Clinical History

A 67-year-old man underwent an uncomplicated arthroscopic surgical procedure on his left shoulder for shoulder pain. In the next 1 to 2 weeks he began to experience fluctuating dysarthria, ptosis, and intermittent diplopia. He noted blurring of his vision when reading or driving, with occasional double vision. He also noted that either or both of his eyelids would droop when he was tired. He had some difficulty swallowing liquids. The symptoms were present throughout the day, but tended to fluctuate in nature and were typically worse toward the afternoon and evening. He also reported feeling generalized fatigue and some weakness in his arms and legs. He had no sensory complaints or pain.

Physical Examination

The patient's neurologic examination demonstrated mild bilateral ptosis that seemed to worsen slightly with sustained upgaze. There were no definite extraocular movement abnormalities. Strength was normal except for mild weakness in his orbicularis oculi and oris muscles, and in the proximal shoulder muscles bilaterally. Deep tendon reflexes, gait, sensory, and coordination were normal.

Differential Diagnosis

This patient seemed to have a generalized process, primarily causing weakness in a cranial-cervical distribution. In this patient with fatigable weakness, double vision, and bulbar symptoms, the primary concern was a neuromuscular junction disorder such as myasthenia gravis. Other generalized neuromuscular conditions, such as a myopathy, polyradiculopathy, or motor neuron disorder, were also considered, and can be associated with fatigue or an increased sense of weakness after activity or later in the day. In this case, it is unclear whether or how the patient's antecedent surgery contributed to his symptoms, but the stress of the surgery could have been a trigger for unmasking certain conditions, including myasthenia gravis, an inflammatory polyradiculopathy, or a subclinical myopathy.

Electrodiagnostic Summary and Interpretation

The electrodiagnostic studies (NCSs and needle examination) are shown in **Tables 17** and **18**. The median sensory and ulnar motor conduction studies were normal. Repetitive stimulation studies were performed at 2 Hz before and after 1 minute of exercise in the left spinal accessory and facial nerves. No abnormal decrement in the CMAP amplitude or area was seen in the spinal accessory nerve (maximum decrement

Table 17 Case 9: nerve conduction studies				
Stimulate (Record)	Amplitude (mV or μV) (Normal)	Velocity (m/s) (Normal)	Distal Latency (ms) (Normal)	F-Wave Latency (ms) (Estimate)
Median (index), s	23 (>15)	57 (>56)	3.2 (<3.6)	
Ulnar (hypothenar), m	7.2 (>6.0)	52 (>51)	3.4 (<3.6)	28 (27)
Facial (nasalis), m[a]	1.5 (>1.8)		2.0 (<4.1)	
Spinal accessory, m (trapezius)[a]	4.5		2.5	

[a] 2-Hz repetitive stimulation performed.

Table 18
Case 9: needle examination

Muscle	Insertional Activity	Fibrillation Potentials	MUP
Deltoid	NL	0	NL
First dorsal interosseous	NL	0	NL
Frontalis	NL	0	Varying
Orbicularis oculi	NL	0	Varying

Abbreviation: NL, normal findings.

between the first and fourth stimulus was 8%), but a mild degree of abnormal decrement (maximum of 12%) was seen in the facial nerve. After 1 minute of exercise, the maximum degree of decrement was 9% in the spinal accessory nerve and 20% in the facial nerve (**Fig. 4**). The needle examination demonstrated varying (unstable) MUPs in the orbicularis oculi and frontalis, but not in limb muscles. The mild abnormalities on repetitive stimulation studies and needle examination of cranial muscles were suggestive of a mild defect of neuromuscular transmission, consistent with a neuromuscular junction disorder such as myasthenia gravis.

Case Comment

This type of case, a patient with mild weakness in cranial and proximal muscles, can be challenging from an electrodiagnostic standpoint. In these patients, the main differential diagnosis is a neuromuscular junction disorder, unusual distribution myopathy (eg, mitochondrial, facioscapulohumeral muscular dystrophy, and so forth), motor neuron disorder, or polyradiculopathy. The study began with one routine motor and sensory NCS in the arm, both of which were normal as was expected. Even though the patient had no sensory symptoms and no distal weakness, the performance of at least a few routine studies can help to identify or exclude a process such as a polyradiculoneuropathy (in which there may be abnormal sensory responses, or conduction velocity slowing or increased temporal dispersion on the motor studies) as well as a motor neuron disorder (in which the CMAP amplitudes may be low). In addition, low CMAP amplitudes may also increase the suspicion for the less common types of

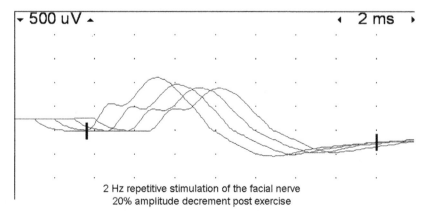

2 Hz repetitive stimulation of the facial nerve
20% amplitude decrement post exercise

Fig. 4. Facial nerve repetitive stimulation at 2 Hz at 3 minutes after exercise in case 9. There is a 20% decrement in amplitude between the first and the fourth stimulus.

neuromuscular junction disorders, such as LEMS. When this disorder is suspected and low CMAP amplitudes are seen, assessment for facilitation by supramaximally stimulating the motor nerve immediately after 10 seconds of exercise should be performed.

In addition to routine motor and sensory NCSs, repetitive stimulation is important and necessary to evaluate for a neuromuscular junction disorder, such as myasthenia gravis. Choosing the nerve on which to perform repetitive stimulation studies depends on the distribution and extent of clinical involvement. In patients with generalized symptoms, distal nerve-muscle combinations, such as the ulnar or peroneal, are technically the easiest and most reliable nerves to test. However, this patient had only bulbar and proximal weakness and, therefore, repetitive stimulation was performed on the spinal accessory and facial nerves. The repetitive nerve stimulation studies were essentially normal in the spinal accessory, because many consider an abnormal decrement as greater than 10% reduction in amplitude and area between the first and fourth or fifth stimulus. However, any degree of true decrement is technically abnormal; so in this patient the 8% decrement that was consistently present in three trials at rest may have been a clue to a defect in neuromuscular transmission. Caution should always be used when interpreting abnormal decrement to ensure that the study is technically reliable and that the pattern of decrement (largest drop between the first and second stimulus with a tapering pattern) is physiologic. This patient demonstrated more significant (>10%) decrement in the most affected muscles, with repetitive stimulation of the facial nerve. Because the decrement was only mild or borderline at rest, repetitive stimulation studies were performed also after 1 minute of exercise, which may increase the degree of decrement in some patients.

The needle examination focused on not only muscles that were clinically weak but also sampled muscles (such as the first dorsal interosseous) that were clinically spared, to assess for more widespread subclinical involvement. The absence of fibrillation potentials or markedly short-duration or long-duration MUPs essentially excluded a severe myopathy or motor neuron disorder. However, some mild myopathies may not demonstrate prominent needle examination abnormalities, but these conditions would also not be expected to produce decrement on repetitive stimulation either. The only finding on the needle examination in the clinically weak muscles was abnormal MUP variation (unstable or varying MUPs), which is the typical finding in neuromuscular junction disorders. Unstable MUPs can also be seen in myopathies and neurogenic disorders, but those conditions would also be associated with other configurational changes in the MUPs. The unstable MUPs in conjunction with the abnormal repetitive stimulation were consistent with a neuromuscular junction disorder.

In this patient, had the routine needle examination been normal, single-fiber EMG would have been performed as the most sensitive test for a defect of neuromuscular transmission. Single-fiber EMG should be performed if there is a high clinical index of suspicion or if ptosis and/or diplopia are the only clinical symptoms, and the routine studies are normal.

As a final note, patients who are being studied for a neuromuscular junction disorder should not take pyridostigmine (Mestinon) for at least 4 to 8 hours before electrodiagnostic testing, because the medication may improve and mask abnormal decrement, producing a false-negative study. This patient was being treated for presumed myasthenia gravis with pyridostigmine before confirmation with the EMG study. When he arrived at the laboratory on the morning of the test, he had indicated that he had taken his pyridostigmine 1 hour before. The test was delayed until later in the afternoon to avoid false-negative results.

CASE 10. A VETERINARIAN WITH PROGRESSIVE WEAKNESS
Clinical History

A 35-year-old left-handed veterinarian presented with a 3-year history of slowly progressive weakness. The weakness initially began in her right hand and gradually worsened to involve both upper and lower extremities. She required the use of a walker to assist with ambulation. She reported mild dysphagia, but no ptosis, diplopia, dysarthria, or respiratory symptoms. She described no pain or sensory complaints.

Physical Examination

Her neurologic examination demonstrated generalized weakness of moderate severity in her arms and legs, right side worse than left, with increased tone in the right lower extremity, brisk deep tendon reflexes, and bilateral Babinski signs. She had atrophy of her intrinsic hand muscles bilaterally and fasciculations in many muscles. Her speech was notable for a subtle spastic dysarthria, and tongue strength was mildly weak. Sensory examination was normal.

Differential Diagnosis

The primary concern in this case, given the combination of upper and lower motor neuron examination findings, is progressive motor neuron disease such as amyotrophic lateral sclerosis (ALS). Other possibilities include multiple cervical, thoracic, and lumbosacral radiculopathies, a polyradiculopathy, or a severe neuromuscular junction disorder or myopathy. However, the upper motor neuron signs would not be typical of these other possibilities, unless she had two processes.

Electrodiagnostic Summary and Interpretation

The electrodiagnostic studies (NCSs and needle examination) are shown in **Tables 19** and **20**. The NCSs of the right upper and lower limbs revealed an absent median motor response and low ulnar and tibial motor CMAP amplitudes. No conduction velocity slowing, conduction blocks, or abnormal temporal dispersion were seen. Needle examination demonstrated fibrillation potentials in most muscles studied with fasciculation potentials in many muscles. In addition, there was reduced recruitment of long-duration, high-amplitude, and frequently polyphasic and varying MUPs in most muscles. The findings were those of a diffuse neurogenic disorder affecting anterior

Table 19
Case 10: nerve conduction studies

Stimulate (Record)	Amplitude (mV or µV) (Normal)	Velocity (m/s) (Normal)	Distal Latency (ms) (Normal)	F-Wave Latency (ms) (Estimate)
Ulnar, m (hypothenar)	3.8 (>6)	65 (>51)	3.0 (<3.6)	24 (28)
Ulnar, s anti (fifth)	66 (>10)	64 (54)	2.8 (<3.1)	
Median, m (thenar)	NR	NR	NR	
Median, s anti (index)	64 (>15)	57 (>56)	2.7 (<3.6)	
Peroneal, m (extensor digitorum brevis)	4.8 (>2)	48 (>41)	5.4 (6.6)	45 (43)
Superficial peroneal, s (ankle)	17 (>0)		3.7 (<6.1)	
Tibial, m (abductor hallucis)	1.9 (4)	41 (>40)	5.2 (<6.1)	52 (49)

Abbreviation: NR, no response.

Table 20
Case 10: needle examination

Muscle	Insertional Activity	Fibrillation Potentials	Fasciculation Potentials	MUP	Recruitment (Reduced)	Duration (Long)	Amplitude (High)	Phases
Biceps[a]	Inc	2+	1+		2+	2+	2+	
Triceps[a]	Inc	3+	0		2+	2+	2+	25%
First dorsal interosseous	Inc	2+	0		2+	2+	2+	
Vastus lateralis[a]	Inc	2+	1+		1+	2+	2+	
Tibialis anterior[a]	Inc	1+	0		2+	2+	2+	
Lateral gastrocnemius	Inc	1+	1+		1+	2+	1+	
T7 paraspinal	Inc	1+	0		1+	±	±	25%

Abbreviation: Inc, increased.
[a] Varying MUP.

horn cells or their axons affecting the cervical, thoracic, and lumbosacral segments, consistent with a progressive motor neuron disease such as ALS.

Case Comment

This case demonstrates electrodiagnostic features that are seen with progressive motor neuron disease (eg, ALS). The motor NCSs in the upper and lower extremities demonstrated low CMAP amplitudes, indicating axonal loss. Careful observation of the waveforms was important to assess for abnormal temporal dispersion or conduction block (which were not seen in this case), which would be seen in some inflammatory/demyelinating polyradiculopathies, such as chronic inflammatory demyelinating polyradiculopathy or multifocal motor neuropathy with conduction block, both of which can have some clinical similarities to ALS. The sensory NCSs were normal, which would be expected in motor neuron disease unless there was a concomitant peripheral neuropathy or mononeuropathy.

The needle examination approach was based on clinical findings. The needle examination included examination of 2 to 3 muscles in the cervical, thoracic, and lumbar region that were not innervated by the same root or nerve, to assess for a diffuse process. The findings of fibrillation potentials and long-duration MUPs with reduced recruitment in a widespread distribution were consistent with a severe, diffuse neurogenic process. Varying or unstable MUPs are common in progressive neurogenic disorders, such as ALS, but are often overlooked when the examiner is focusing more on the MUP size and recruitment pattern. Muscles selected were those likely to be abnormal. Thoracic paraspinal muscles were examined to demonstrate involvement of the disease process in this segment, and the presence of abnormalities in these muscles helps to exclude multiple chronic cervical and lumbosacral radiculopathies. Of note, fasciculation potentials were also present in several muscles sampled, a finding which is nonspecific but consistent with motor neuron disease.

The combination of findings fit with progressive motor neuron disease. However, taken in isolation the EMG findings could also be seen with a severe axonal polyradiculopathy and therefore must be interpreted in the context of the clinical features. In severe polyradiculopathies, deep tendon reflexes are typically reduced or absent rather than hyperactive, as in this case of ALS. In addition, there is often some degree of subjective or objective sensory loss in polyradiculopathies, despite the normal sensory NCSs.

SUMMARY

These 10 cases demonstrate the approaches taken in the EMG laboratory to certain common and uncommon clinical problems. Although the approach to any one patient may vary to some extent by different laboratories or electromyographers and needs to be individualized toward the clinical problem and findings on the examination, the general guidelines as have been described in these cases and elsewhere can assist in identifying the appropriate localization and diagnosis of each type of clinical problem.[4]

REFERENCES

1. Vennix MJ, Hirsh DD, Chiou-Tan FY, et al. Predicting acute denervation in carpal tunnel syndrome. Arch Phys Med Rehabil 1998;79:306–12.
2. Levin KH. L5 radiculopathy with reduced superficial peroneal sensory responses: intraspinal and extraspinal causes. Muscle Nerve 1998;21:3–7.
3. Rubin DI. Neuralgic amyotrophy: clinical manifestations and evaluation. Neurologist 2001;7:350–6.
4. Rubin DI, Daube JR. Application of clinical neurophysiology: assessing peripheral neuromuscular symptom complexes. In: Daube JR, Rubin DI, editors. Clinical neurophysiology. 3rd edition. New York: Oxford University Press; 2009. p. 801–37.

Index

Note: Page numbers of article titles are in **boldface** type.

Neurol Clin 30 (2012) 757–779
doi:10.1016/S0733-8619(12)00010-2
0733-8619/12/$ – see front matter © 2012 Elsevier Inc. All rights reserved.

neurologic.theclinics.com

Moving?

Make sure your subscription moves with you!

To notify us of your new address, find your **Clinics Account Number** (located on your mailing label above your name), and contact customer service at:

Email: journalscustomerservice-usa@elsevier.com

800-654-2452 (subscribers in the U.S. & Canada)
314-447-8871 (subscribers outside of the U.S. & Canada)

Fax number: 314-447-8029

Elsevier Health Sciences Division
Subscription Customer Service
3251 Riverport Lane
Maryland Heights, MO 63043

*To ensure uninterrupted delivery of your subscription, please notify us at least 4 weeks in advance of move.

Printed and bound by CPI Group (UK) Ltd, Croydon, CR0 4YY

03/10/2024

01040448-0010